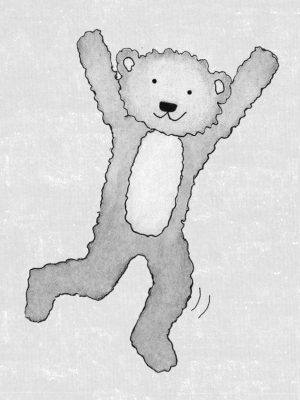

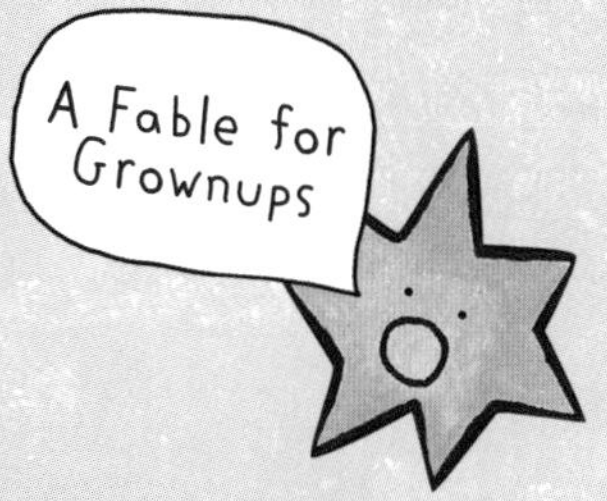

A Fable for Grownups

Bipolar Bear
and the Terrible,
Horrible, No Good,
Very Bad Health
Insurance

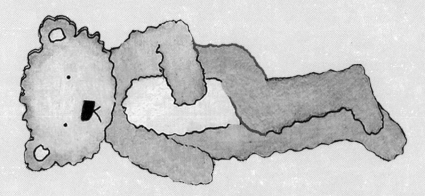

KATHLEEN FOUNDS

graphic mundi

Library of Congress Cataloging-in-Publication Data

Names: Founds, Kathleen, author, artist.
Title: Bipolar bear and the terrible, horrible, no good, very bad health insurance : a fable for adults / Kathleen Founds.
Description: University Park, Pennsylvania : Graphic Mundi, [2022]
Summary: "A graphic novel about navigating the US medical insurance system and receiving fair and adequate coverage for mental illness. Based on the author's own experience in being treated for bipolar disorder"—Provided by publisher.
Identifiers: LCCN 2022006338 | ISBN 9781637790359 (paperback)
Subjects: LCSH: Bears—Comic books, strips, etc. | Manic-depressive illness—Comic books, strips, etc. | Health insurance—United States—Comic books, strips, etc. | Medical care—United States—Comic books, strips, etc. | LCGFT: Graphic novels.
Classification: LCC PN6727.F6798 B57 2022 | DDC 741.5/973—dc23/eng/20220302
LC record available at https://lccn.loc.gov/2022006338

Printed in China
Published by The Pennsylvania State University Press, University Park, PA 16802–1003

10 9 8 7 6 5 4 3 2 1

graphic mundi
drawing our worlds together

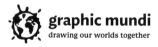

Graphic Mundi is an imprint of The Pennsylvania State University Press.

The Pennsylvania State University Press is a member of the Association of University Presses.

It is the policy of The Pennsylvania State University Press to use acid-free paper. Publications on uncoated stock satisfy the minimum requirements of American National Standard for Information Sciences—Permanence of Paper for Printed Library Material, ANSI Z39.48–1992.

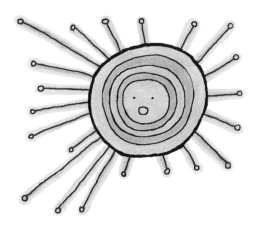

dedication:

For all who:

Brave the slough of despond,

Wander the labyrinth of health insurance claims, &

Endure the shackles of crushing debt.

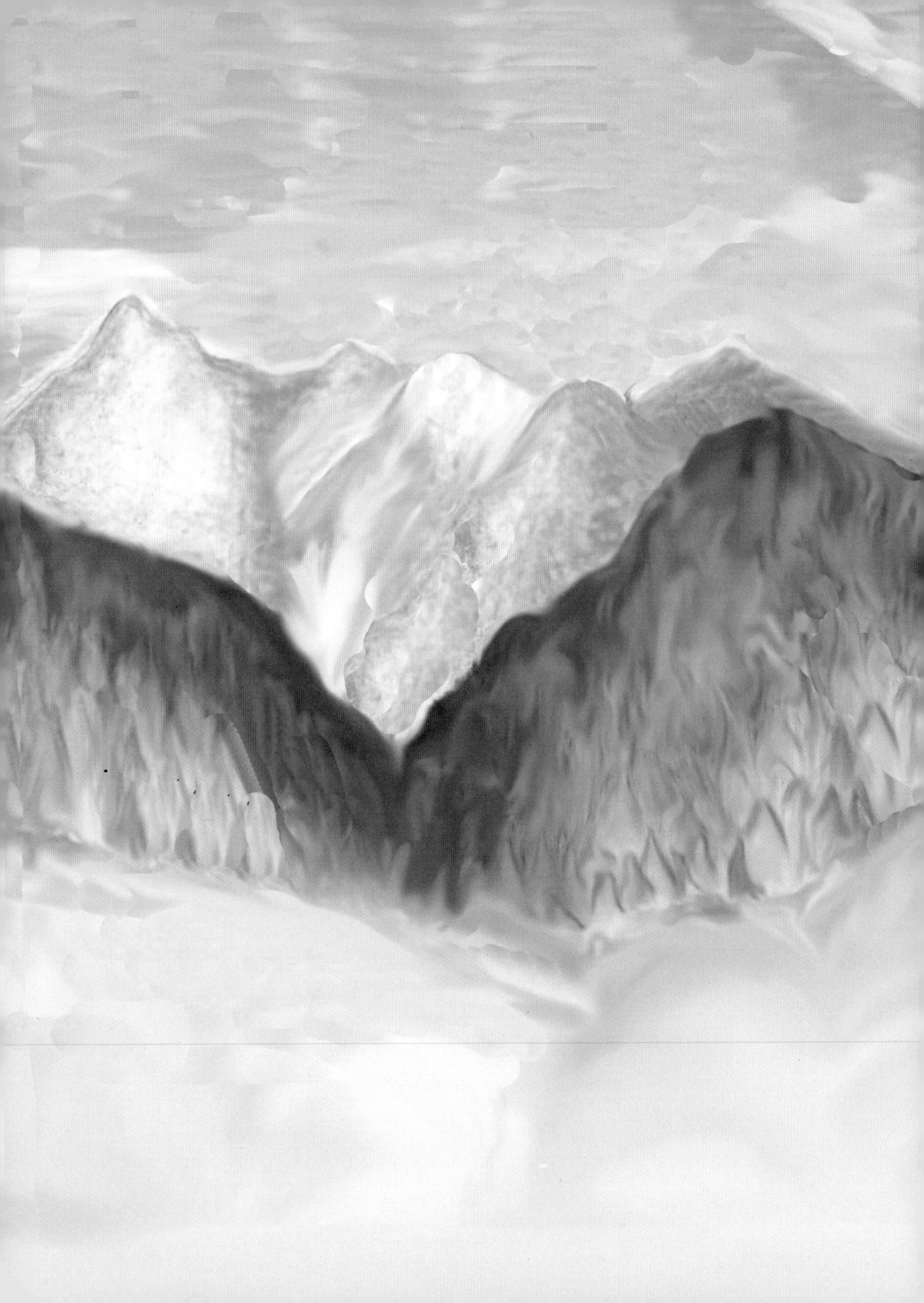

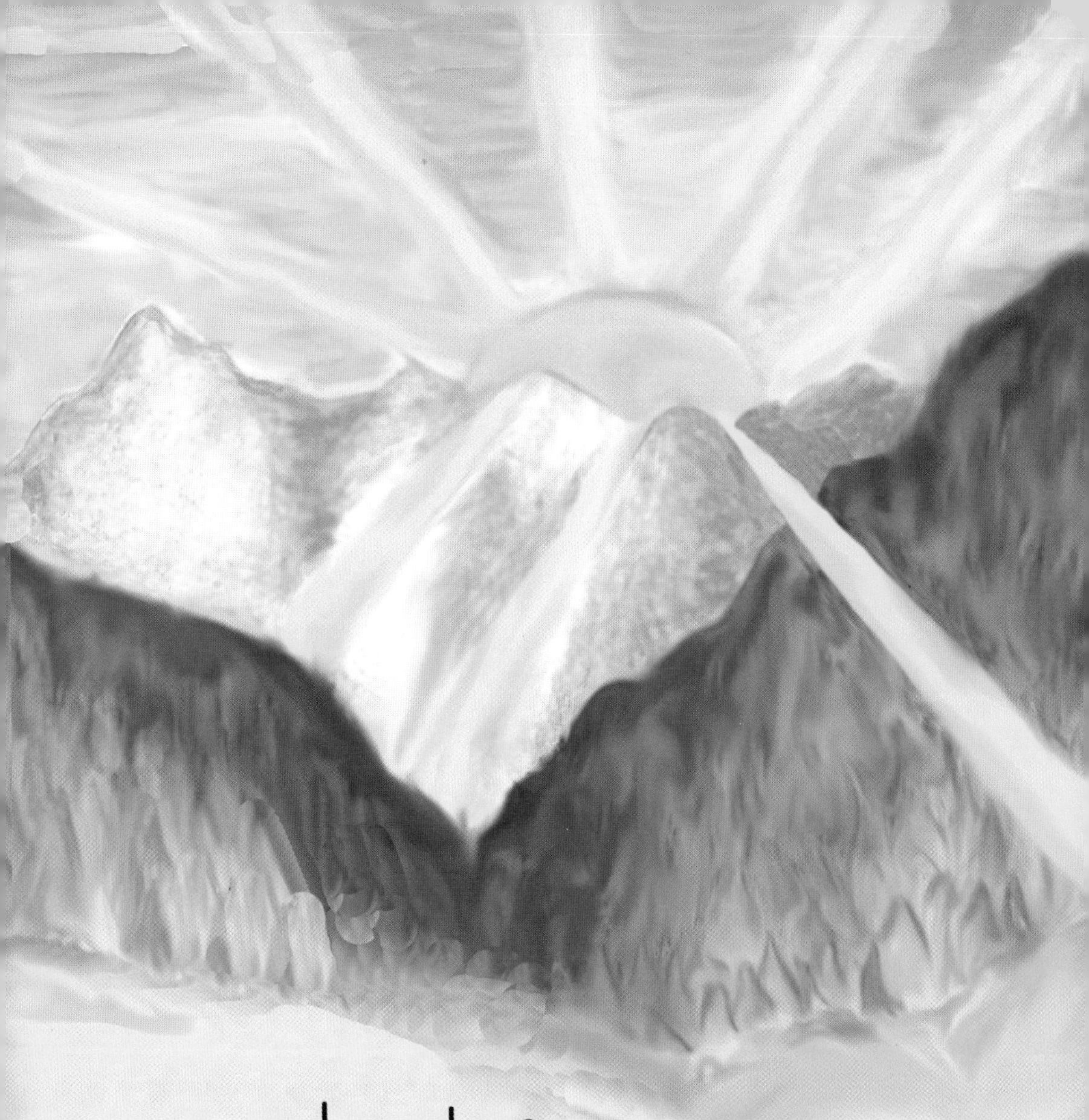

chapter one:

The Quest

Theodore was a bear.

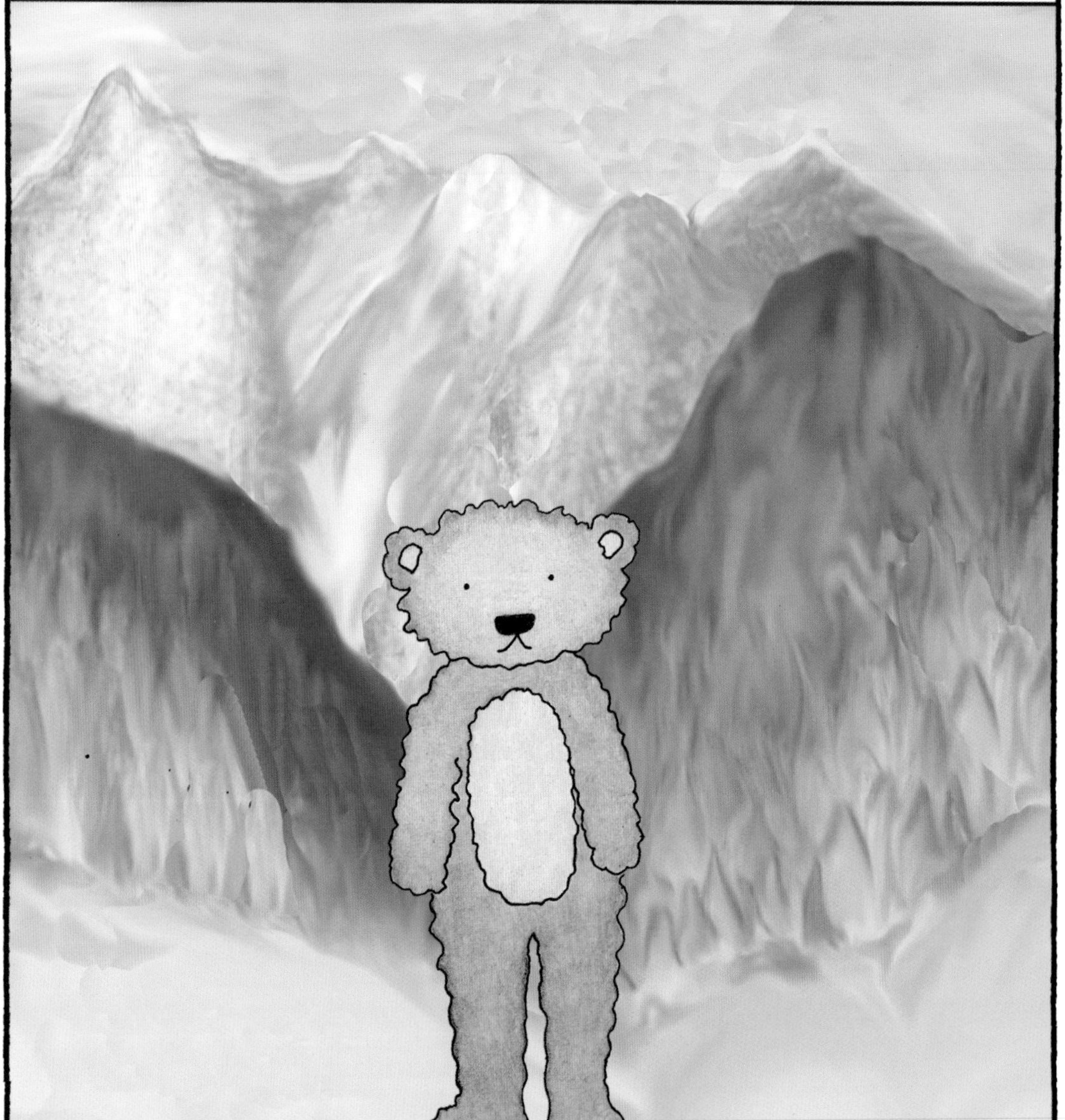

Most of the time, he lived an ordinary life.

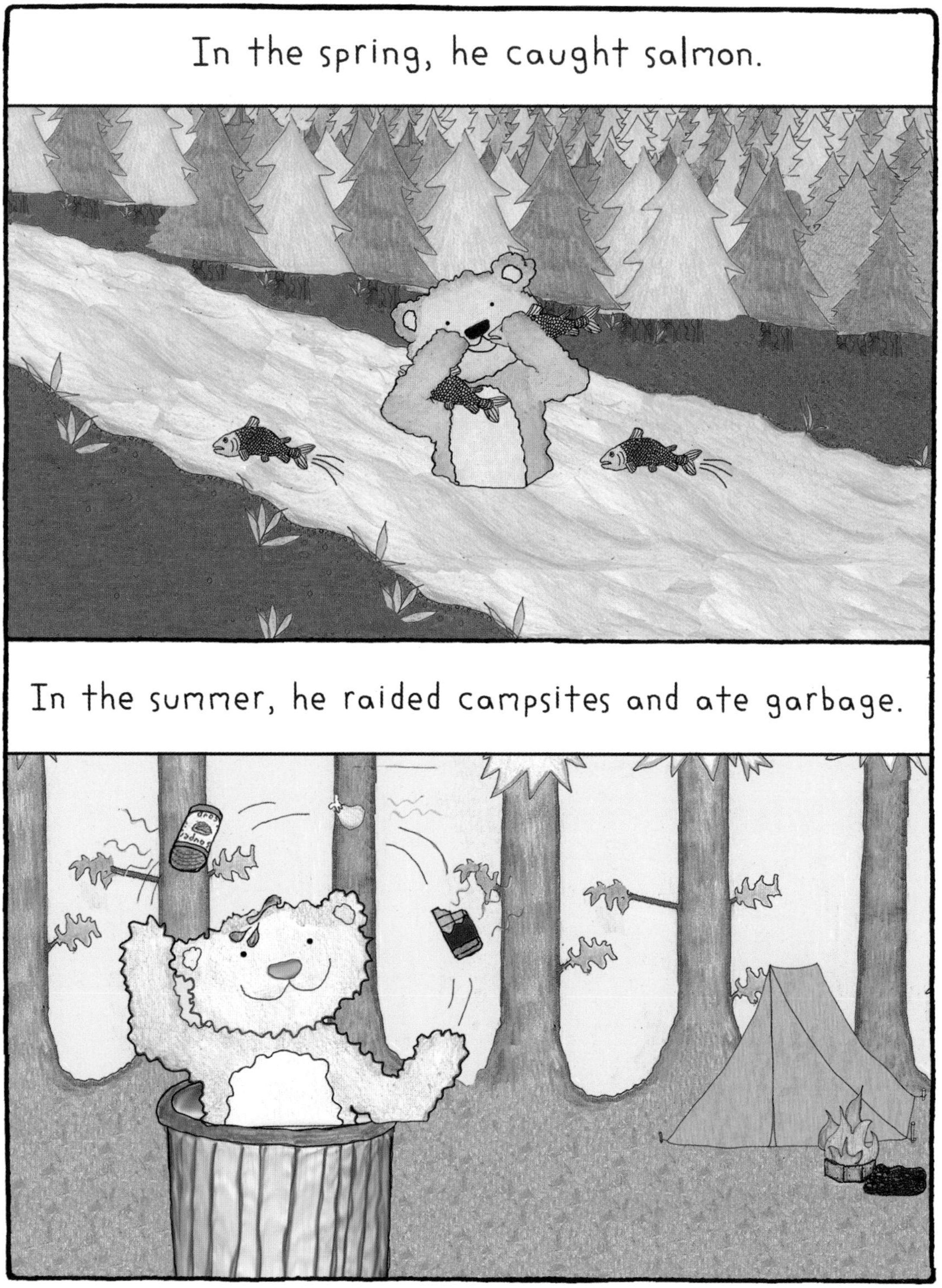
In the spring, he caught salmon.
In the summer, he raided campsites and ate garbage.

In the fall, he gorged on berries and honey.

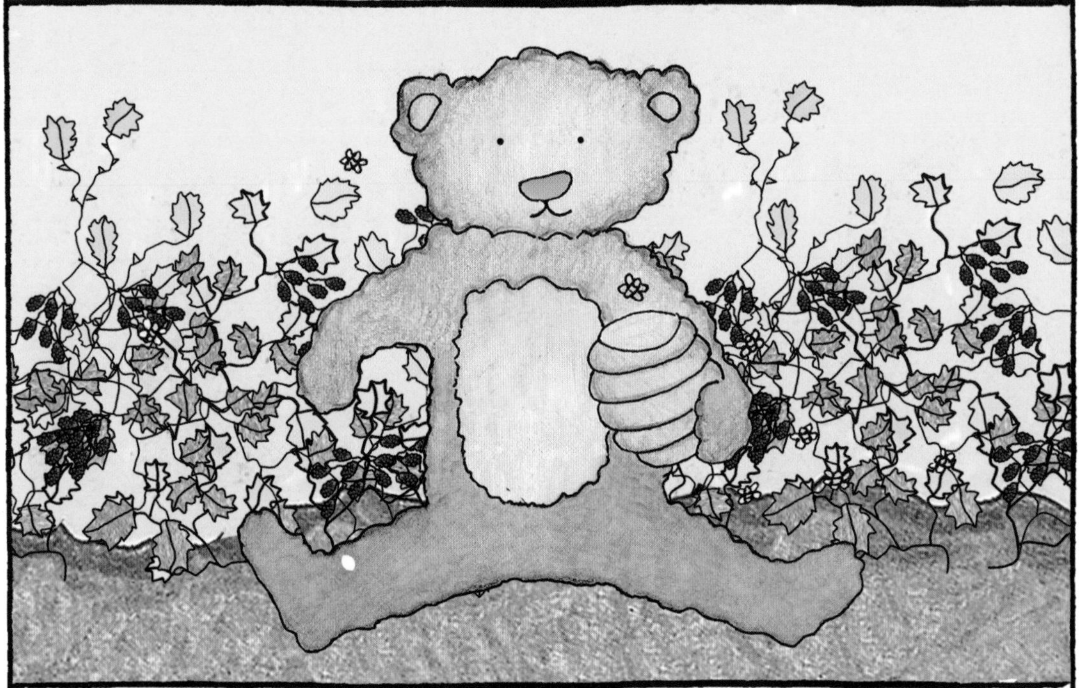

In the winter, he hibernated.

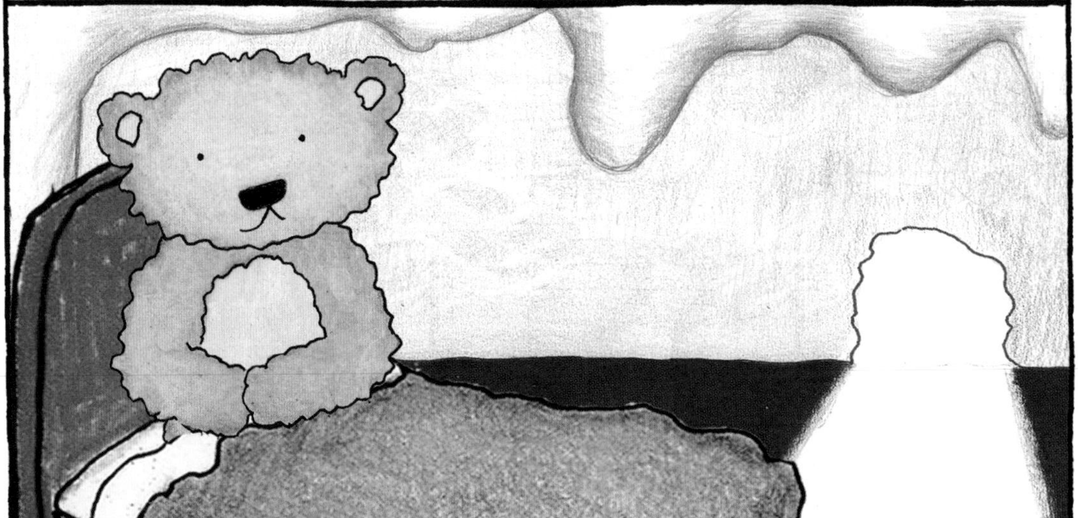

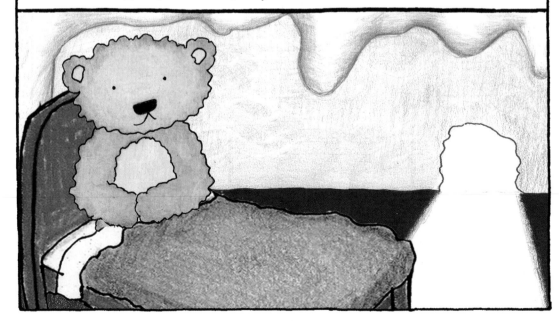

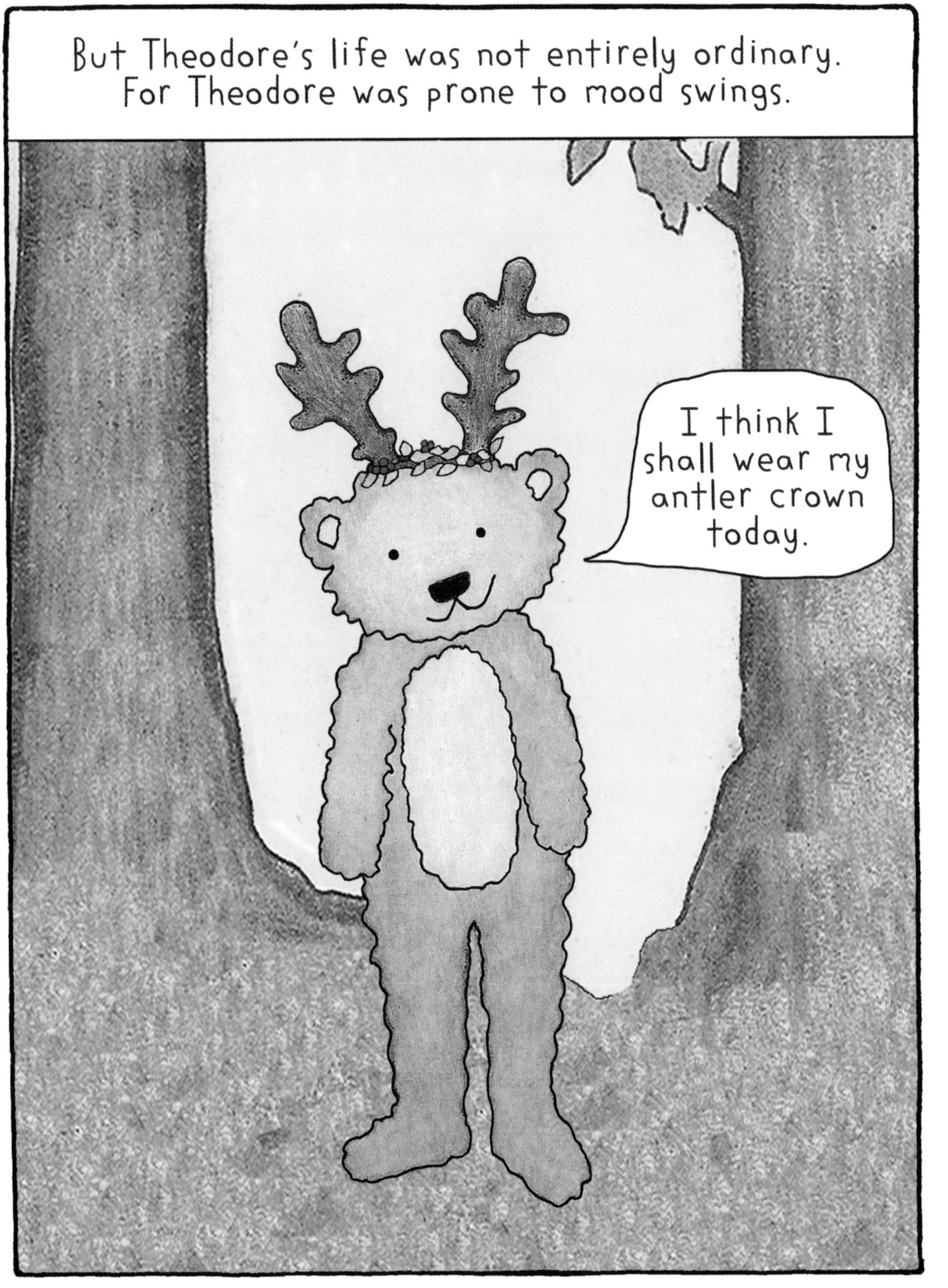
But Theodore's life was not entirely ordinary. For Theodore was prone to mood swings.
I think I shall wear my antler crown today.

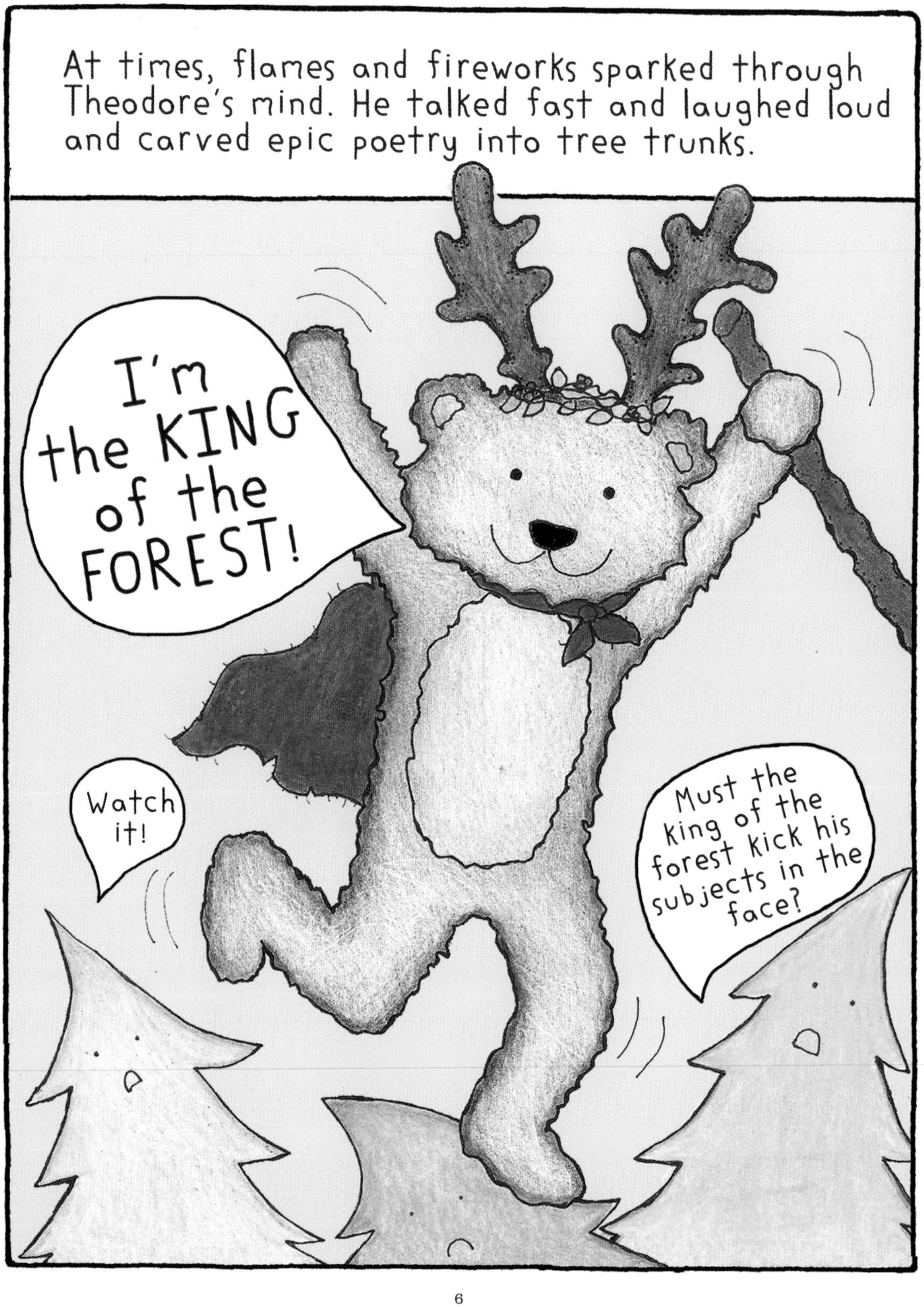
At times, flames and fireworks sparked through Theodore's mind. He talked fast and laughed loud and carved epic poetry into tree trunks.
I'm the KING of the FOREST!
Watch it!
Must the king of the forest kick his subjects in the face?

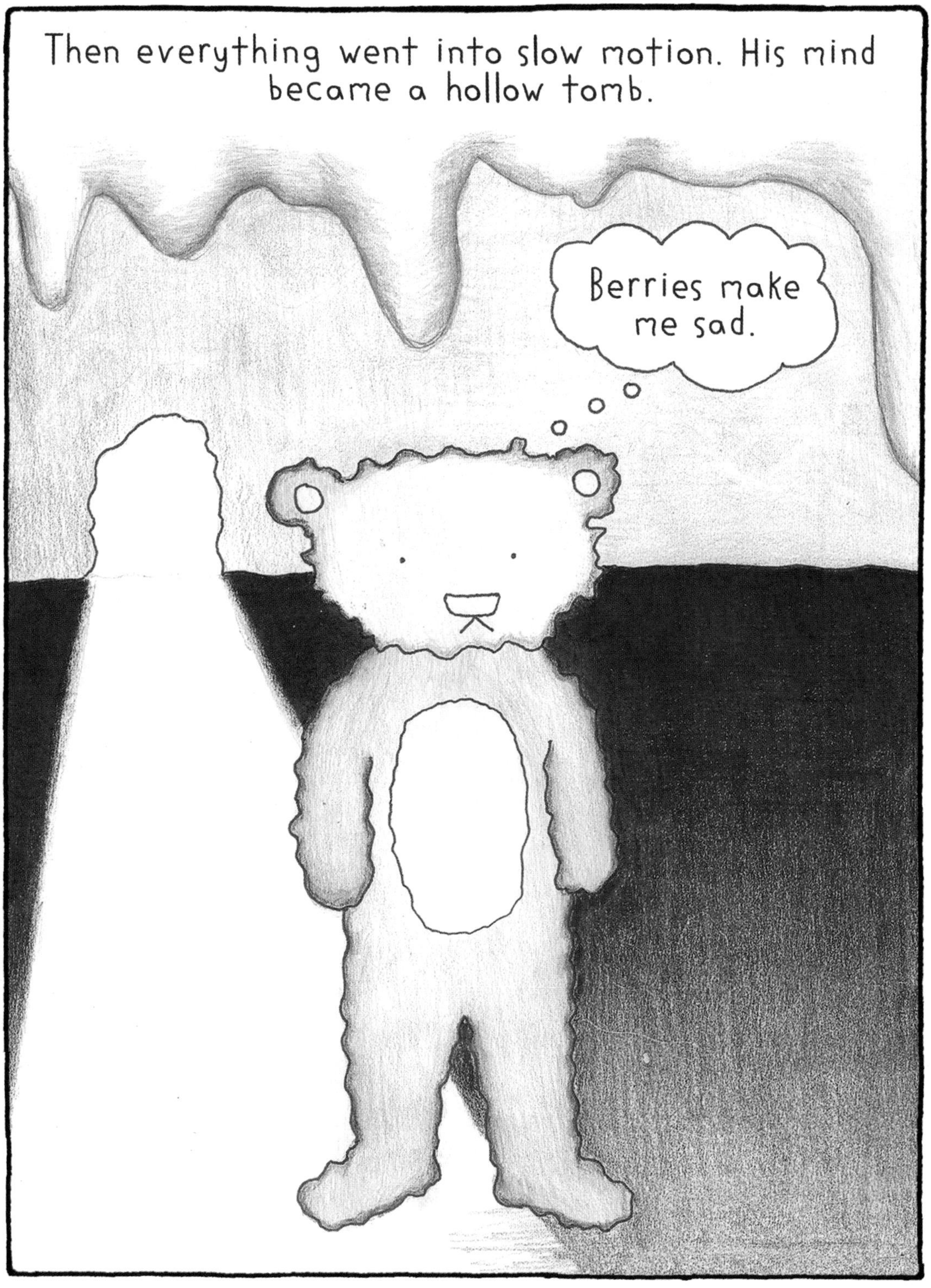
Then everything went into slow motion. His mind became a hollow tomb.
Berries make me sad.

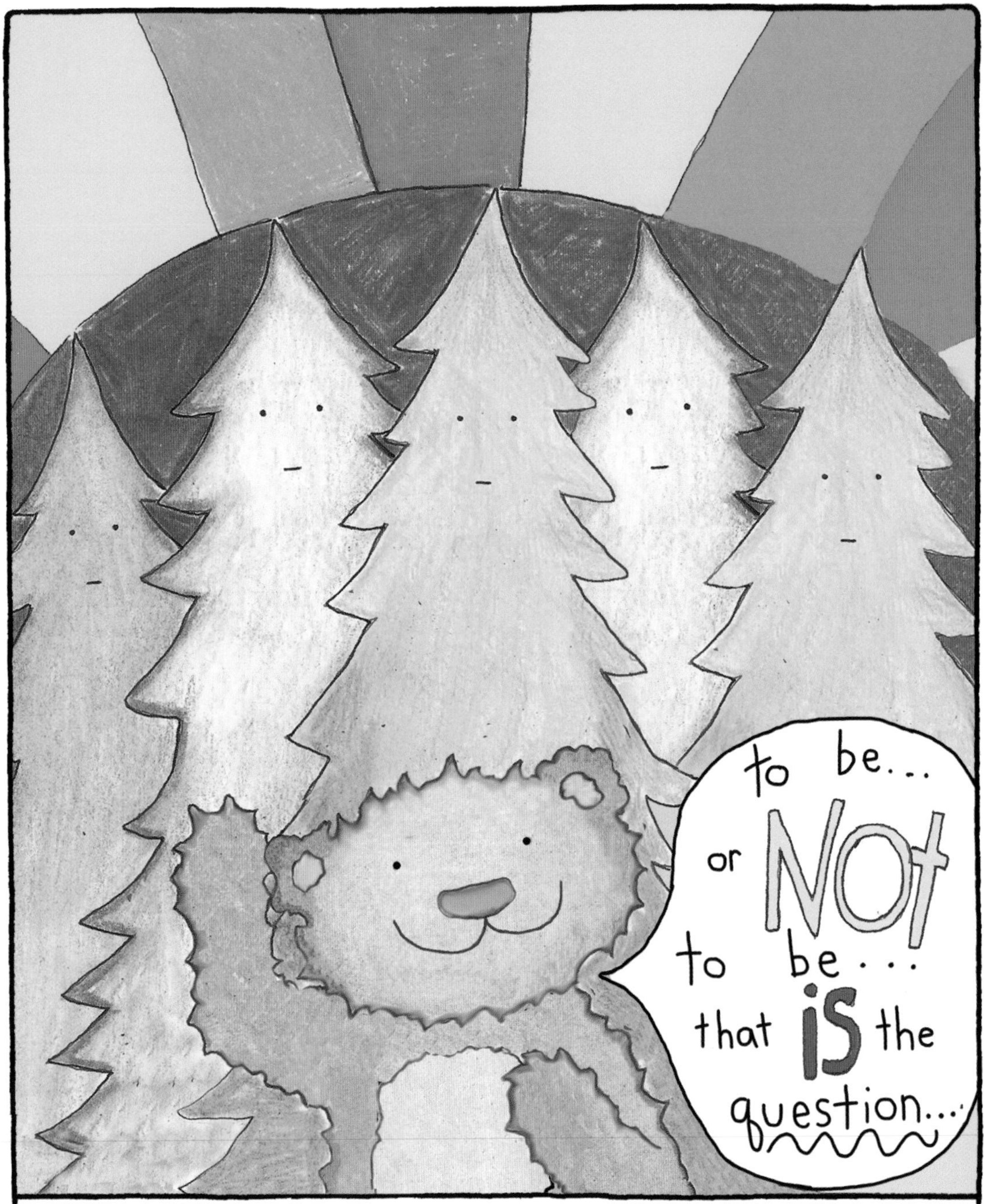
to be... or NOT to be... that IS the question....

When he was up, he performed tragicomic monologues before a captive audience of trees.

When he was down, he drew sad faces on rocks and turtle shells.

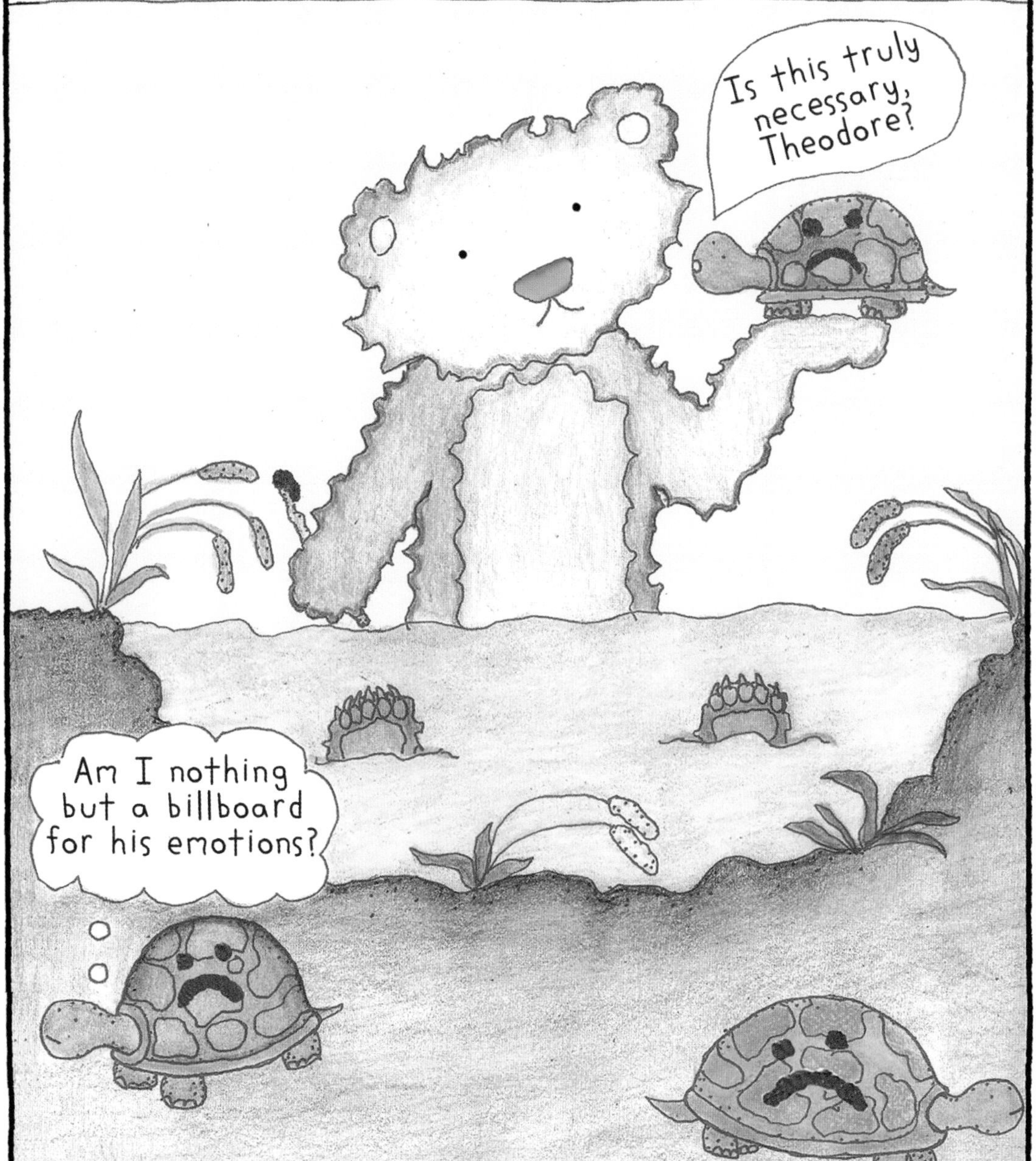

Is this truly necessary, Theodore?
Am I nothing but a billboard for his emotions?

When he was up, he stayed up all night conversing with the stars.

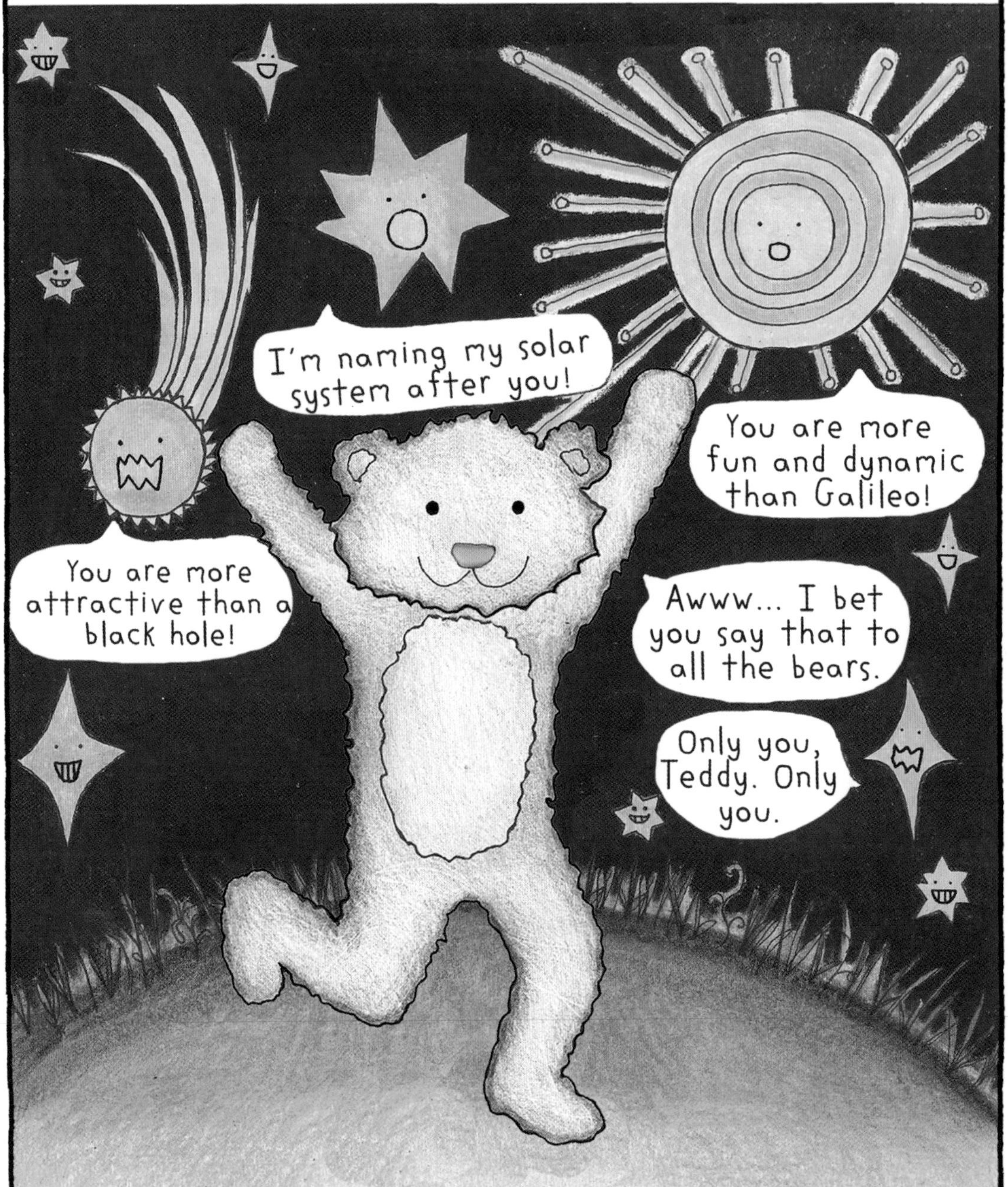

I'm naming my solar system after you!
You are more fun and dynamic than Galileo!
You are more attractive than a black hole!
Awww... I bet you say that to all the bears.
Only you, Teddy. Only you.

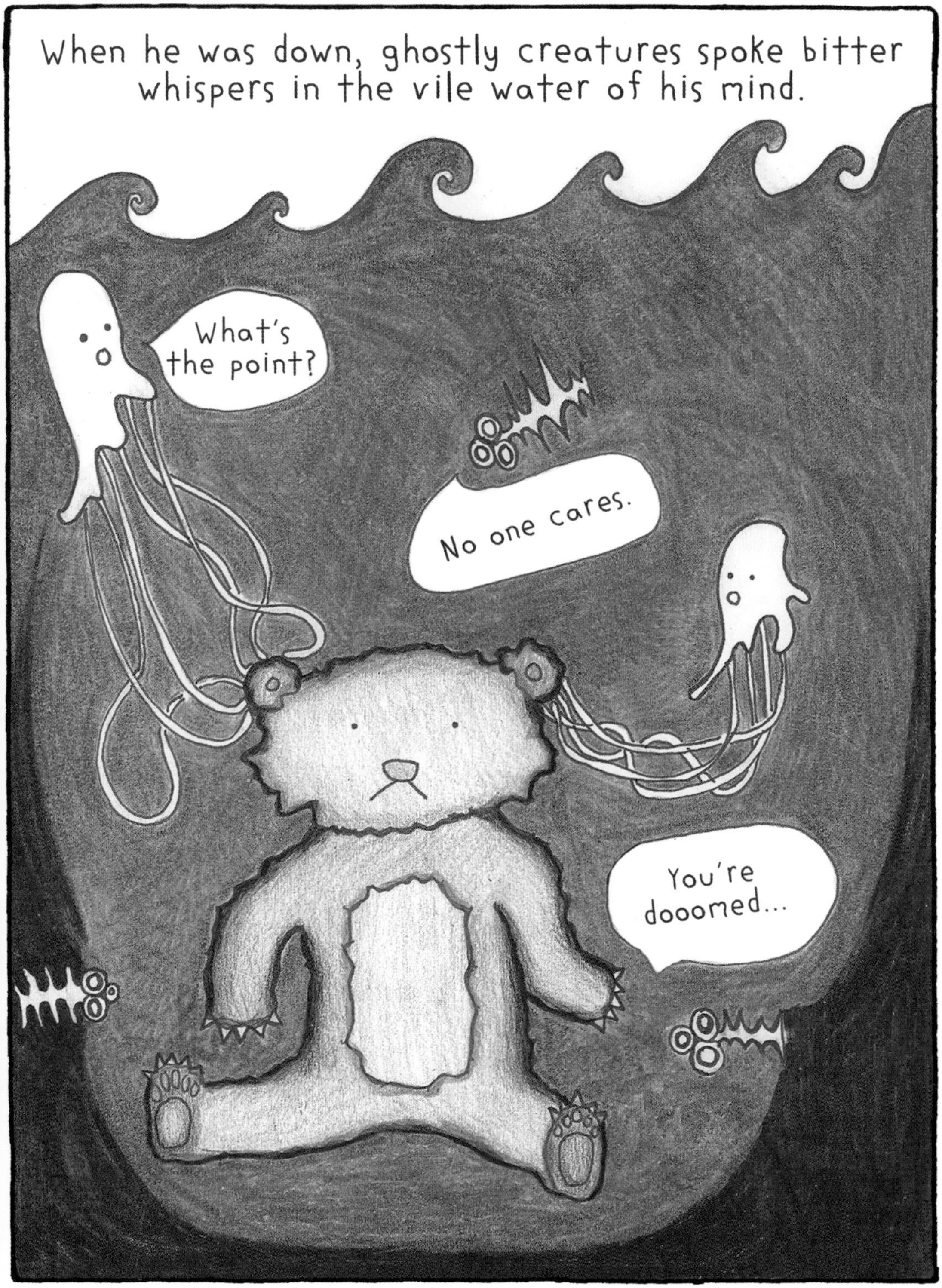
When he was down, ghostly creatures spoke bitter whispers in the vile water of his mind.
What's the point?
No one cares.
You're dooomed...

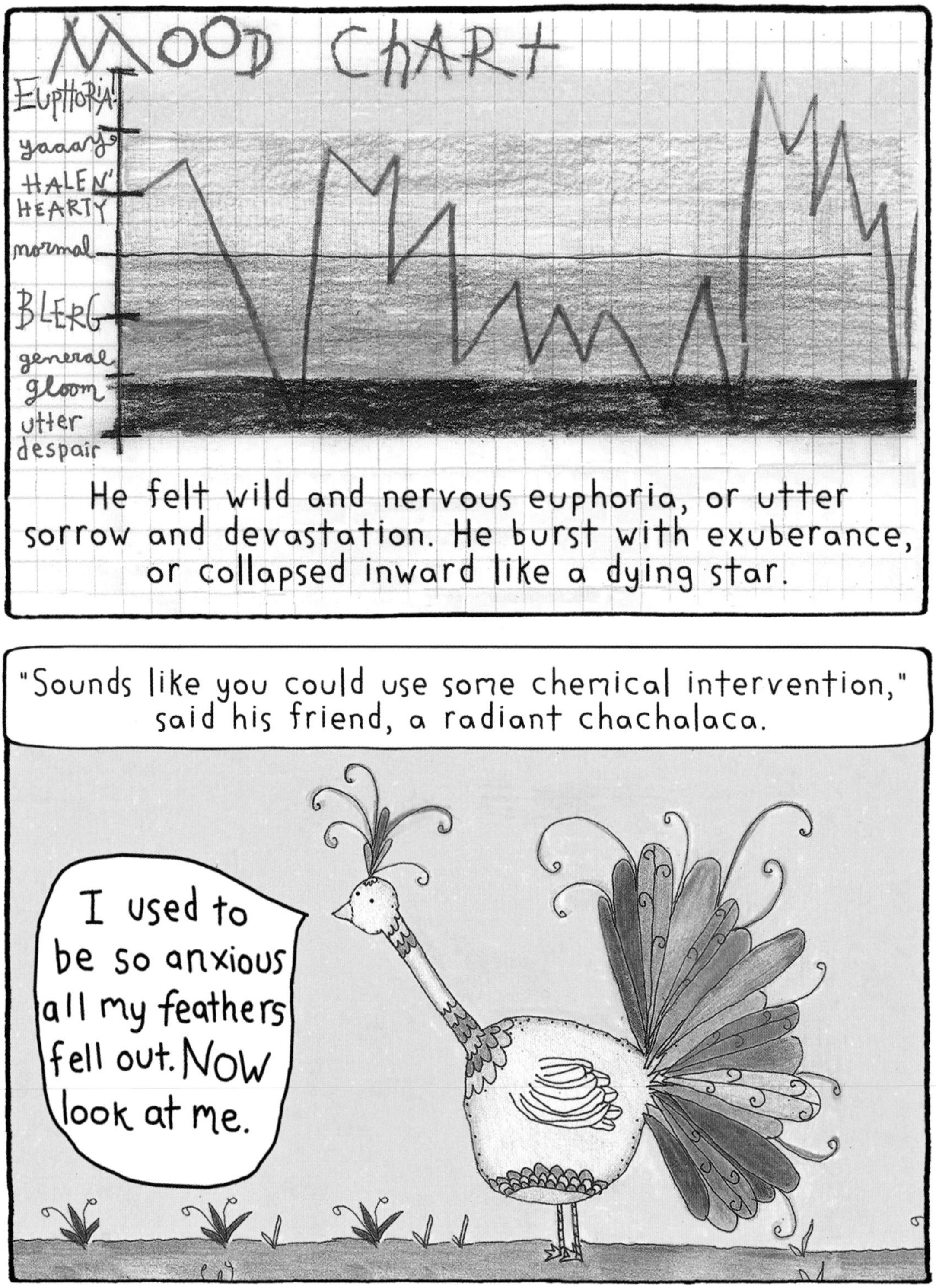
MOOD CHART
EUPHORIA!
yaaay
HALE N' HEARTY
normal
BLERG
general gloom
utter despair
He felt wild and nervous euphoria, or utter sorrow and devastation. He burst with exuberance, or collapsed inward like a dying star.
"Sounds like you could use some chemical intervention," said his friend, a radiant chachalaca.
I used to be so anxious all my feathers fell out. NOW look at me.

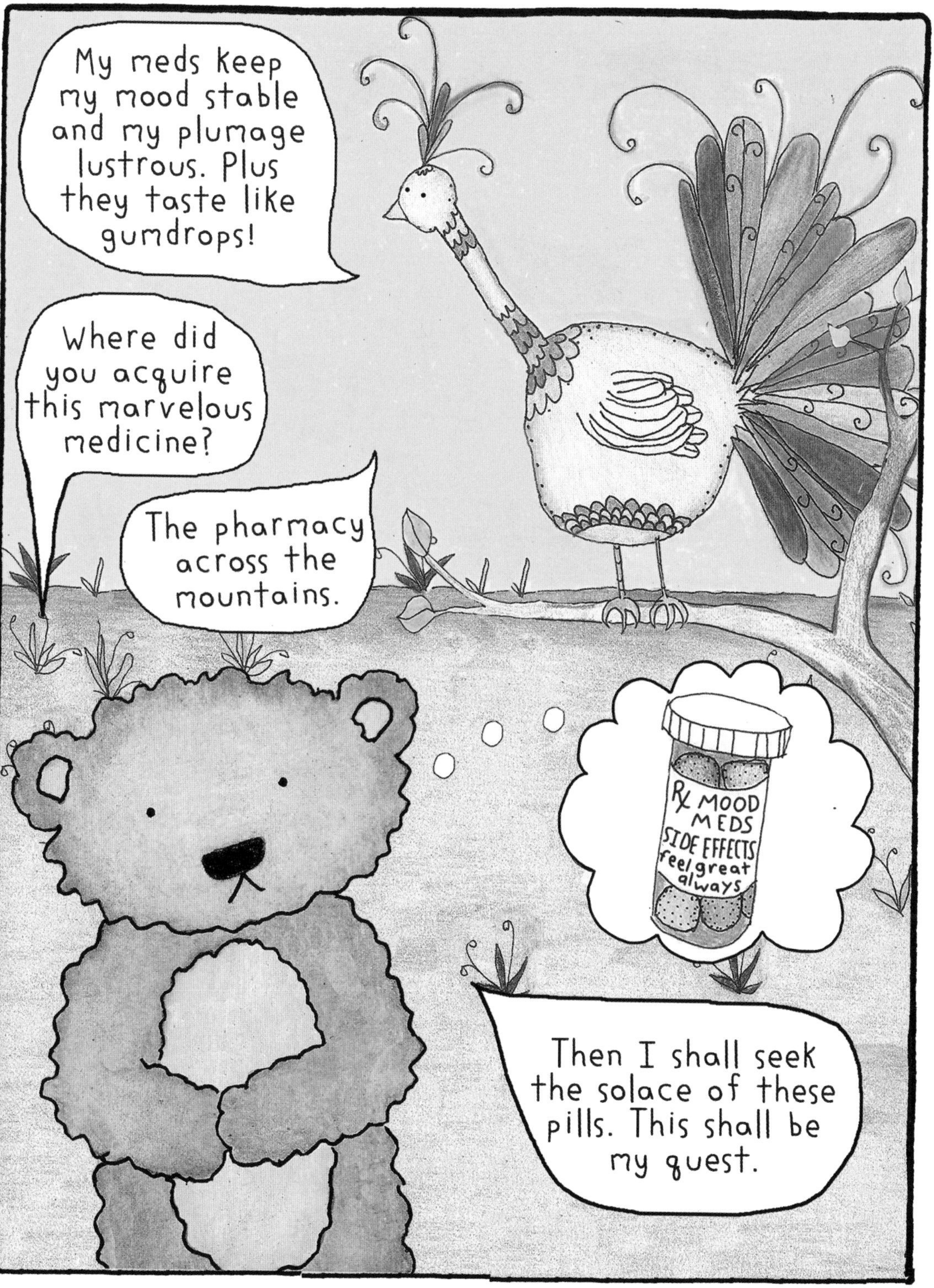
My meds keep my mood stable and my plumage lustrous. Plus they taste like gumdrops!
Where did you acquire this marvelous medicine?
The pharmacy across the mountains.
RX MOOD MEDS SIDE EFFECTS feel great always
Then I shall seek the solace of these pills. This shall be my quest.

Theodore packed five dried salmon, his top hat, and a pair of overalls. Then he climbed the purple mountains that ringed his forest and descended into the desert below.

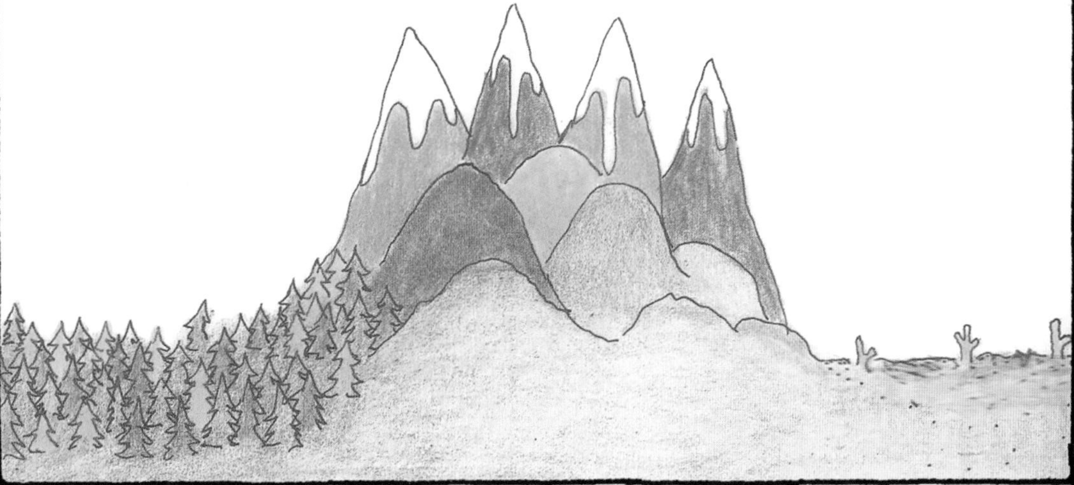

The sun shimmered down like honey. He wandered the expanse of scalding sand, cursing himself for not bringing a canteen of water. He longed to tear off his fur coat.

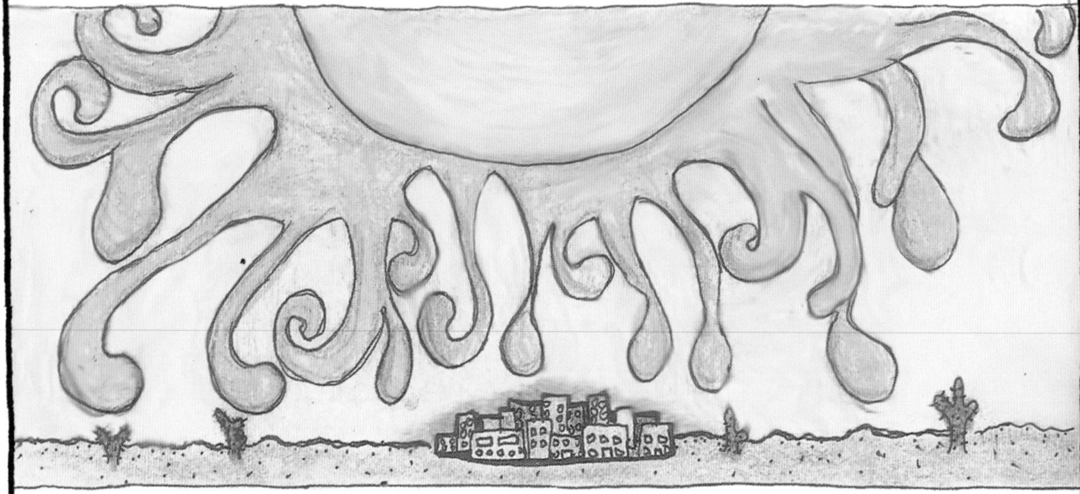

The town glimmered in the distance like a mirage.

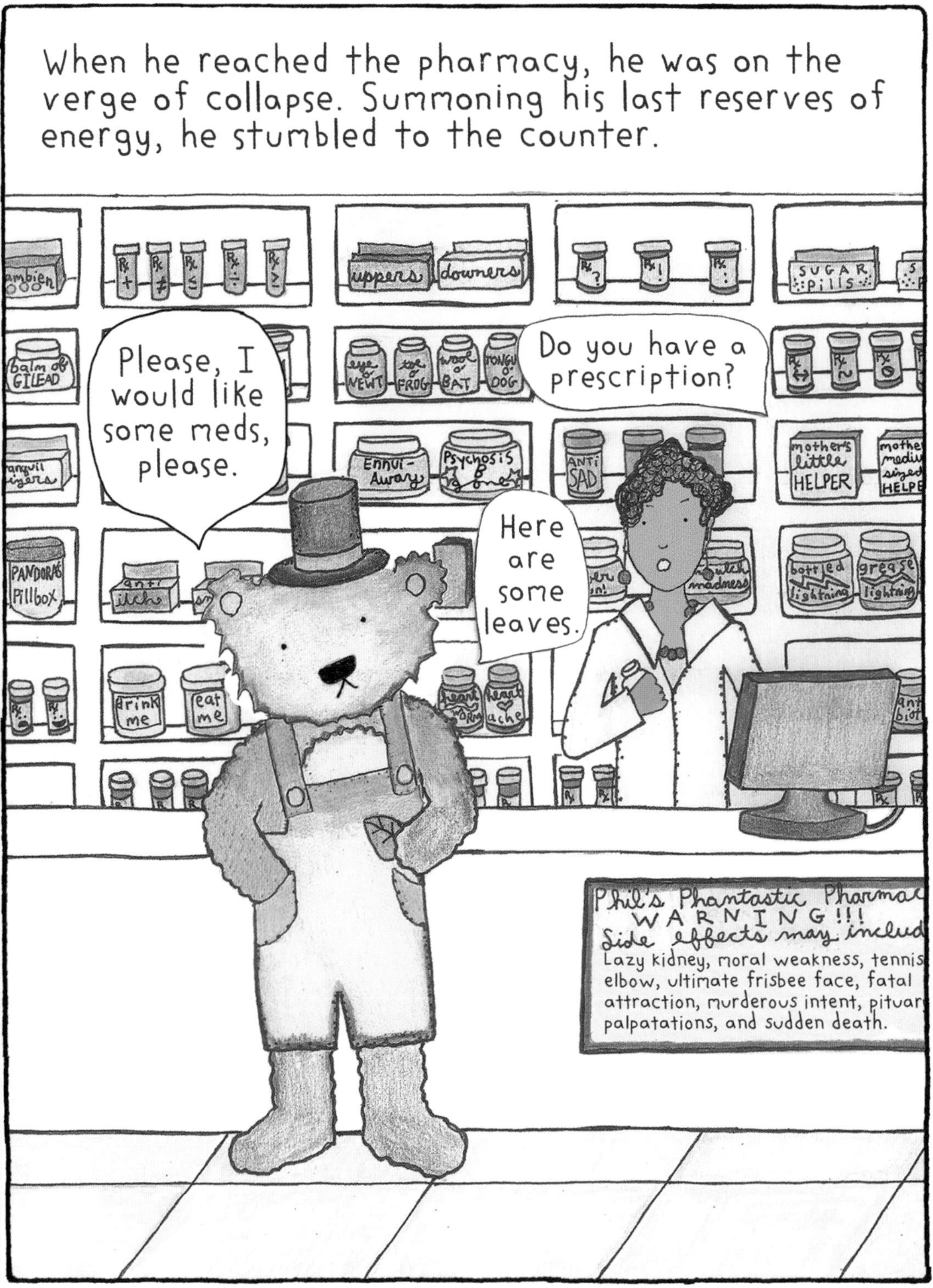
When he reached the pharmacy, he was on the verge of collapse. Summoning his last reserves of energy, he stumbled to the counter.
Please, I would like some meds, please.
Do you have a prescription?
Here are some leaves.
uppers
downers
SUGAR pills
balm of GILEAD
eye of NEWT
toe of FROG
wool of BAT
Ennui-Away
Psychosis B Gone
ANTI SAD
mother's little HELPER
PANDORA'S Pillbox
drink me
eat me
bottled lightning
grease lightning
Phil's Phantastic Pharmac
WARNING!!!
Side effects may includ
Lazy kidney, moral weakness, tennis
elbow, ultimate frisbee face, fatal
attraction, murderous intent, pituar
palpatations, and sudden death.

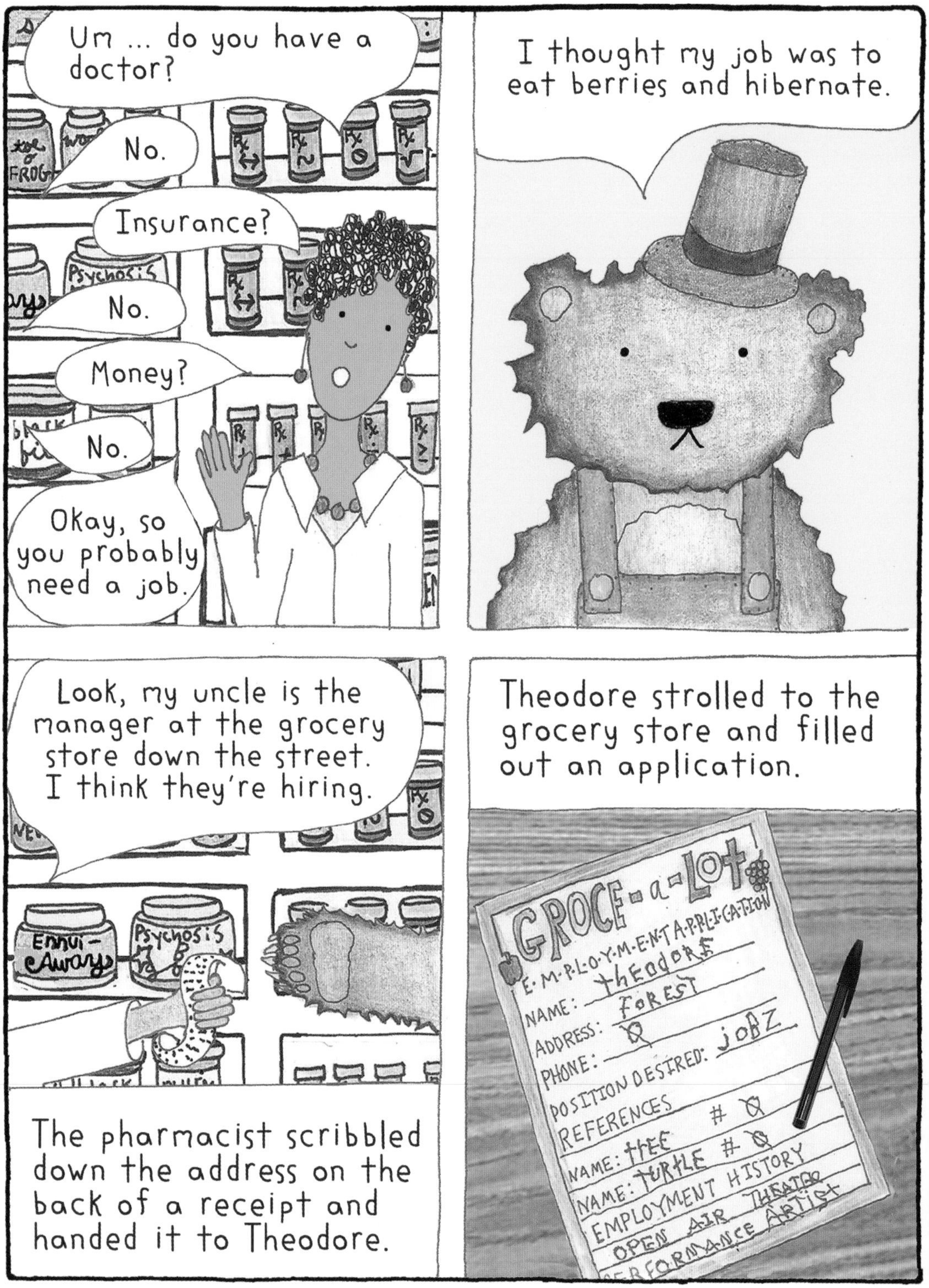

Um ... do you have a doctor?
No.
Insurance?
No.
Money?
No.
Okay, so you probably need a job.
I thought my job was to eat berries and hibernate.
Look, my uncle is the manager at the grocery store down the street. I think they're hiring.
Psychosis
Ennui-Aways
The pharmacist scribbled down the address on the back of a receipt and handed it to Theodore.
Theodore strolled to the grocery store and filled out an application.
GROCE-a-LOT
EMPLOYMENT APPLICATION
NAME: theodore
ADDRESS: FOREST
PHONE:
POSITION DESIRED: jobZ
REFERENCES
NAME: TREE
NAME: TURTLE
EMPLOYMENT HISTORY
OPEN AIR THEATRE
PERFORMANCE ARTIST

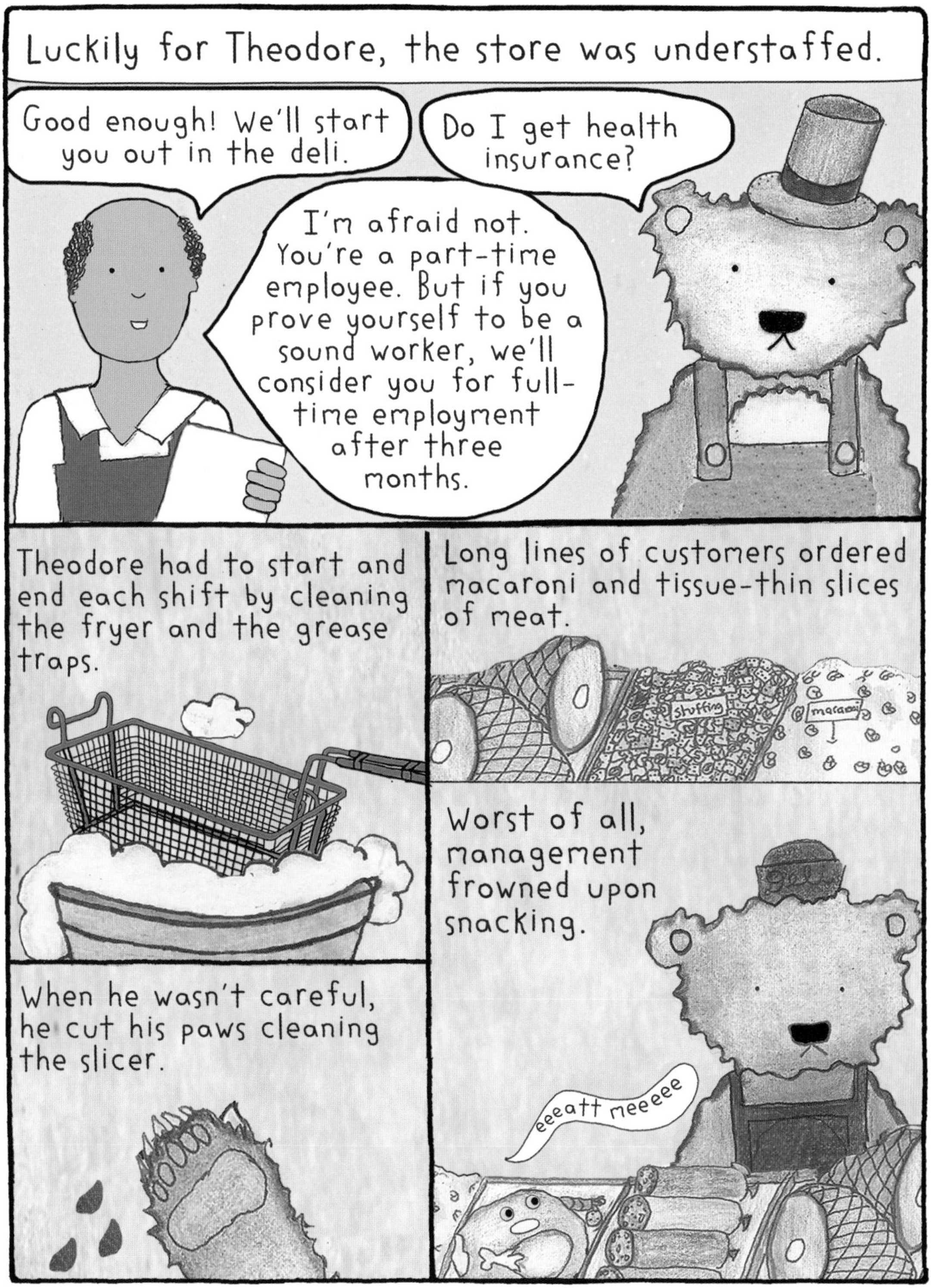

Luckily for Theodore, the store was understaffed.

Good enough! We'll start you out in the deli.

Do I get health insurance?

I'm afraid not. You're a part-time employee. But if you prove yourself to be a sound worker, we'll consider you for full-time employment after three months.

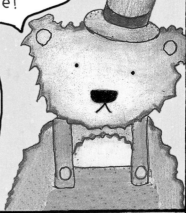

Theodore had to start and end each shift by cleaning the fryer and the grease traps.

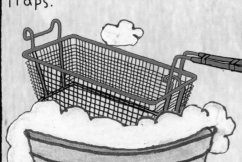

Long lines of customers ordered macaroni and tissue-thin slices of meat.

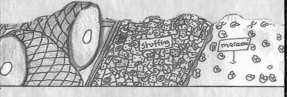

Worst of all, management frowned upon snacking.

When he wasn't careful, he cut his paws cleaning the slicer.

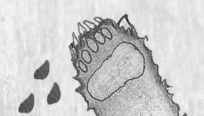

eeeatt meeeee

Because he was so far from home, Theodore had to sleep in a dumpster behind the store.

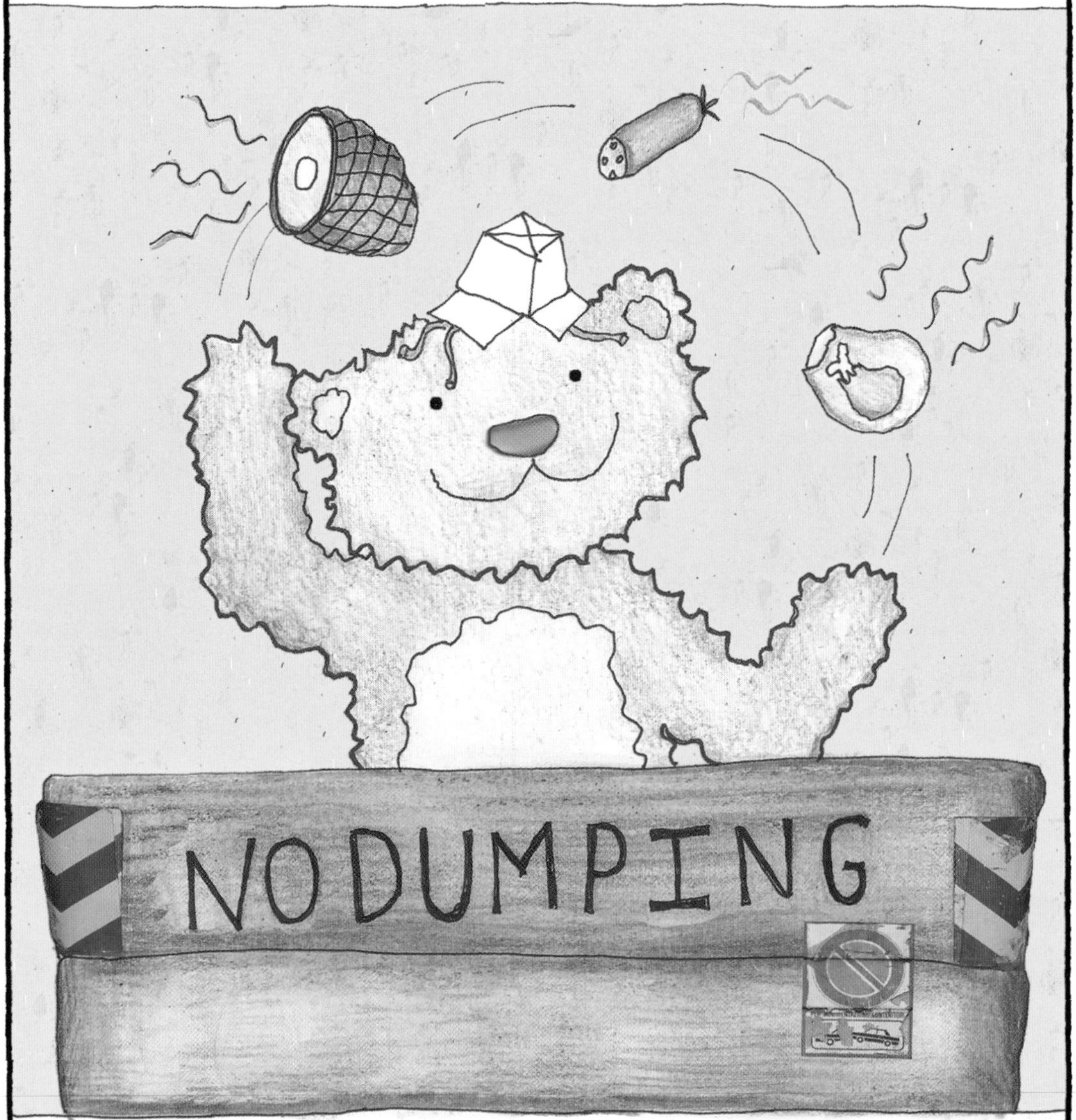
NO DUMPING

And while he enjoyed eating his fill of expired ham and smashed crackers . . .

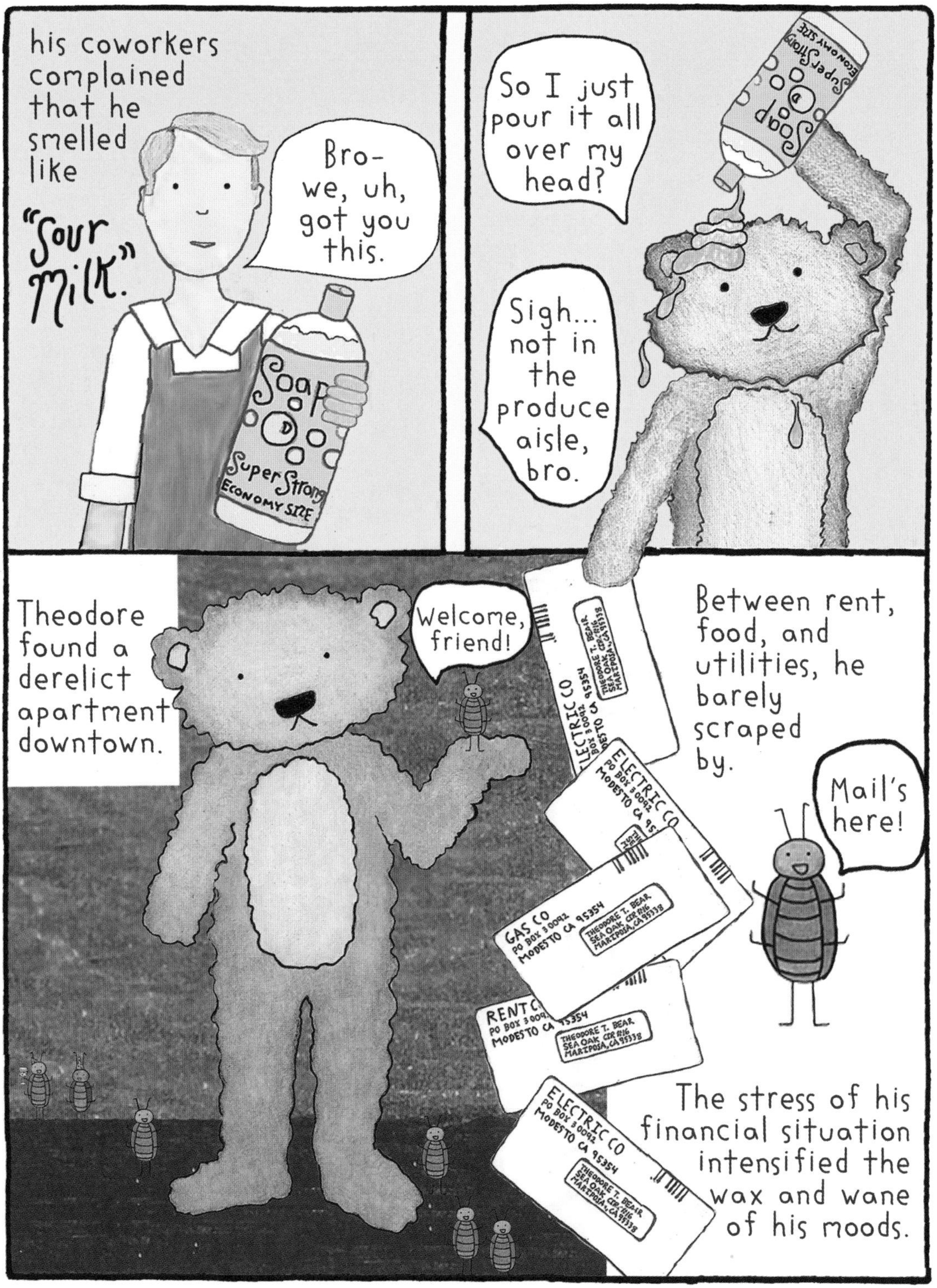
his coworkers complained that he smelled like "Sour Milk."
Bro- we, uh, got you this.
Soap
Super Strong
Economy Size
So I just pour it all over my head?
Sigh... not in the produce aisle, bro.
Theodore found a derelict apartment downtown.
Welcome, friend!
Between rent, food, and utilities, he barely scraped by.
Mail's here!
GAS CO
PO BOX 30092
MODESTO CA 95354
THEODORE T. BEAR
SEA OAK CRK RIG
MARIPOSA, CA 95338
RENT CO
ELECTRIC CO
The stress of his financial situation intensified the wax and wane of his moods.

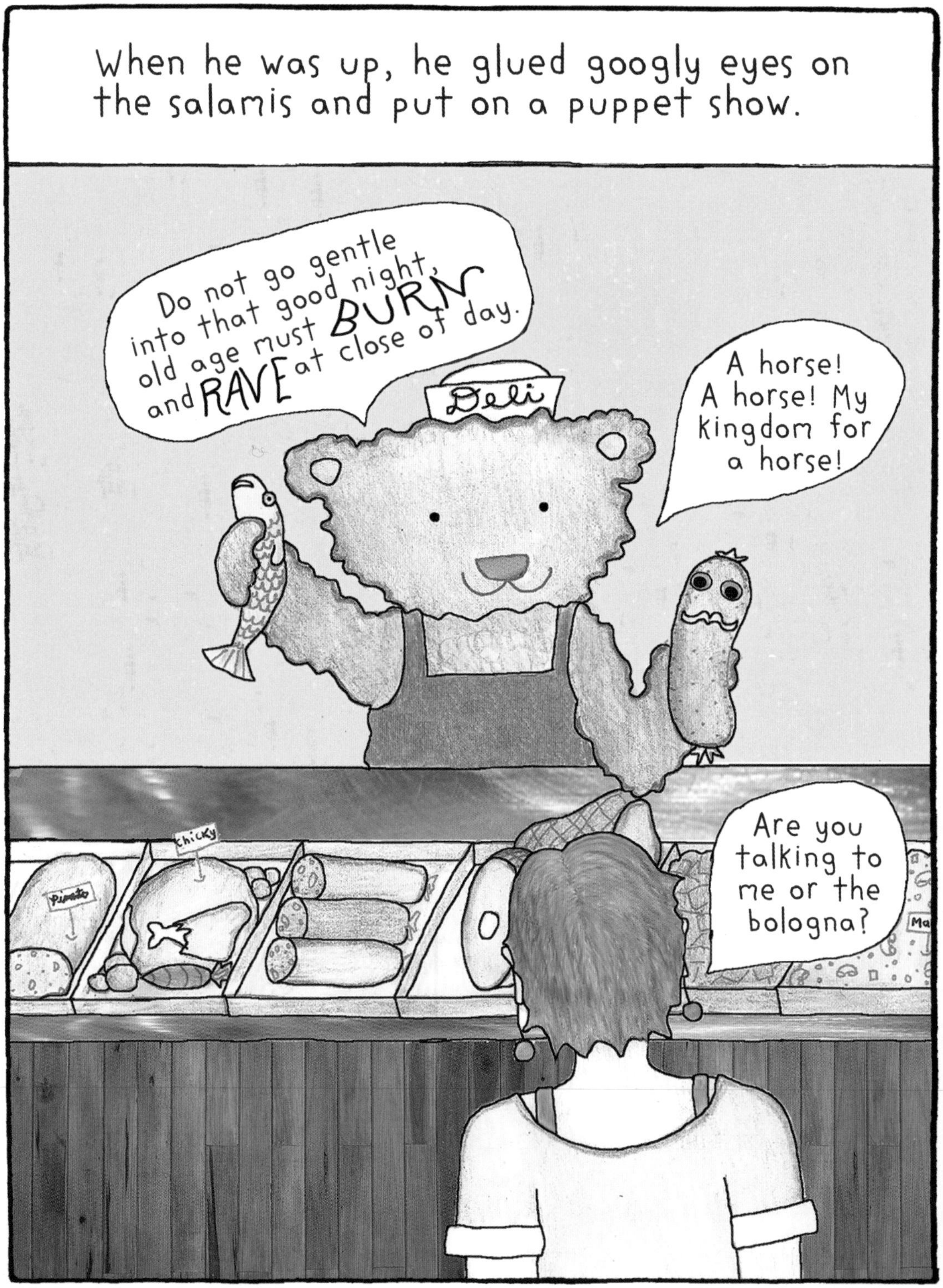
When he was up, he glued googly eyes on the salamis and put on a puppet show.
Do not go gentle into that good night, old age must BURN and RAVE at close of day.
Deli
A horse! A horse! My kingdom for a horse!
Chicky
Are you talking to me or the bologna?

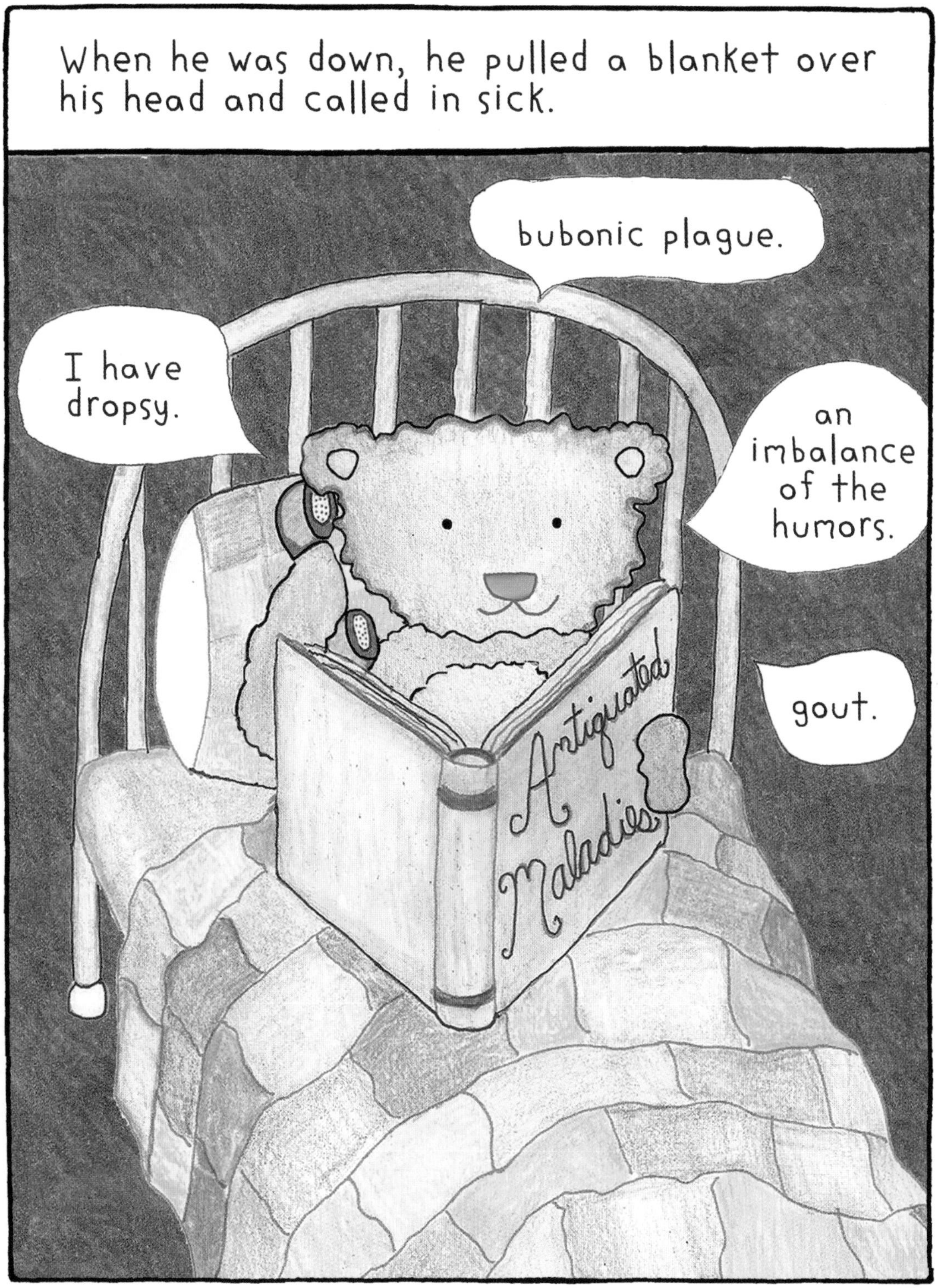
When he was down, he pulled a blanket over his head and called in sick.
I have dropsy.
bubonic plague.
an imbalance of the humors.
gout.
Antiquated Maladies

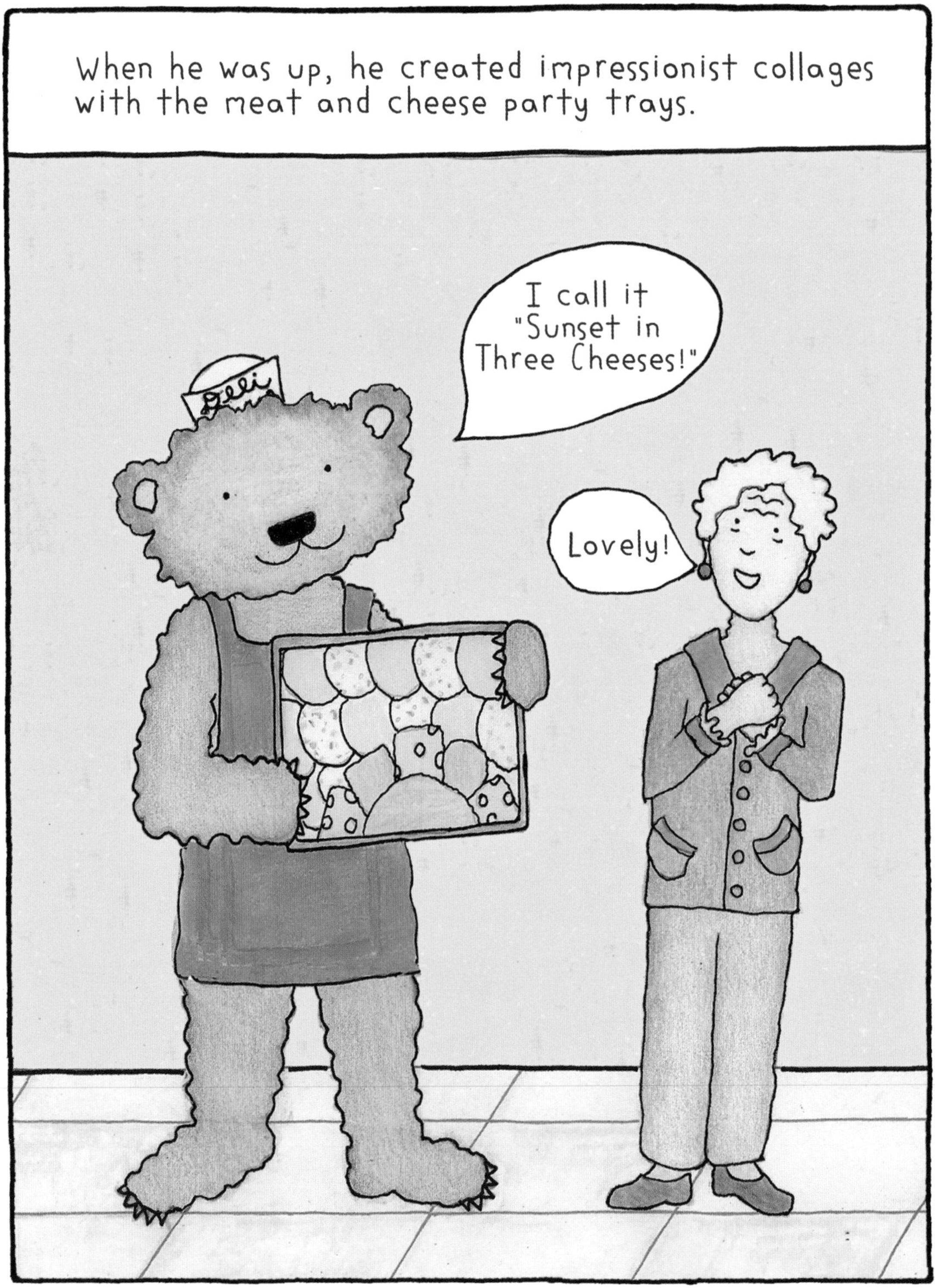
When he was up, he created impressionist collages with the meat and cheese party trays.
Deli
I call it "Sunset in Three Cheeses!"
Lovely!

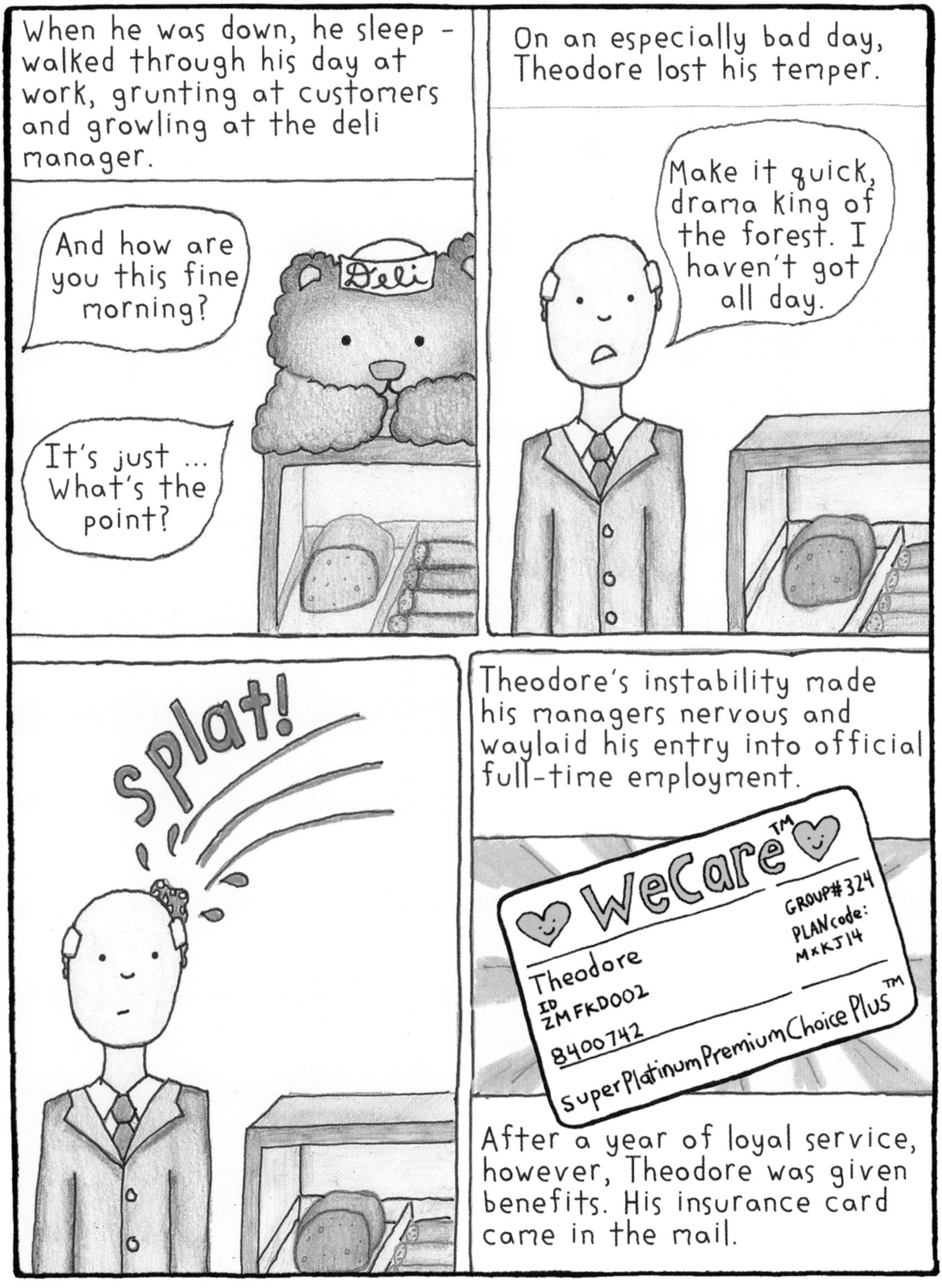
When he was down, he sleep-walked through his day at work, grunting at customers and growling at the deli manager.
Deli
And how are you this fine morning?
It's just ... What's the point?
On an especially bad day, Theodore lost his temper.
Make it quick, drama king of the forest. I haven't got all day.
splat!
Theodore's instability made his managers nervous and waylaid his entry into official full-time employment.
WeCare™
GROUP#324
PLAN code: MxKJ14
Theodore
ID ZMFKD002
8400742
SuperPlatinumPremiumChoicePlus™
After a year of loyal service, however, Theodore was given benefits. His insurance card came in the mail.

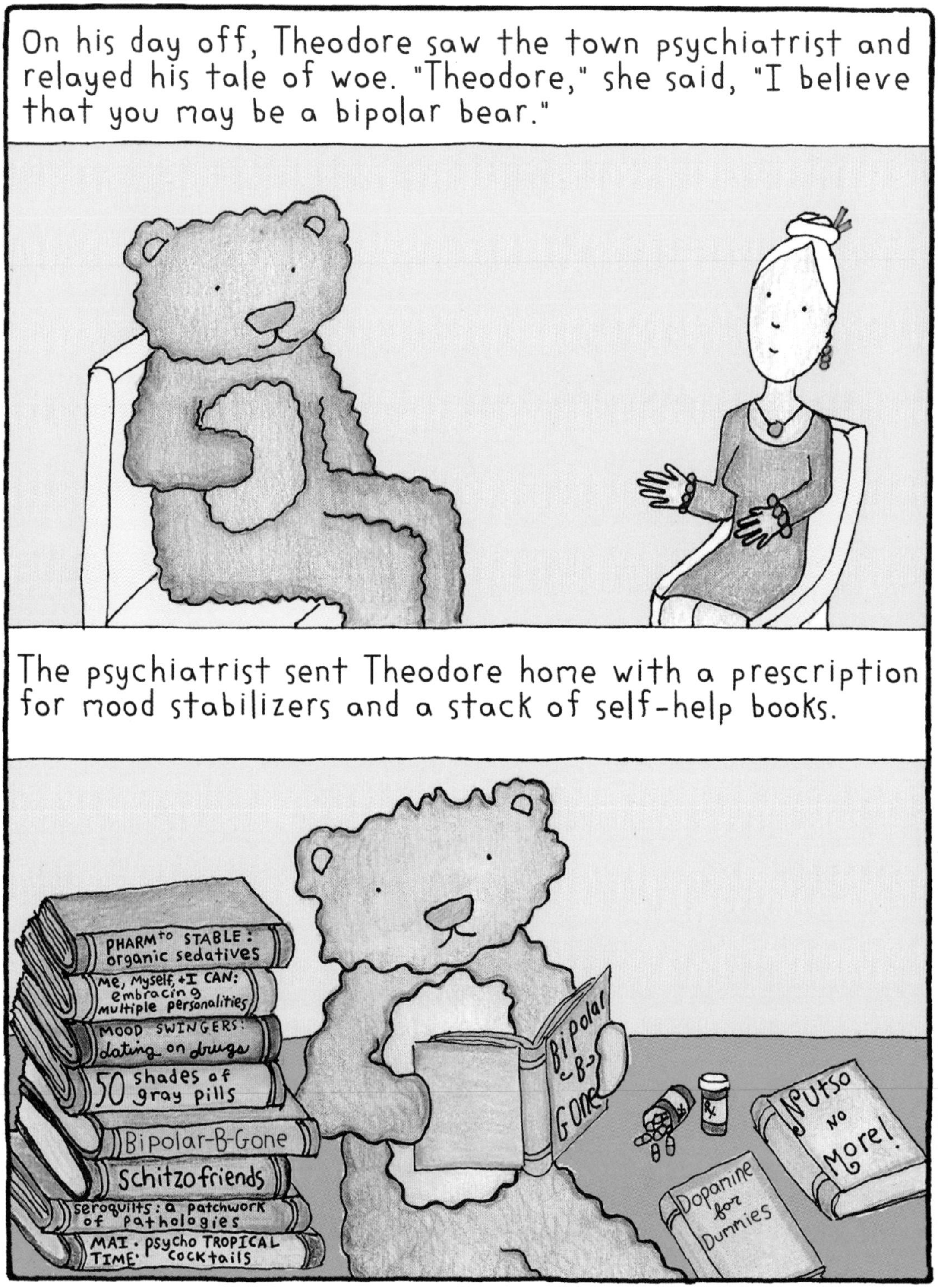
On his day off, Theodore saw the town psychiatrist and relayed his tale of woe. "Theodore," she said, "I believe that you may be a bipolar bear."
The psychiatrist sent Theodore home with a prescription for mood stabilizers and a stack of self-help books.
PHARM to STABLE: organic sedatives
Me, Myself, + I CAN: embracing multiple personalities
MOOD SWINGERS: dating on drugs
50 shades of gray pills
Bipolar-B-Gone
Schitzofriends
Seroquilts: a patchwork of pathologies
MAI TIME • psycho TROPICAL cocktails
Bipolar -B- Gone
Rx
Nutso No More!
Dopamine for Dummies

Theodore tried to follow the psychiatrist's advice. Each morning, he went for a swim in the river. He tried to eat healthy meals.

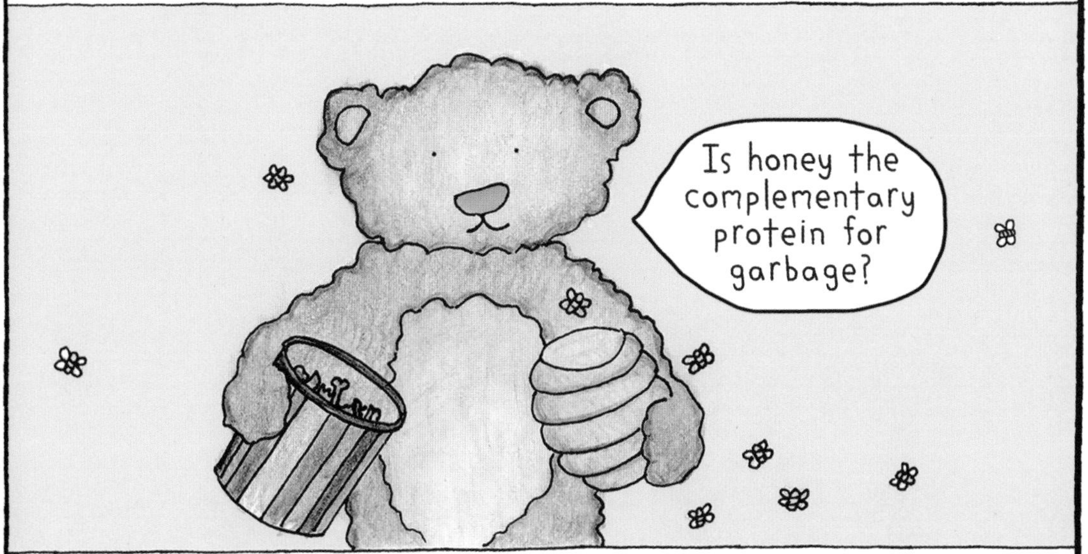
Is honey the complementary protein for garbage?

He took his pills and saw the psychiatrist each week.

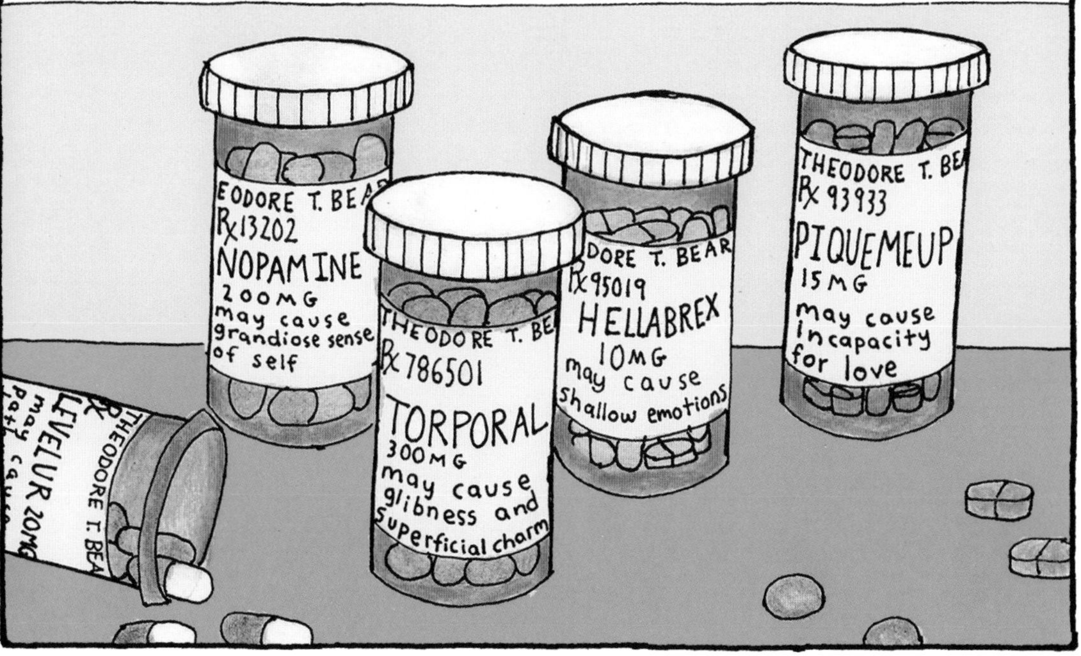
EODORE T. BEA
℞13202
NOPAMINE
200MG
may cause grandiose sense of self
THEODORE T. BE
℞786501
TORPORAL
300MG
may cause glibness and superficial charm
DORE T. BEAR
℞95019
HELLABREX
10MG
may cause shallow emotions
THEODORE T. BEA
℞93933
PIQUEMEUP
15MG
may cause incapacity for love
THEODORE T. BEA
LEVELUR 20MG

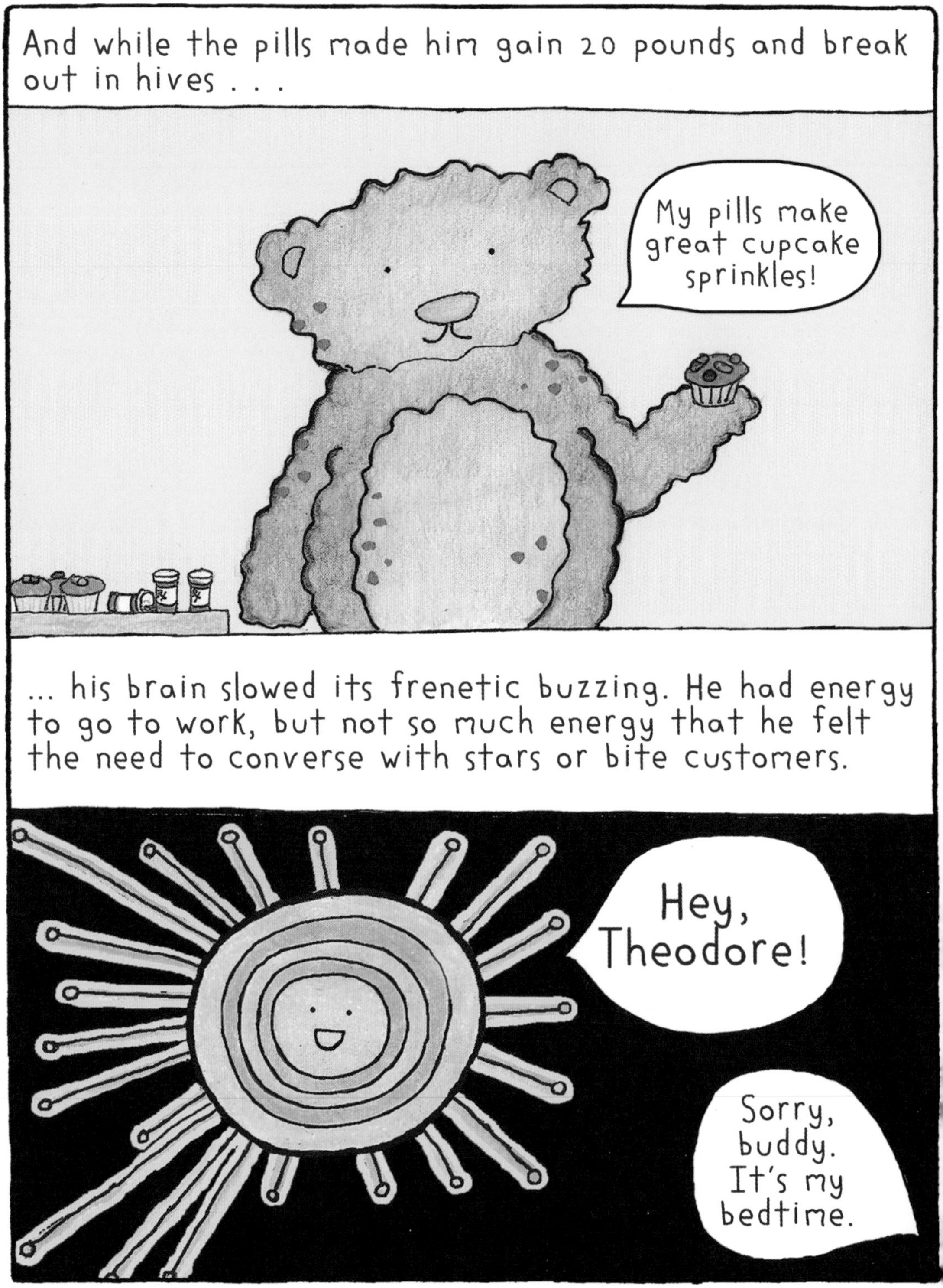
And while the pills made him gain 20 pounds and break out in hives . . .
My pills make great cupcake sprinkles!
... his brain slowed its frenetic buzzing. He had energy to go to work, but not so much energy that he felt the need to converse with stars or bite customers.
Hey, Theodore!
Sorry, buddy. It's my bedtime.

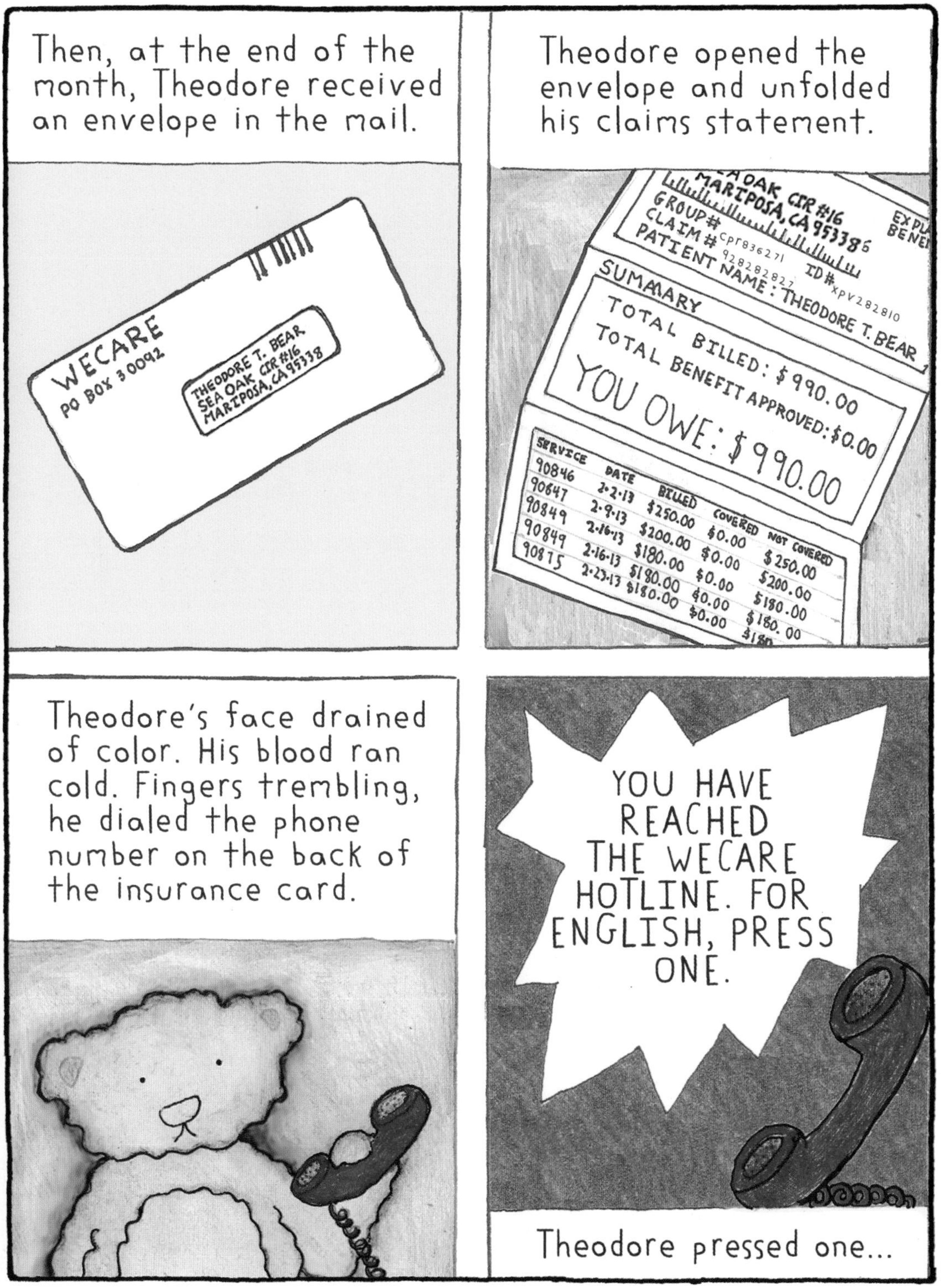
Then, at the end of the month, Theodore received an envelope in the mail.
WECARE
PO BOX 30092
THEODORE T. BEAR
SEA OAK CIR #16
MARIPOSA, CA 95338
Theodore opened the envelope and unfolded his claims statement.
PATIENT NAME: THEODORE T. BEAR
SUMMARY
TOTAL BILLED: $990.00
TOTAL BENEFIT APPROVED: $0.00
YOU OWE: $990.00
Theodore's face drained of color. His blood ran cold. Fingers trembling, he dialed the phone number on the back of the insurance card.
YOU HAVE REACHED THE WECARE HOTLINE. FOR ENGLISH, PRESS ONE.
Theodore pressed one...

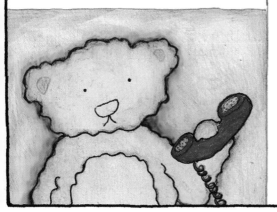

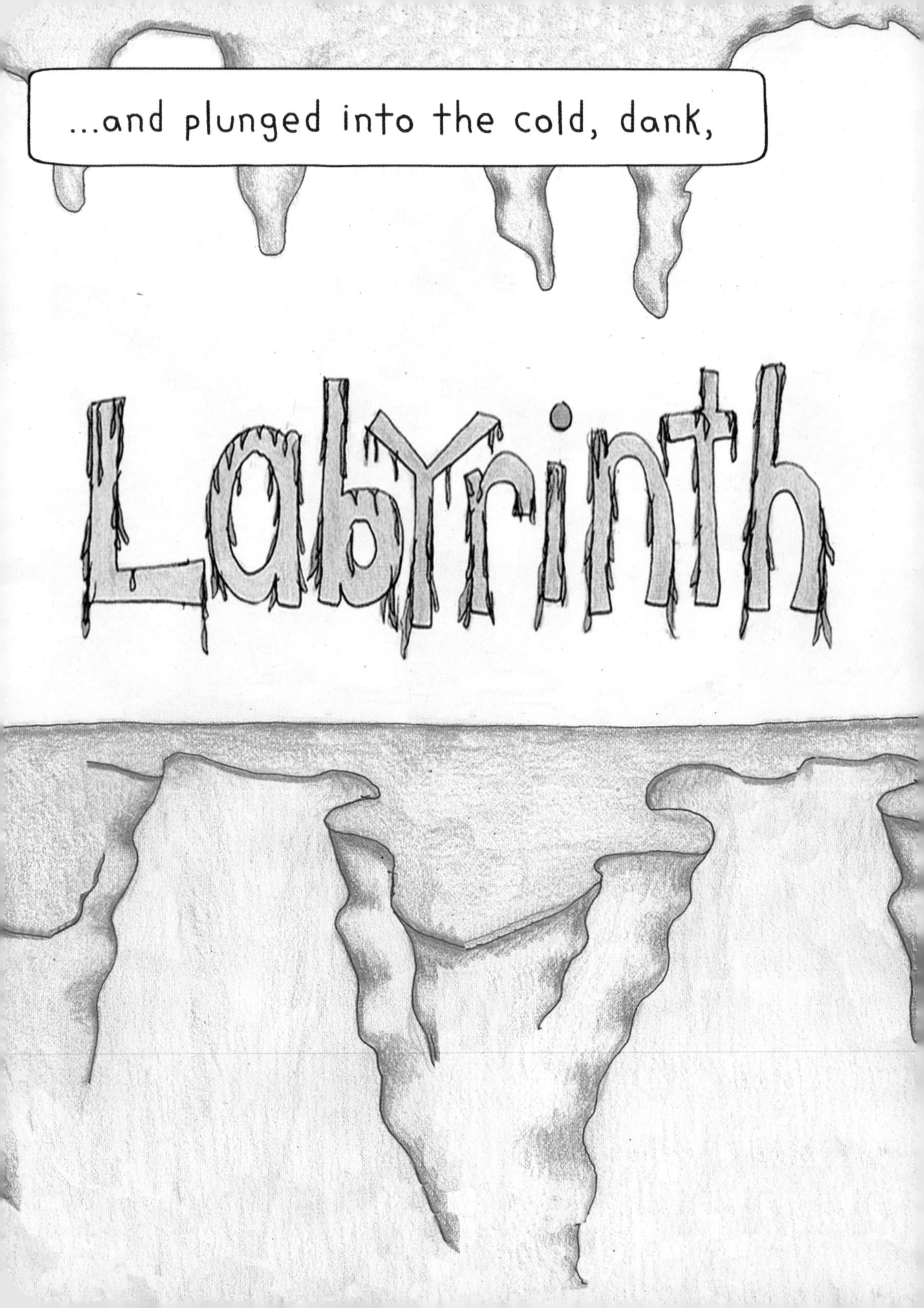
...and plunged into the cold, dank,
Labyrinth

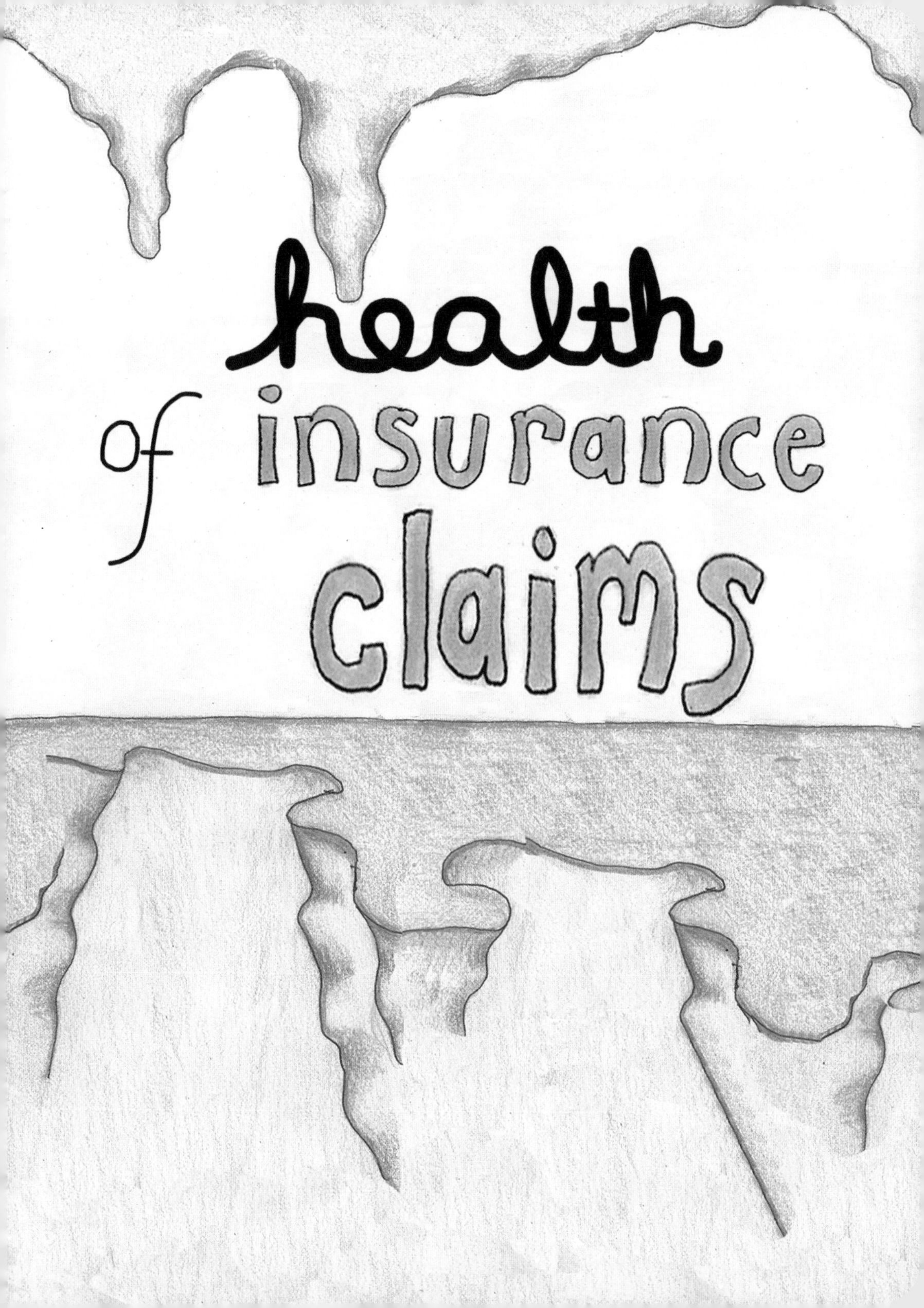
health
of insurance
claims

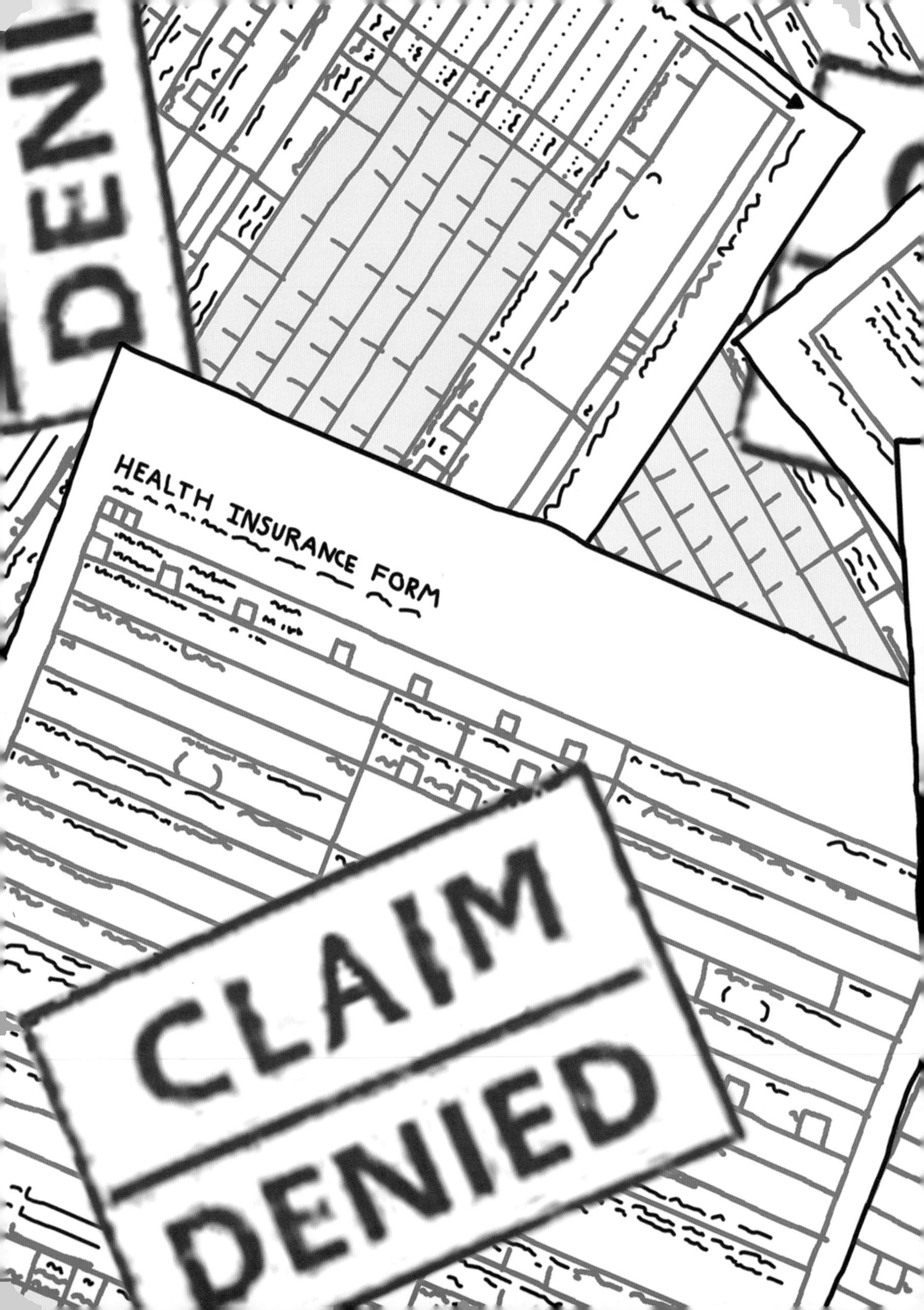
HEALTH INSURANCE FORM
CLAIM
DENIED

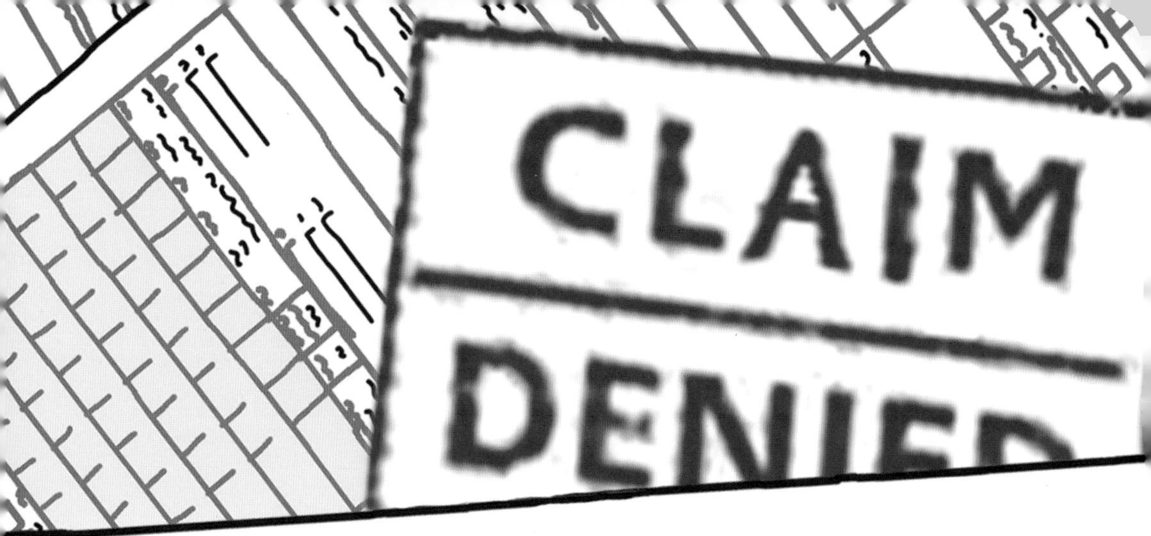
CLAIM

chapter two:

The Labyrinth

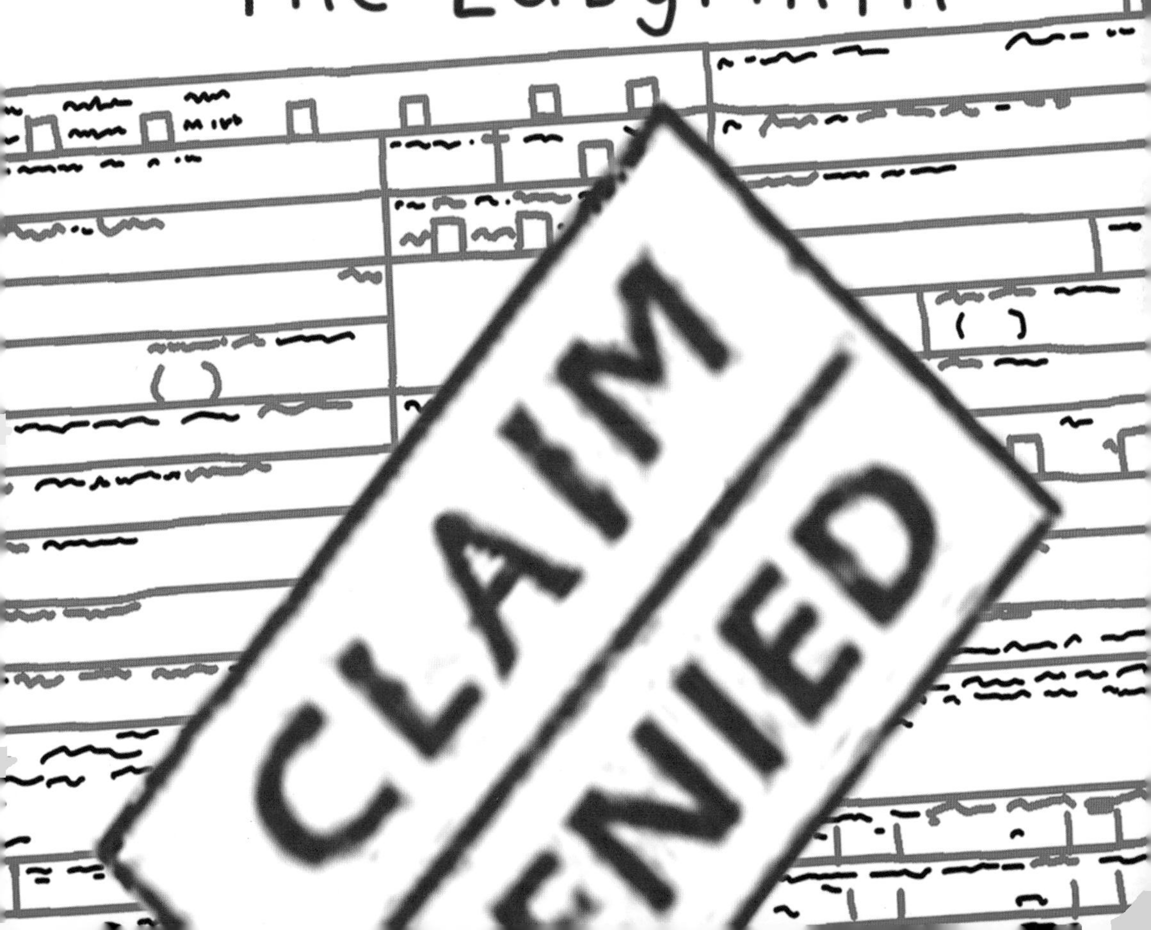
CLAIM

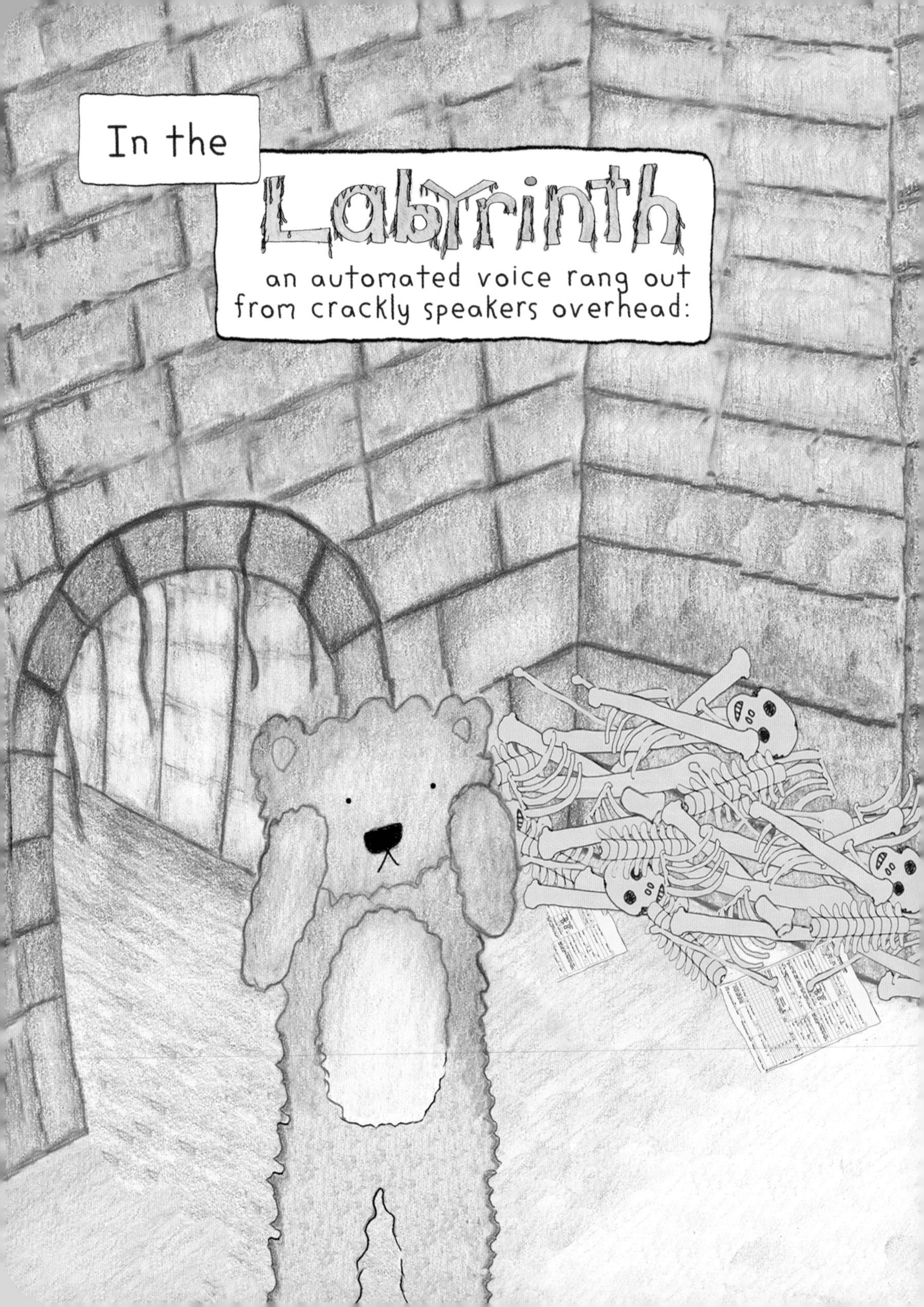
In the
Labyrinth
an automated voice rang out from crackly speakers overhead:

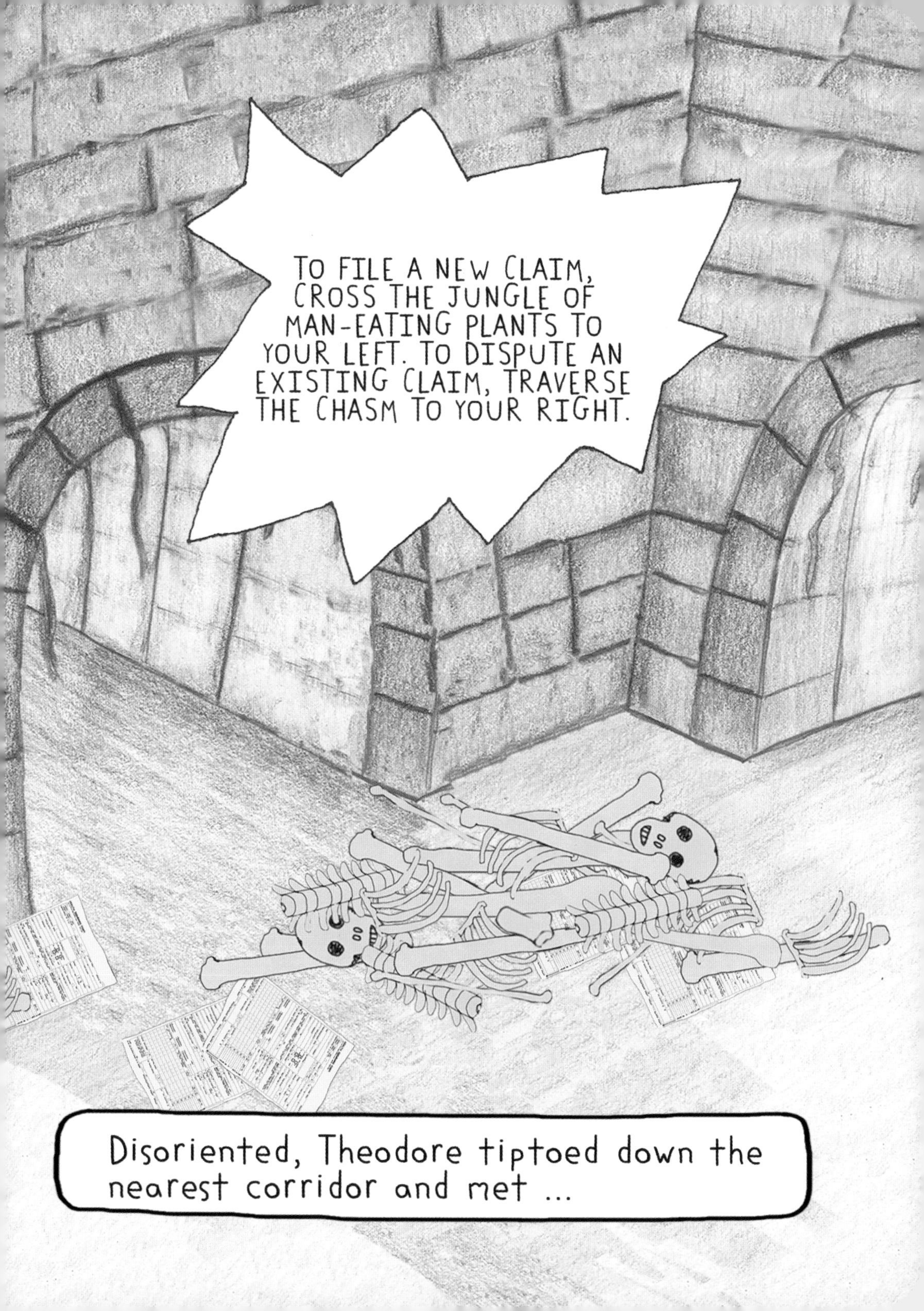
TO FILE A NEW CLAIM, CROSS THE JUNGLE OF MAN-EATING PLANTS TO YOUR LEFT. TO DISPUTE AN EXISTING CLAIM, TRAVERSE THE CHASM TO YOUR RIGHT.
Disoriented, Theodore tiptoed down the nearest corridor and met ...

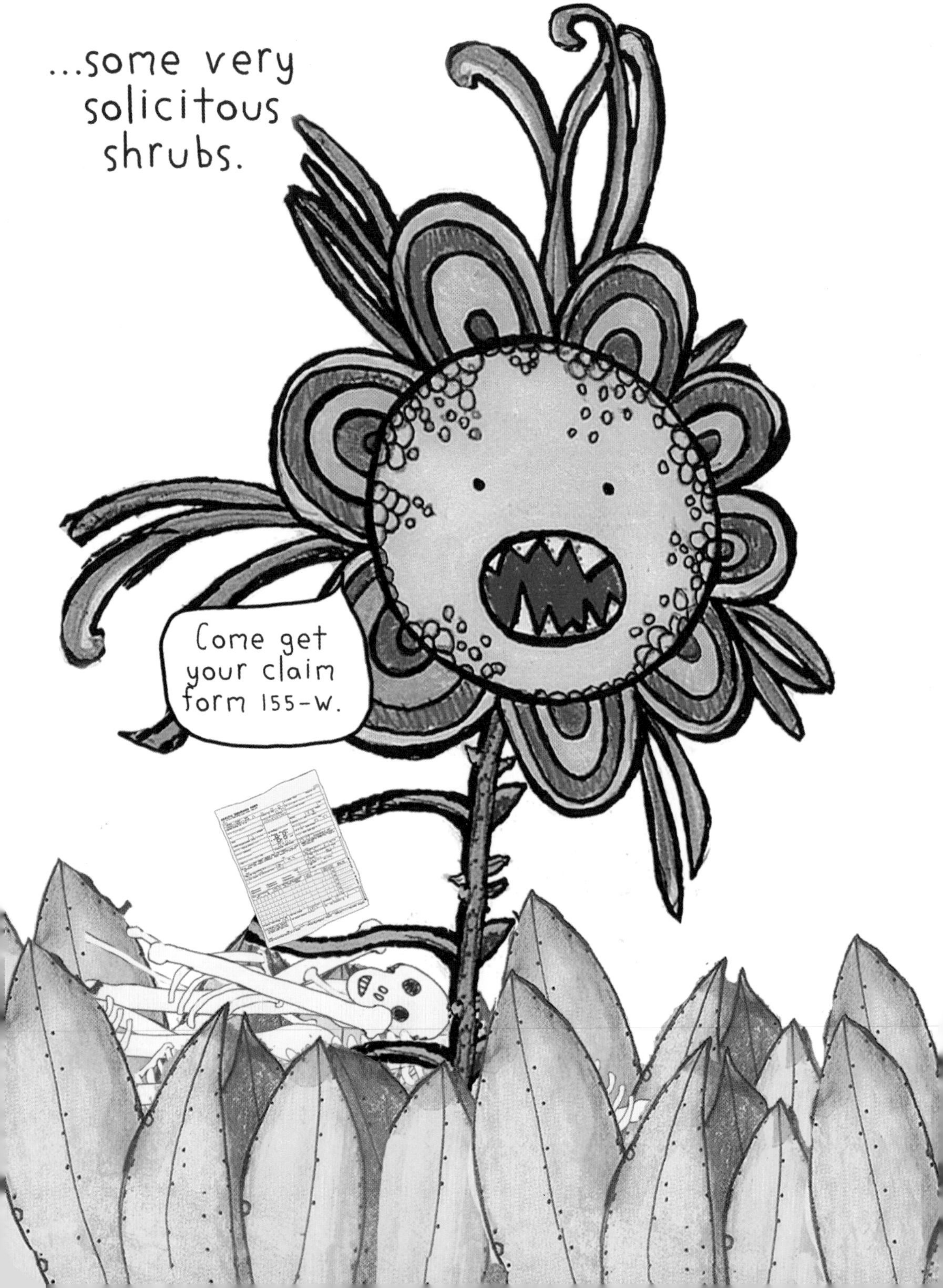
...some very solicitous shrubs.
Come get your claim form 155-W.

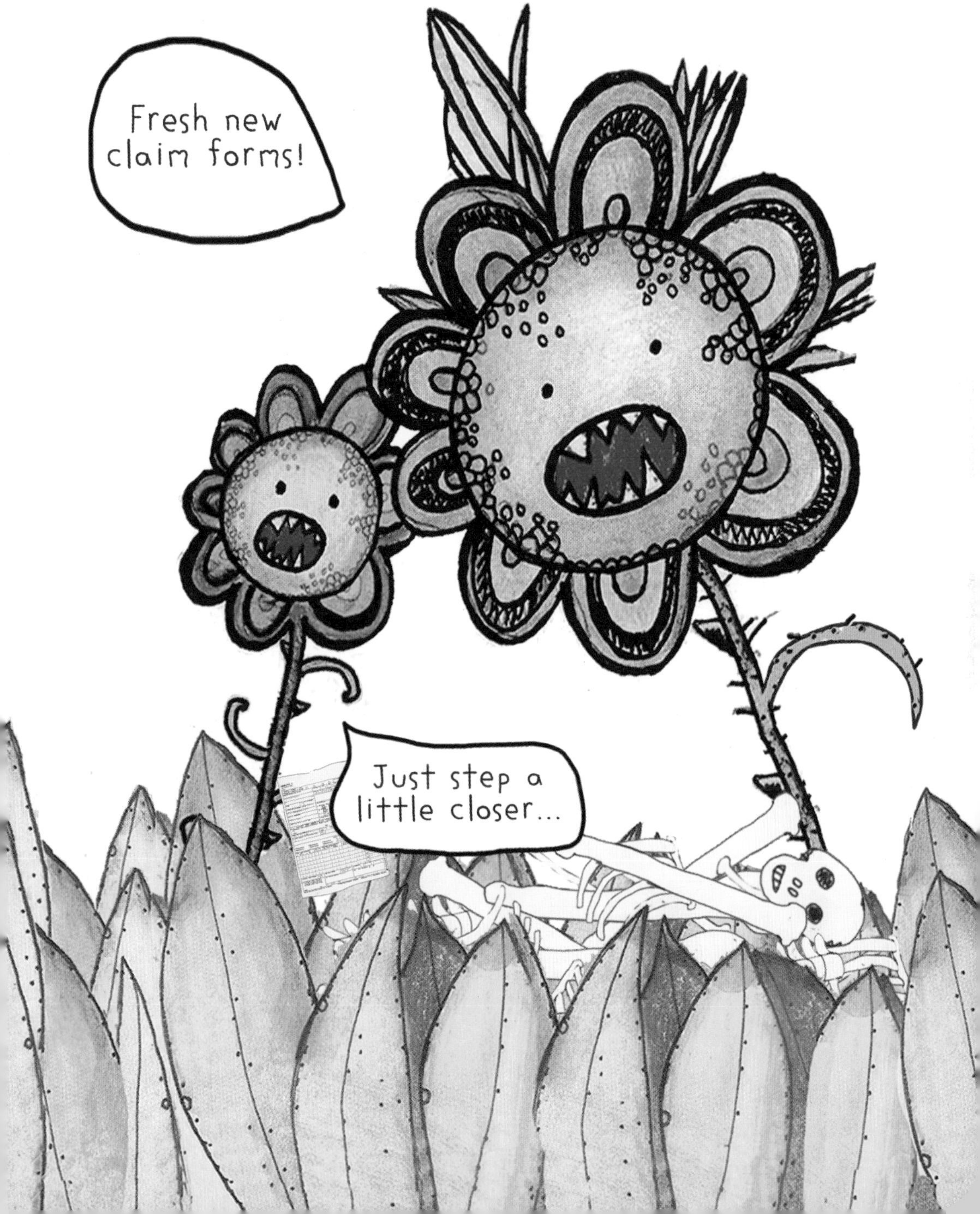
Fresh new claim forms!
Just step a little closer...

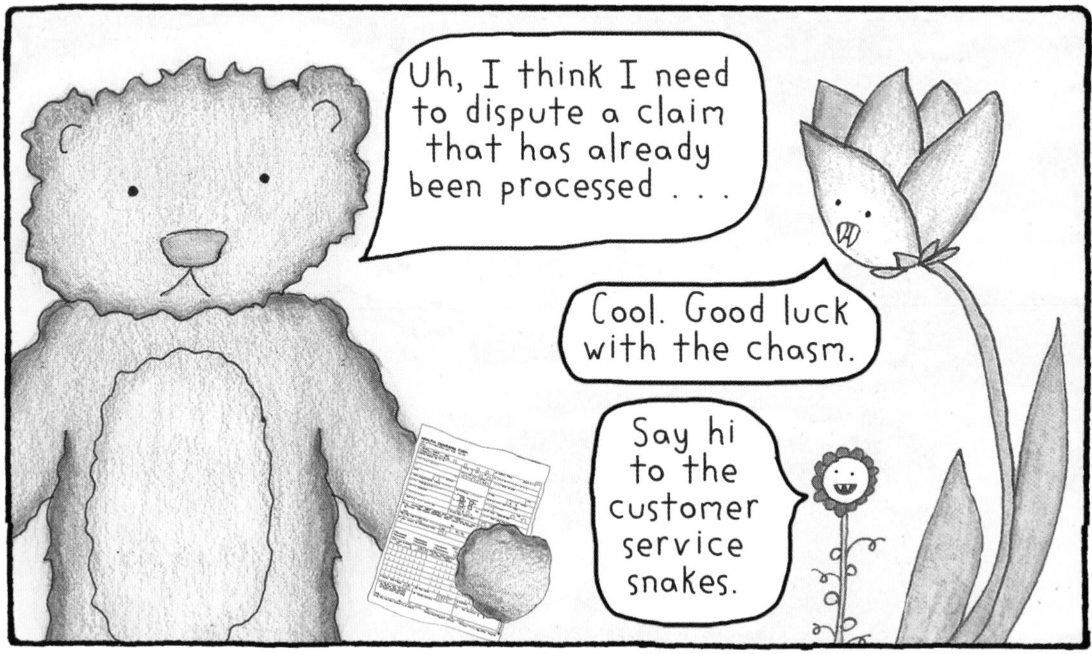
Uh, I think I need to dispute a claim that has already been processed . . .
Cool. Good luck with the chasm.
Say hi to the customer service snakes.

Theodore wandered through the labyrinth until he found the chasm. He peered into the depths...

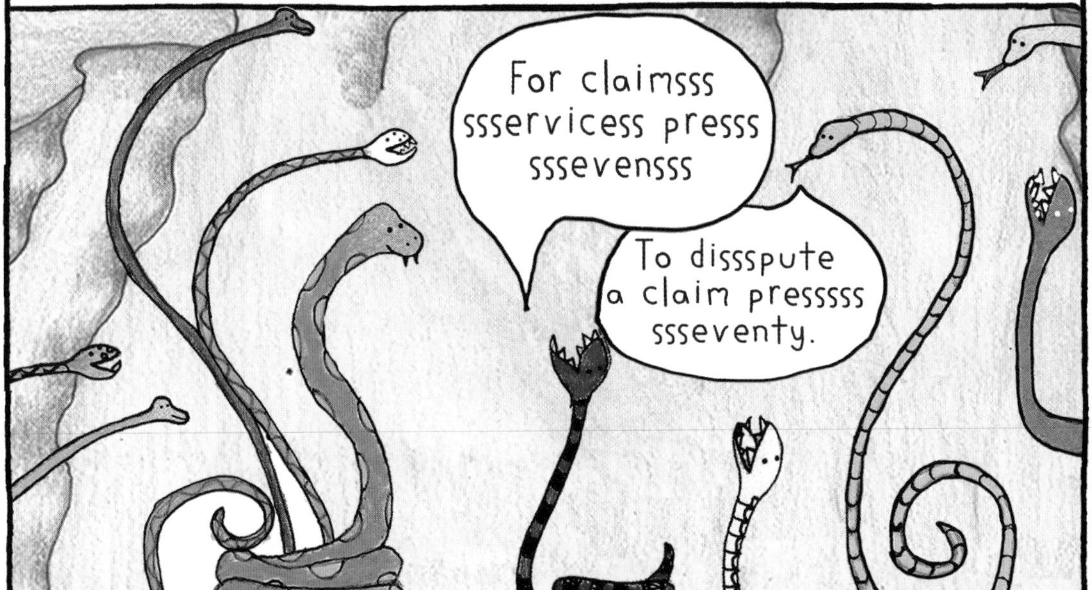
For claimsss ssservicess presss sssevensss
To disssspute a claim presssss sssseventy.

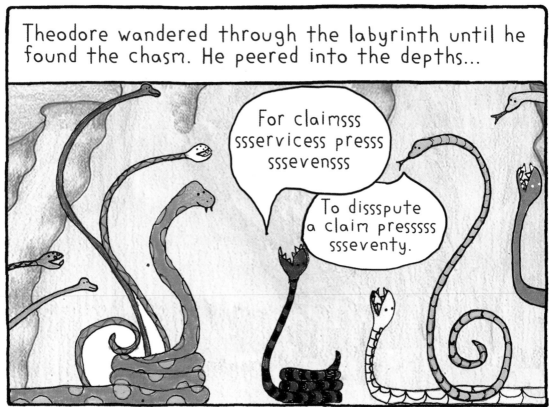

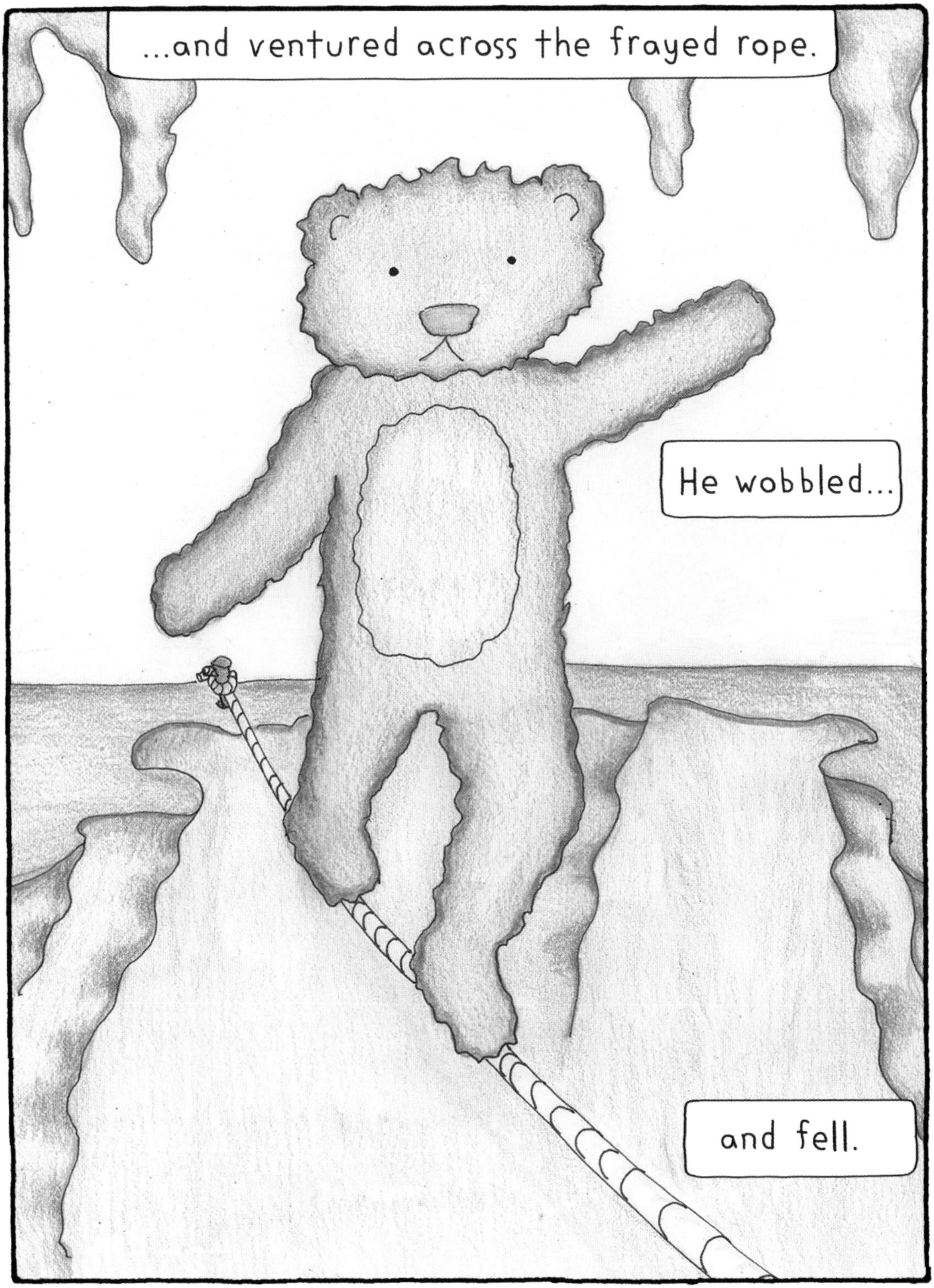
...and ventured across the frayed rope.
He wobbled...
and fell.

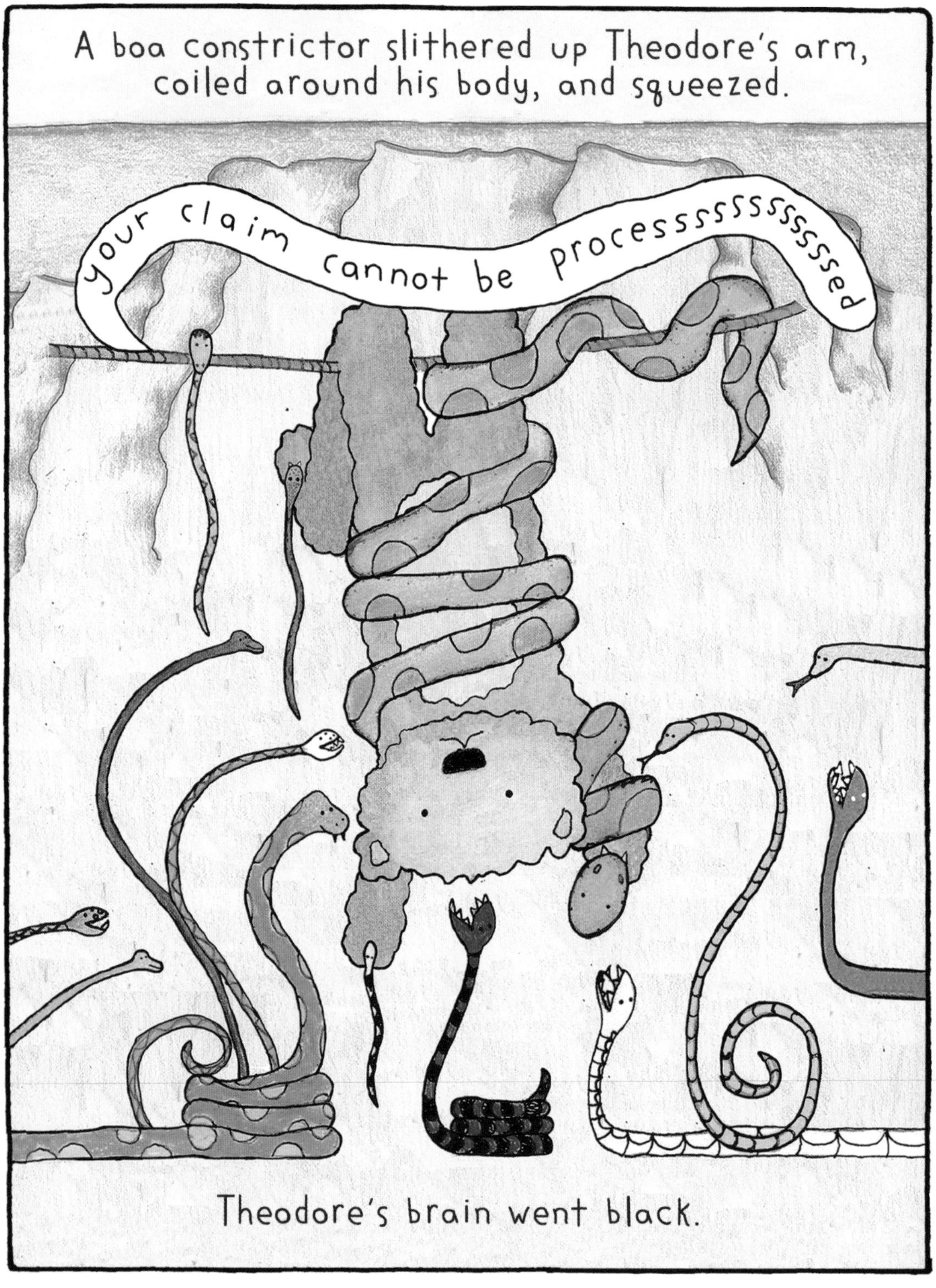
A boa constrictor slithered up Theodore's arm, coiled around his body, and squeezed.
your claim cannot be processssssssssssed
Theodore's brain went black.

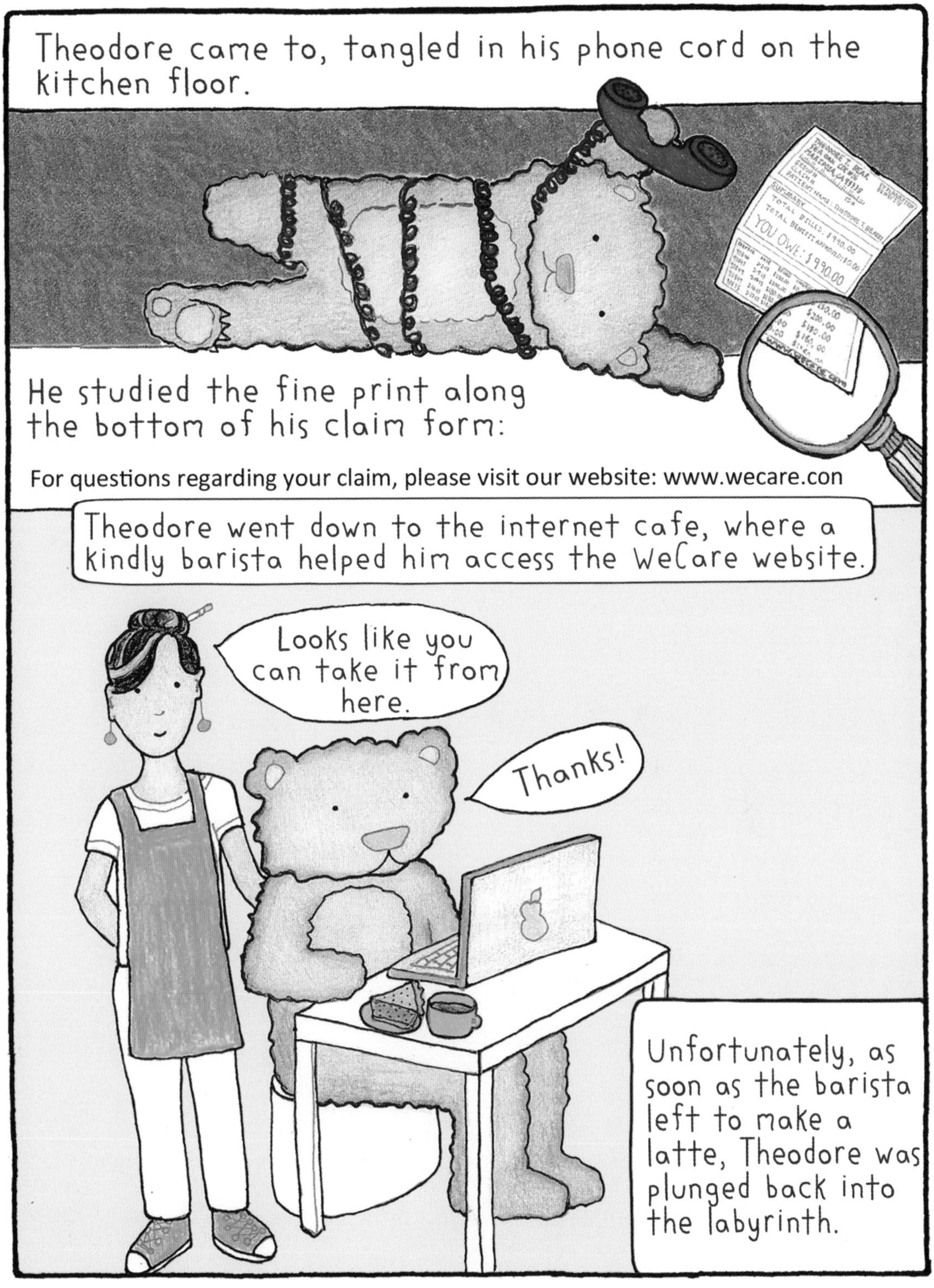

Theodore came to, tangled in his phone cord on the kitchen floor.
YOU OWE: $990.00
He studied the fine print along the bottom of his claim form:
For questions regarding your claim, please visit our website: www.wecare.con
Theodore went down to the internet cafe, where a kindly barista helped him access the WeCare website.
Looks like you can take it from here.
Thanks!
Unfortunately, as soon as the barista left to make a latte, Theodore was plunged back into the labyrinth.

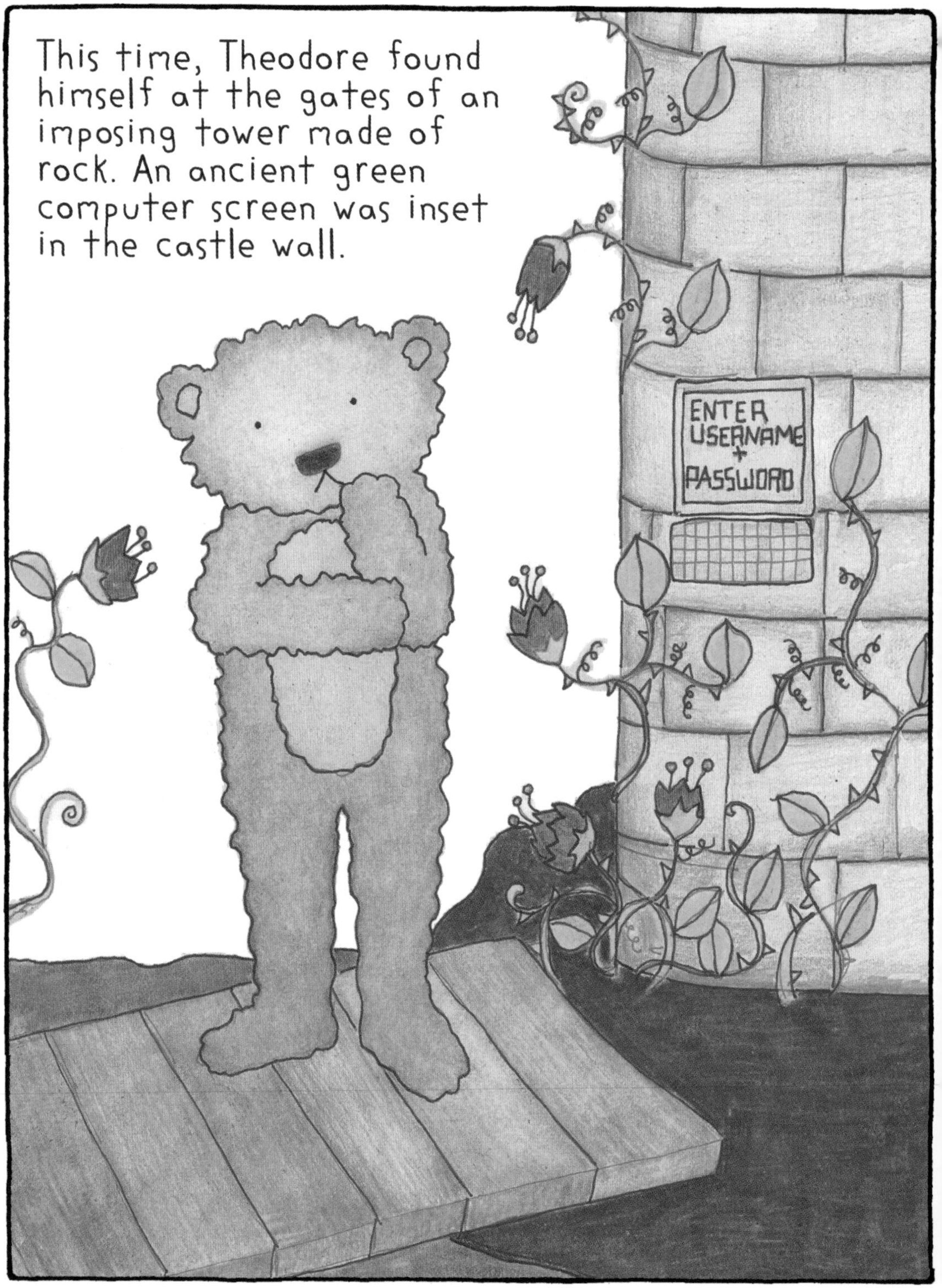
This time, Theodore found himself at the gates of an imposing tower made of rock. An ancient green computer screen was inset in the castle wall.
ENTER USERNAME + PASSWORD

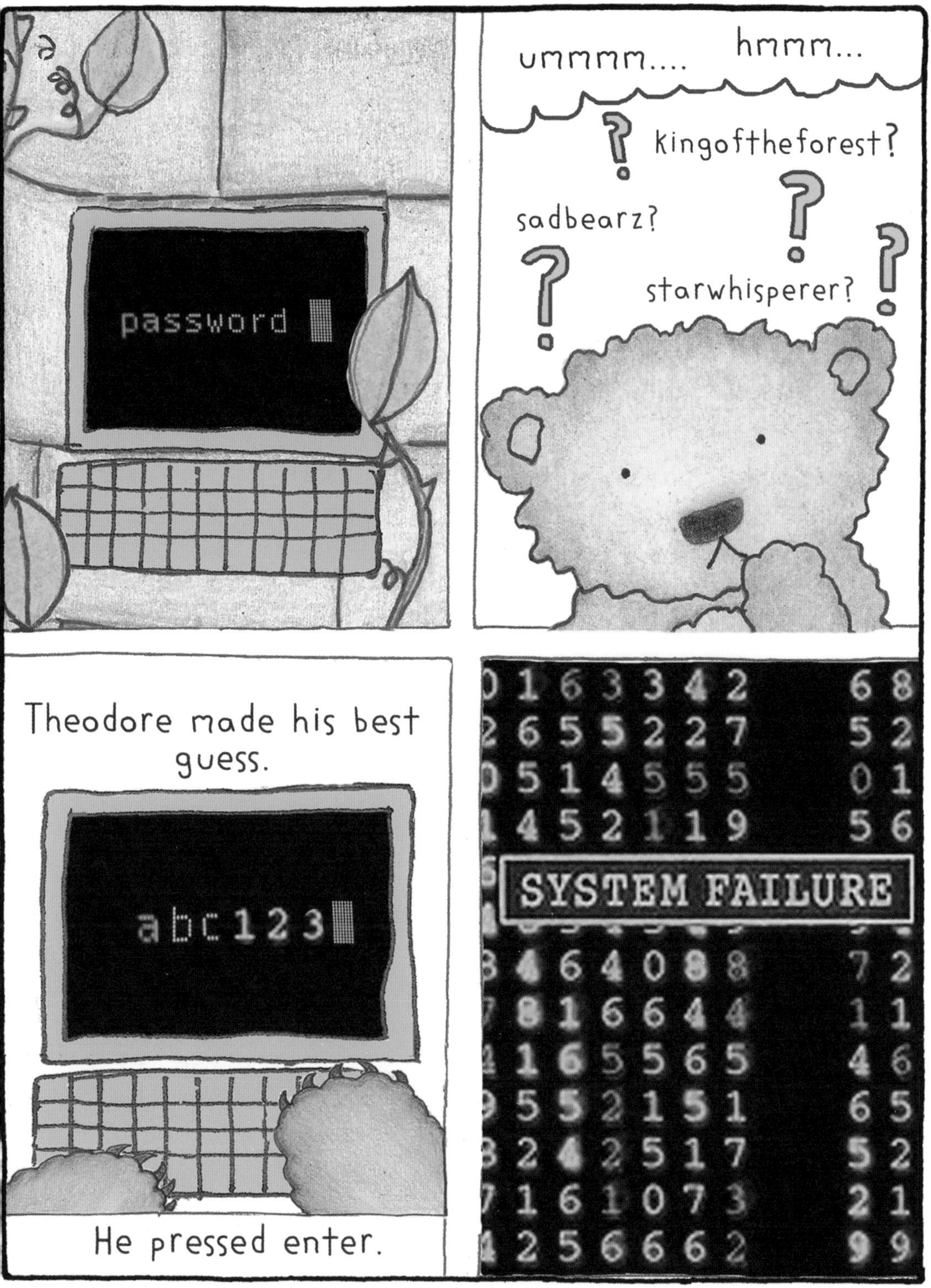
password
ummmm....
hmmm...
kingoftheforest?
sadbearz?
starwhisperer?
Theodore made his best guess.
abc123
He pressed enter.
SYSTEM FAILURE

A trapdoor opened beneath Theodore's feet. He plunged into the moat below, where piranhas nibbled his ears and crocodiles gnashed at his paws.

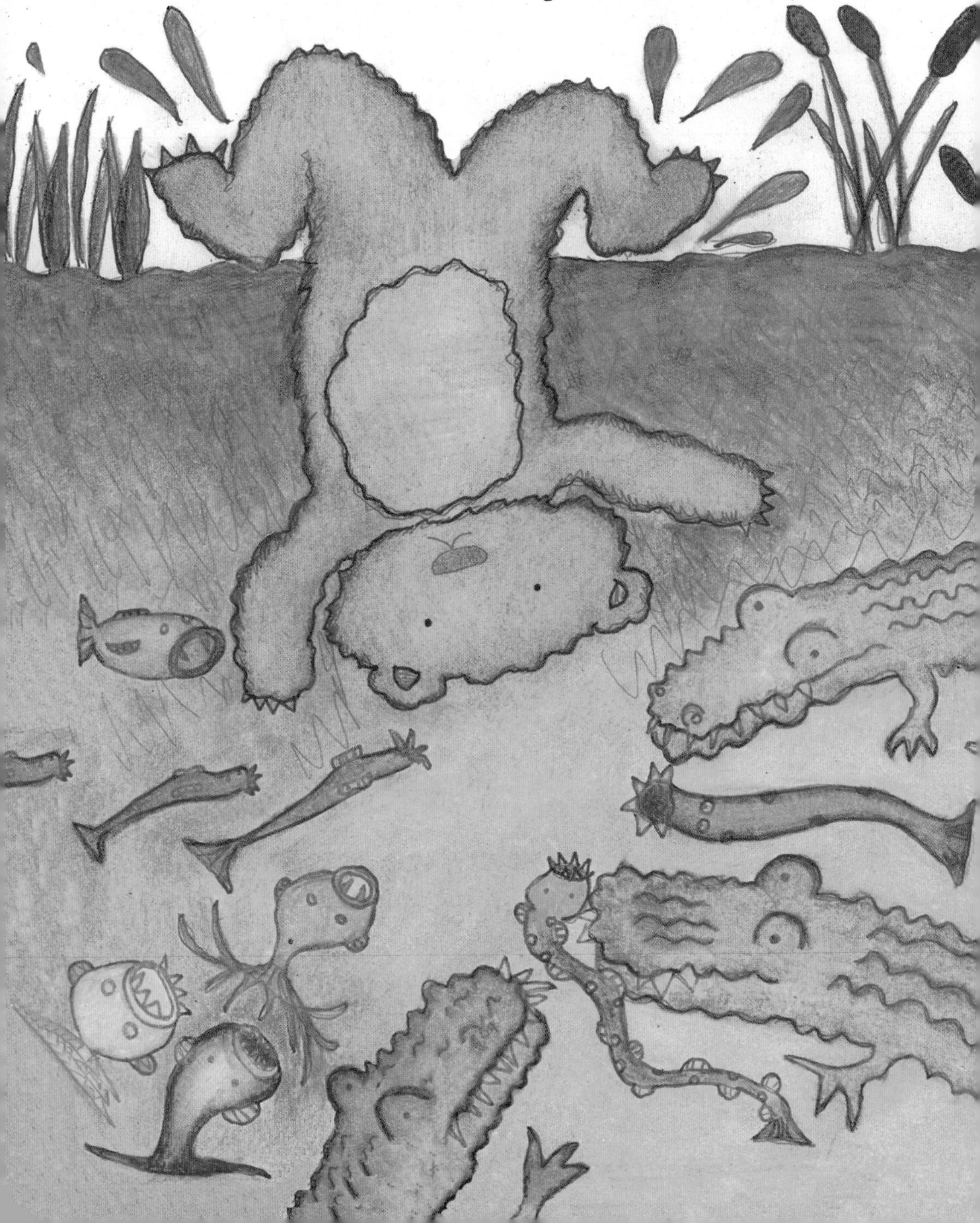

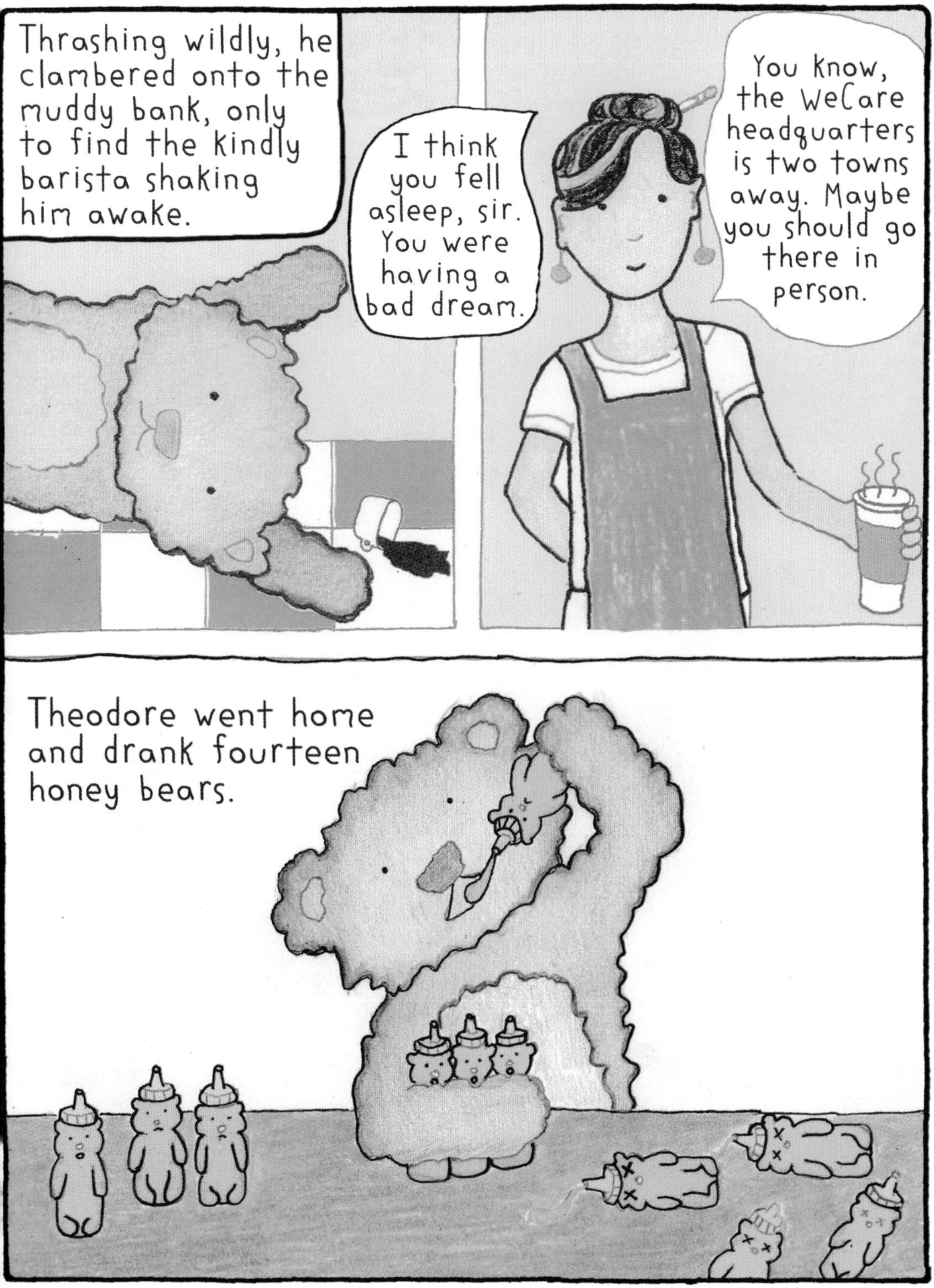
Thrashing wildly, he clambered onto the muddy bank, only to find the kindly barista shaking him awake.
I think you fell asleep, sir. You were having a bad dream.
You know, the WeCare headquarters is two towns away. Maybe you should go there in person.
Theodore went home and drank fourteen honey bears.

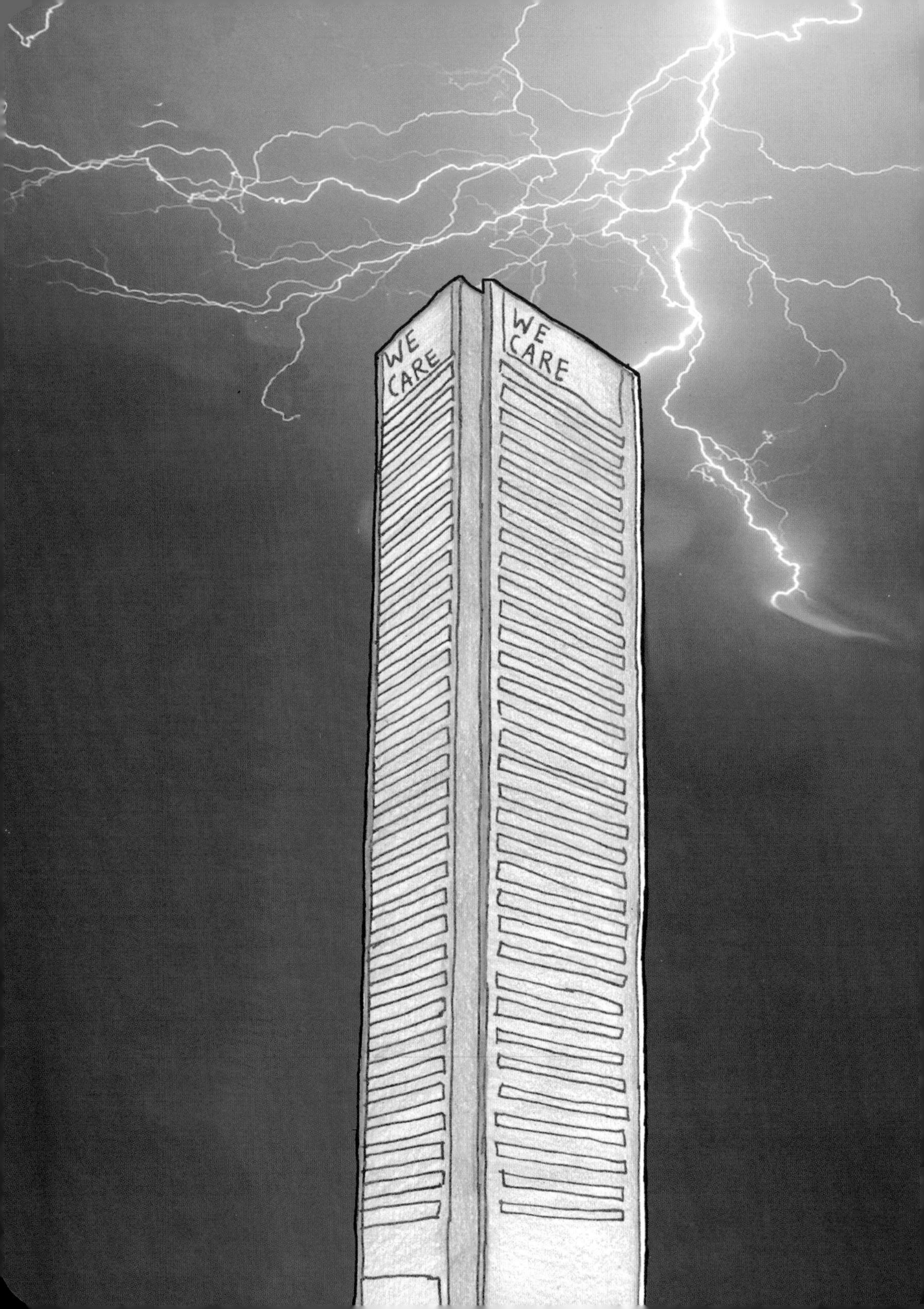
WE CARE
WE CARE

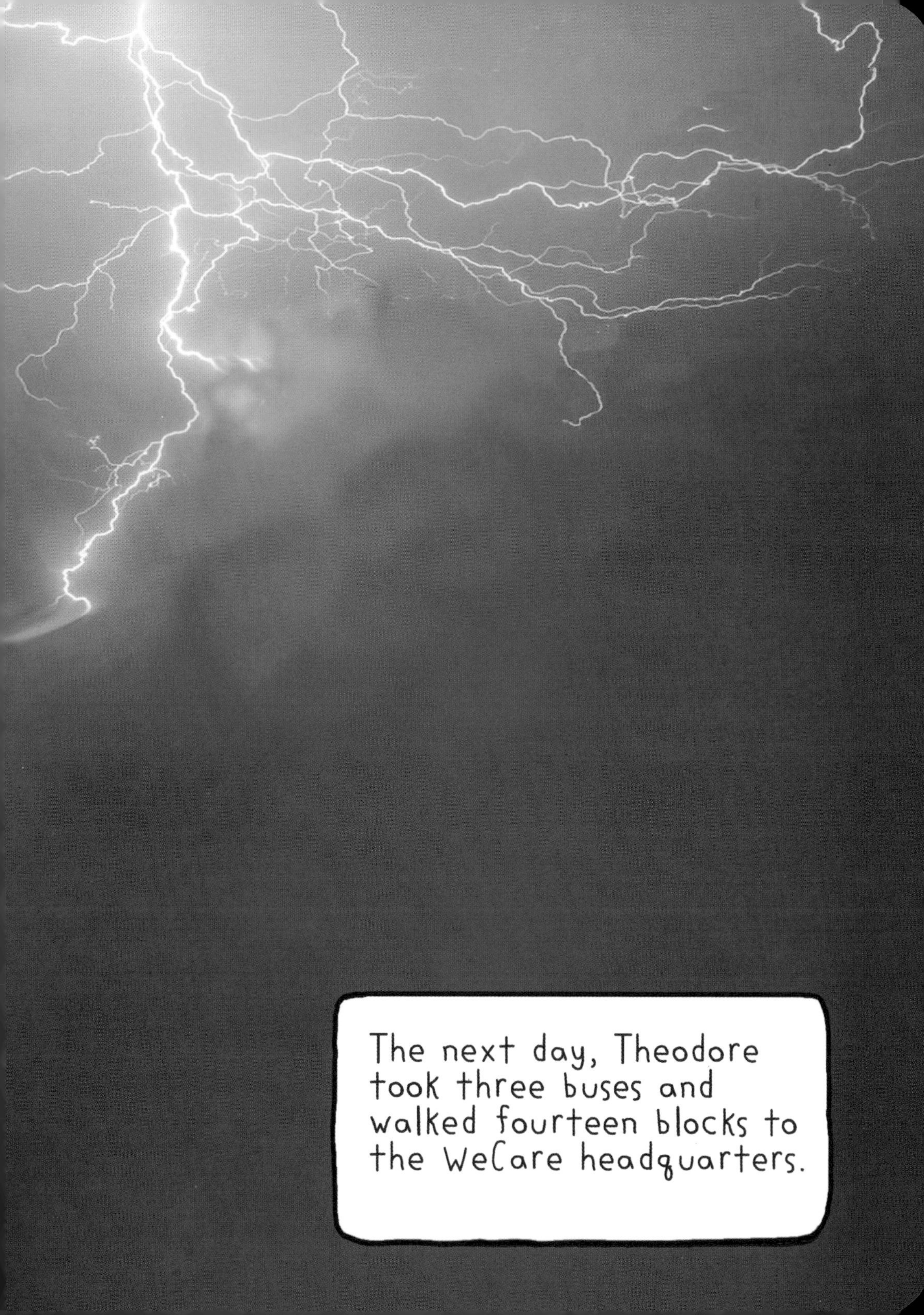
The next day, Theodore took three buses and walked fourteen blocks to the WeCare headquarters.

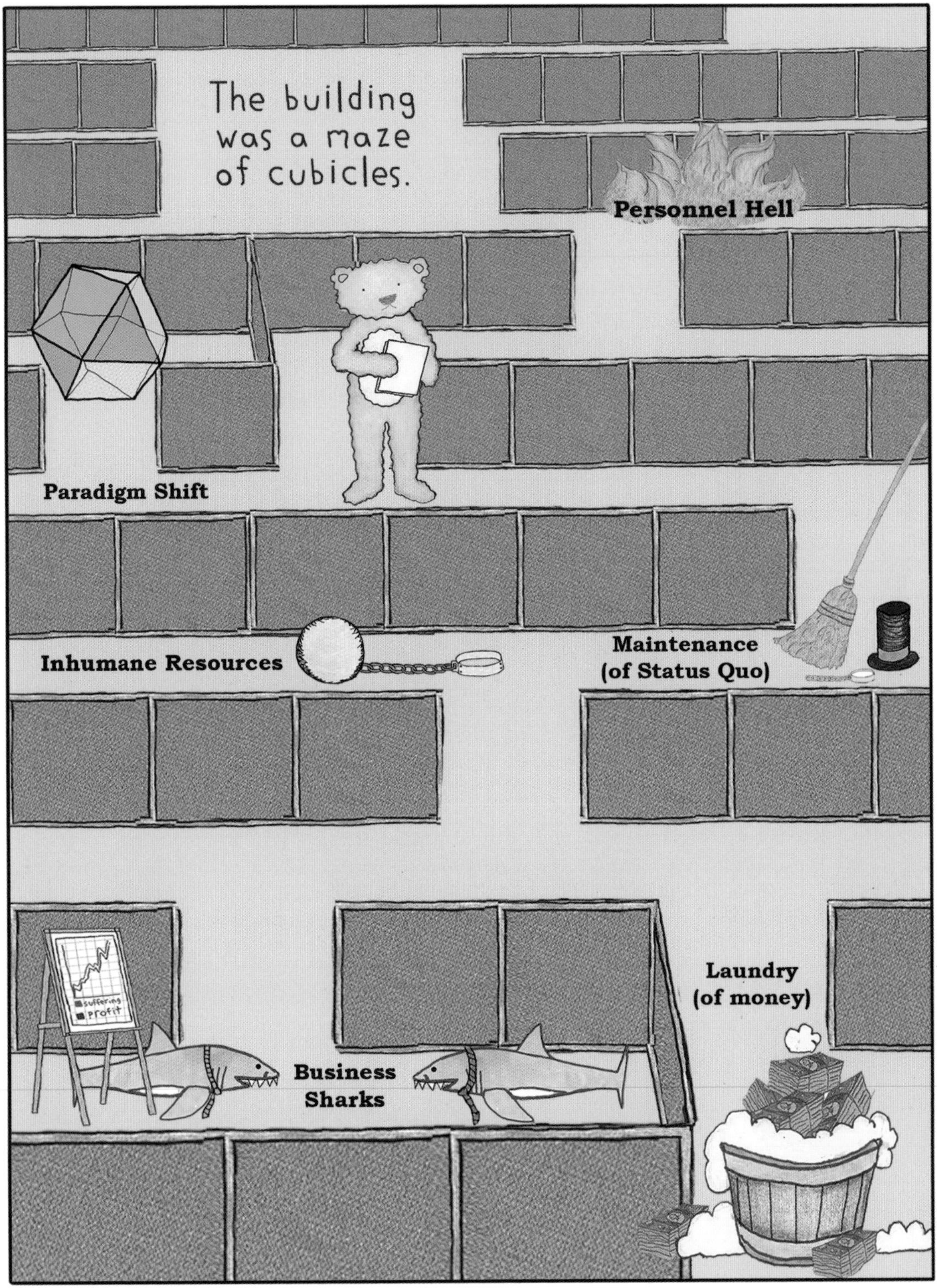
The building was a maze of cubicles.
Personnel Hell
Paradigm Shift
Inhumane Resources
Maintenance (of Status Quo)
Laundry (of money)
suffering
profit
Business Sharks

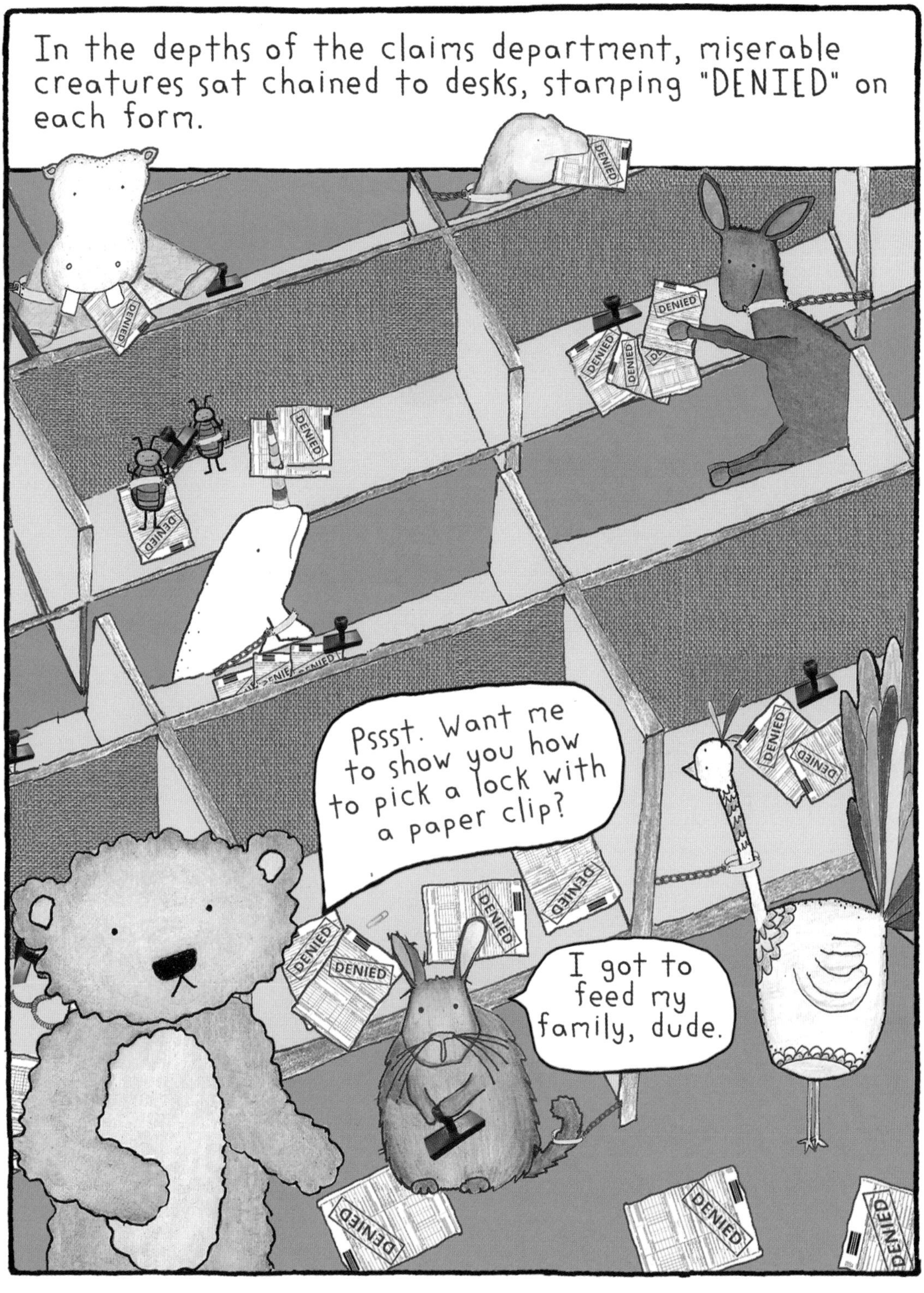
In the depths of the claims department, miserable creatures sat chained to desks, stamping "DENIED" on each form.
Pssst. Want me to show you how to pick a lock with a paper clip?
I got to feed my family, dude.

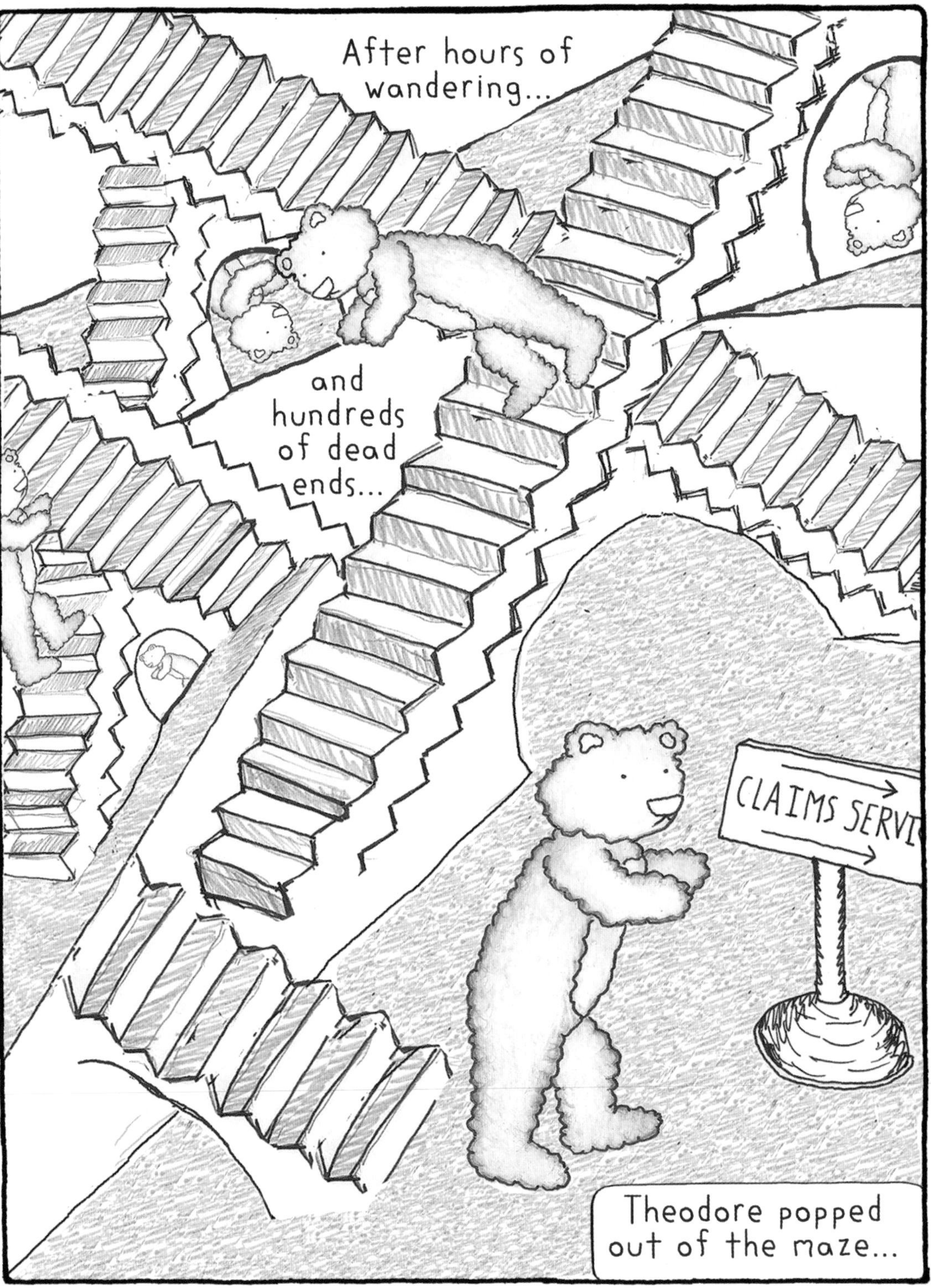
After hours of wandering...
and hundreds of dead ends...
CLAIMS SERVI
Theodore popped out of the maze...

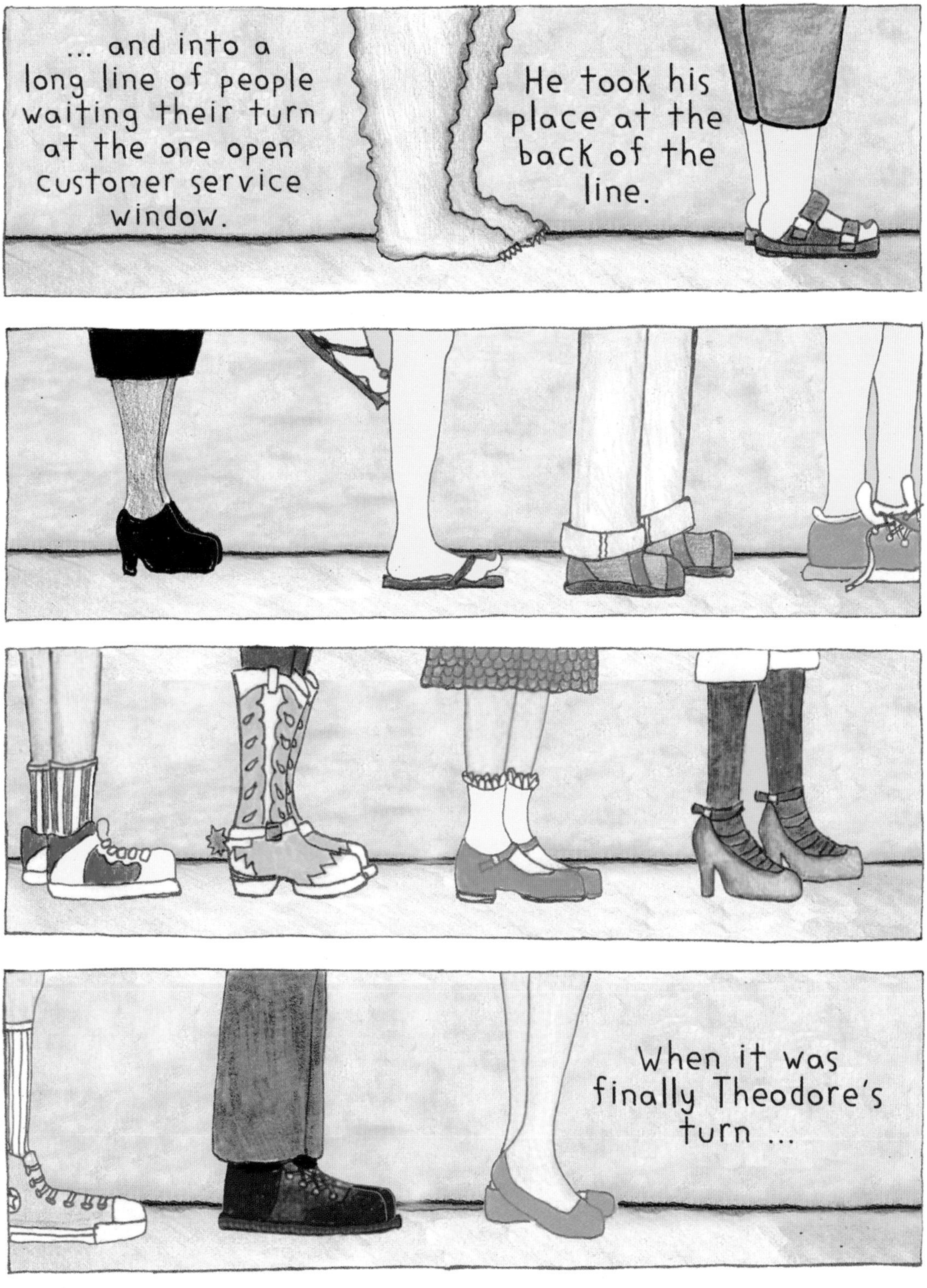
... and into a long line of people waiting their turn at the one open customer service window.
He took his place at the back of the line.
When it was finally Theodore's turn ...

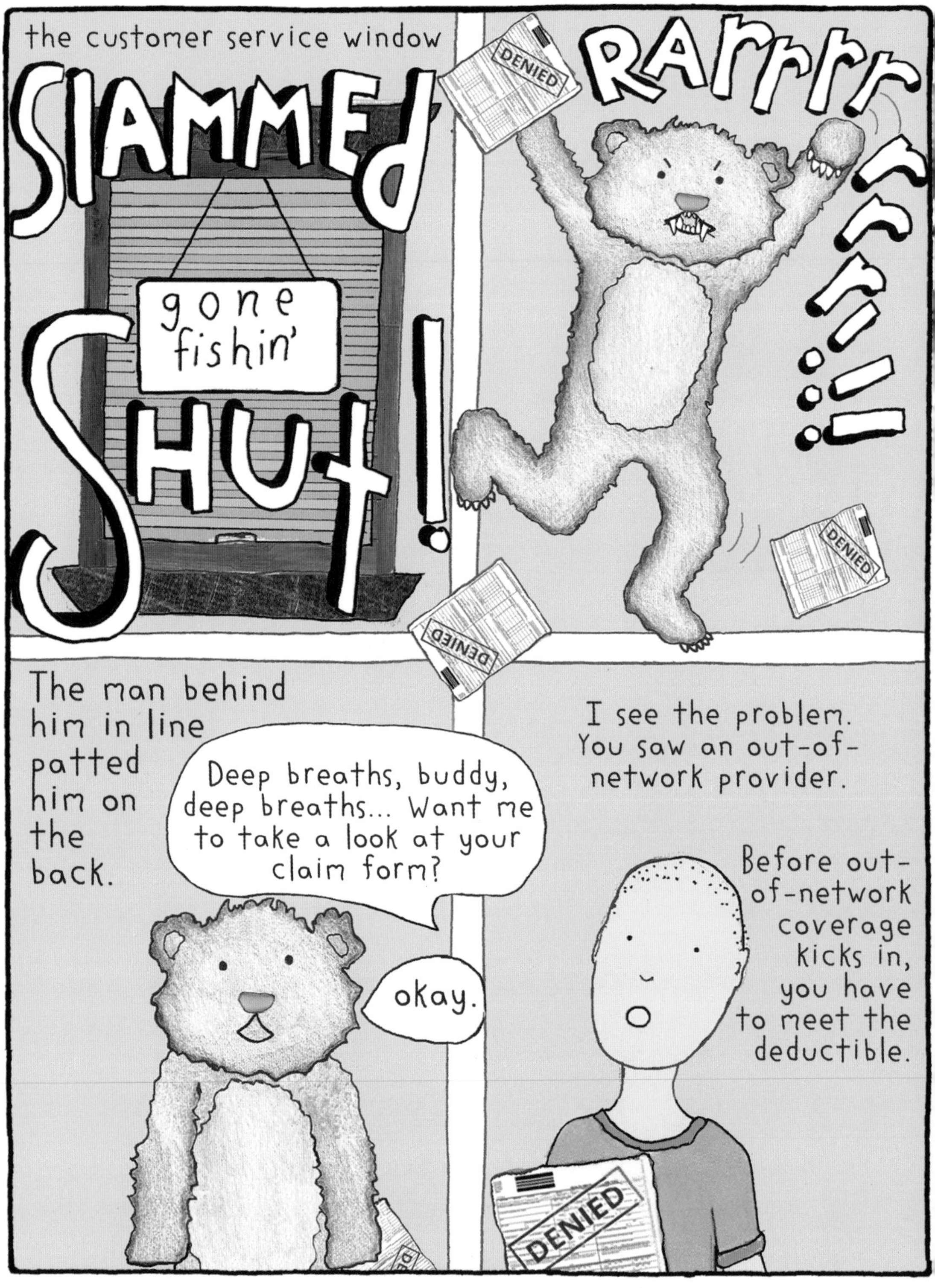
the customer service window
SLAMMED
gone fishin'
SHUT!
DENIED
Rarrrrrrrrrrr!!!!
DENIED
DENIED
DENIED
The man behind him in line patted him on the back.
Deep breaths, buddy, deep breaths... Want me to take a look at your claim form?
okay.
I see the problem. You saw an out-of-network provider.
Before out-of-network coverage kicks in, you have to meet the deductible.
DENIED

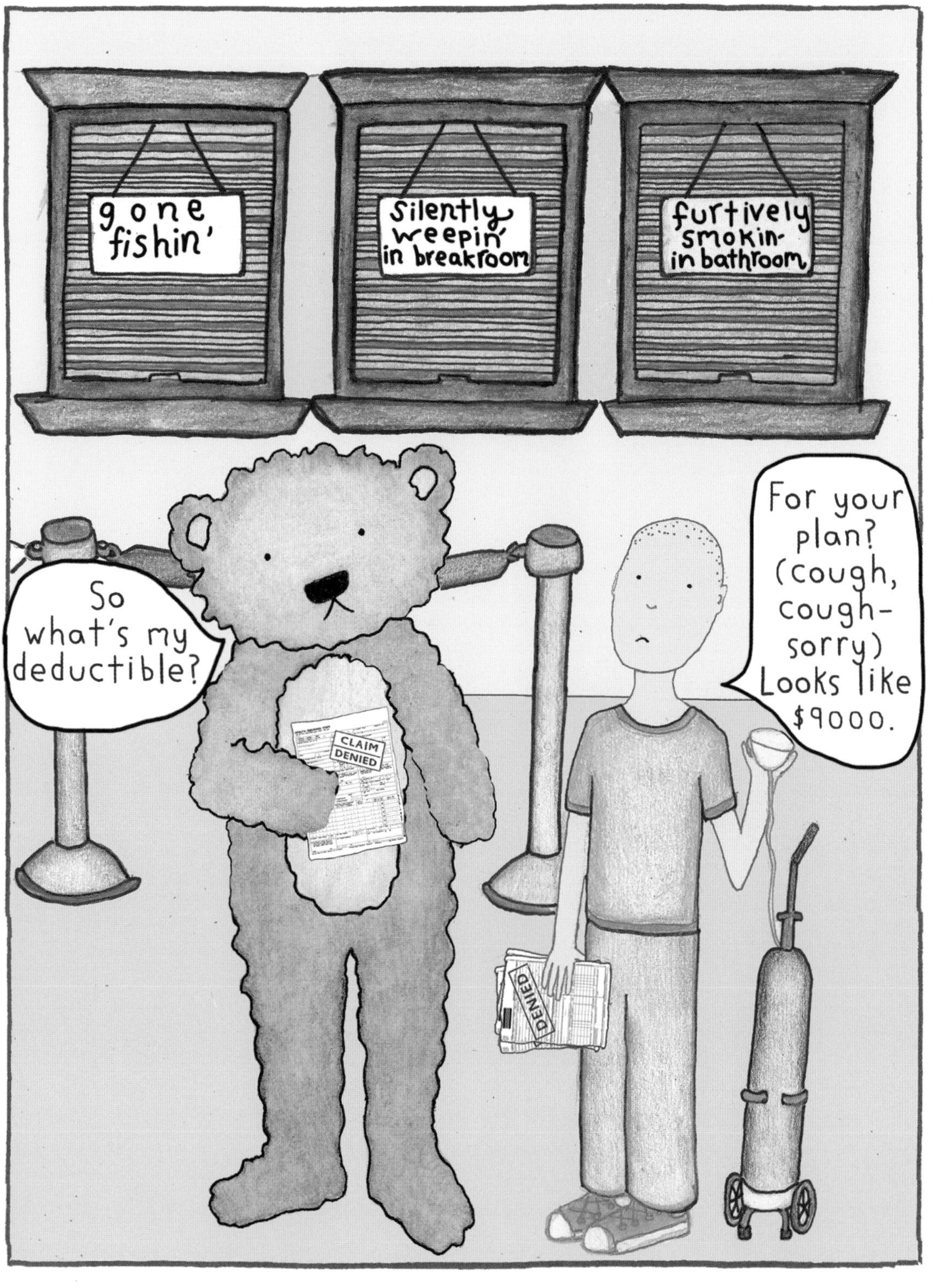
gone fishin'
silently weepin' in breakroom
furtively smokin- in bathroom
So what's my deductible?
For your plan? (cough, cough- sorry) Looks like $9000.
CLAIM DENIED
DENIED

Theodore fainted.

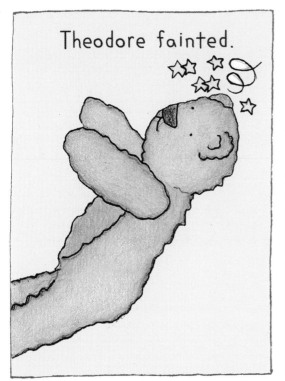

When he awoke, he was alone, and his face was covered in drool. He lay on the carpet. Stale air hummed through the vents.

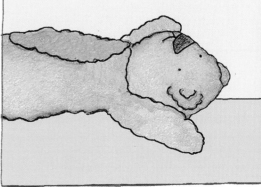

Then Theodore's senses prickled. He sat up, perplexed. The succulent smell of seared salmon was wafting down the stairs.

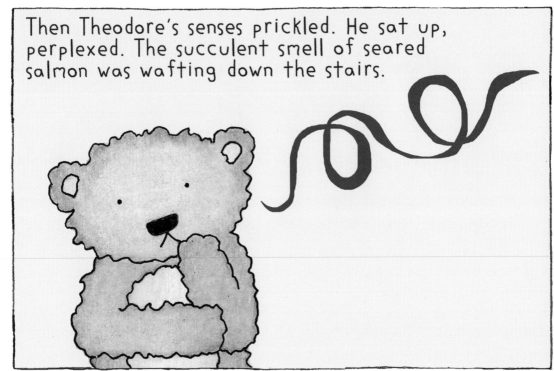

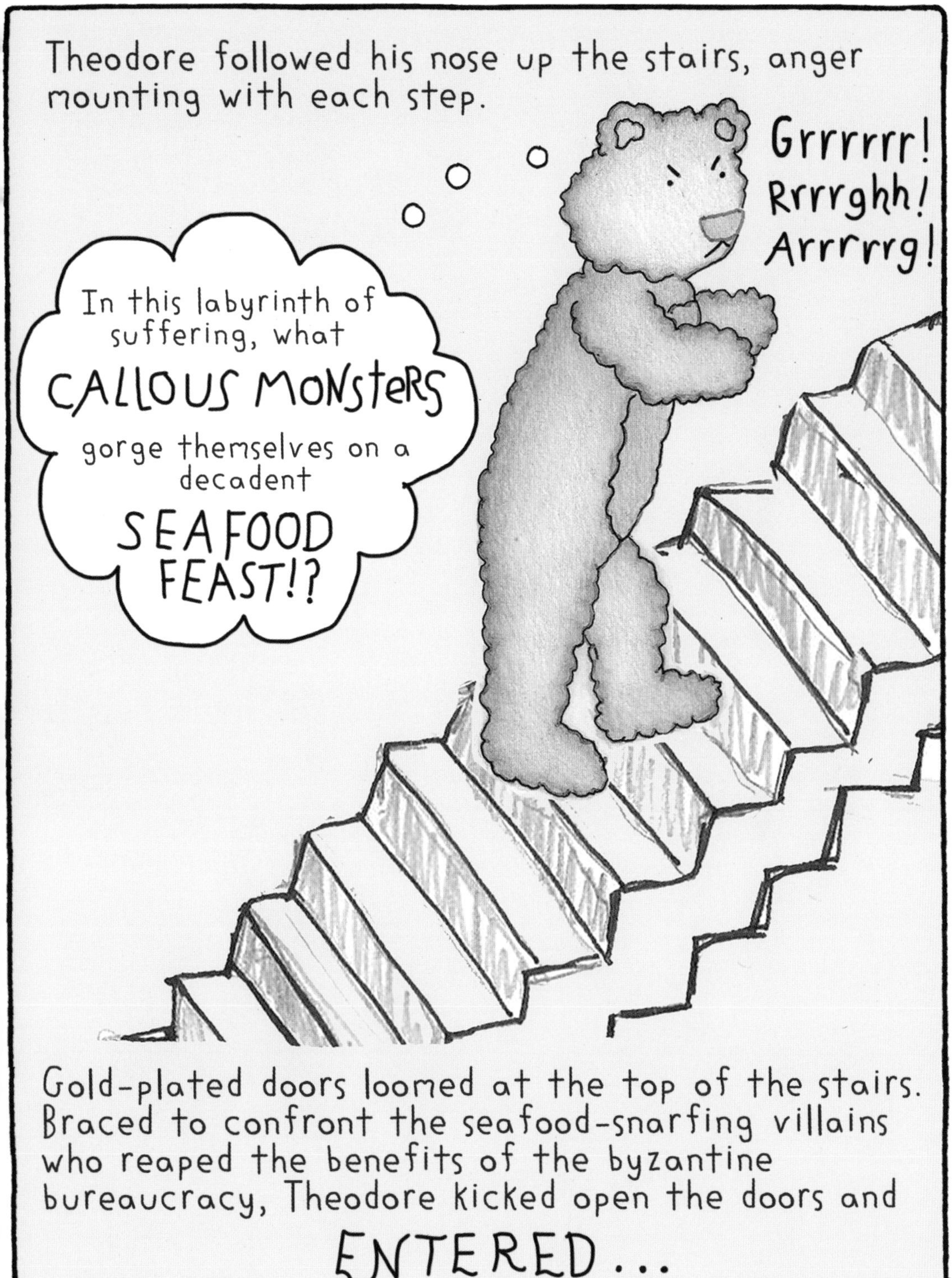
Theodore followed his nose up the stairs, anger mounting with each step.
In this labyrinth of suffering, what CALLOUS MONSTERS gorge themselves on a decadent SEAFOOD FEAST!?
Grrrrrr! Rrrrghh! Arrrrrg!
Gold-plated doors loomed at the top of the stairs. Braced to confront the seafood-snarfing villains who reaped the benefits of the byzantine bureaucracy, Theodore kicked open the doors and
ENTERED...

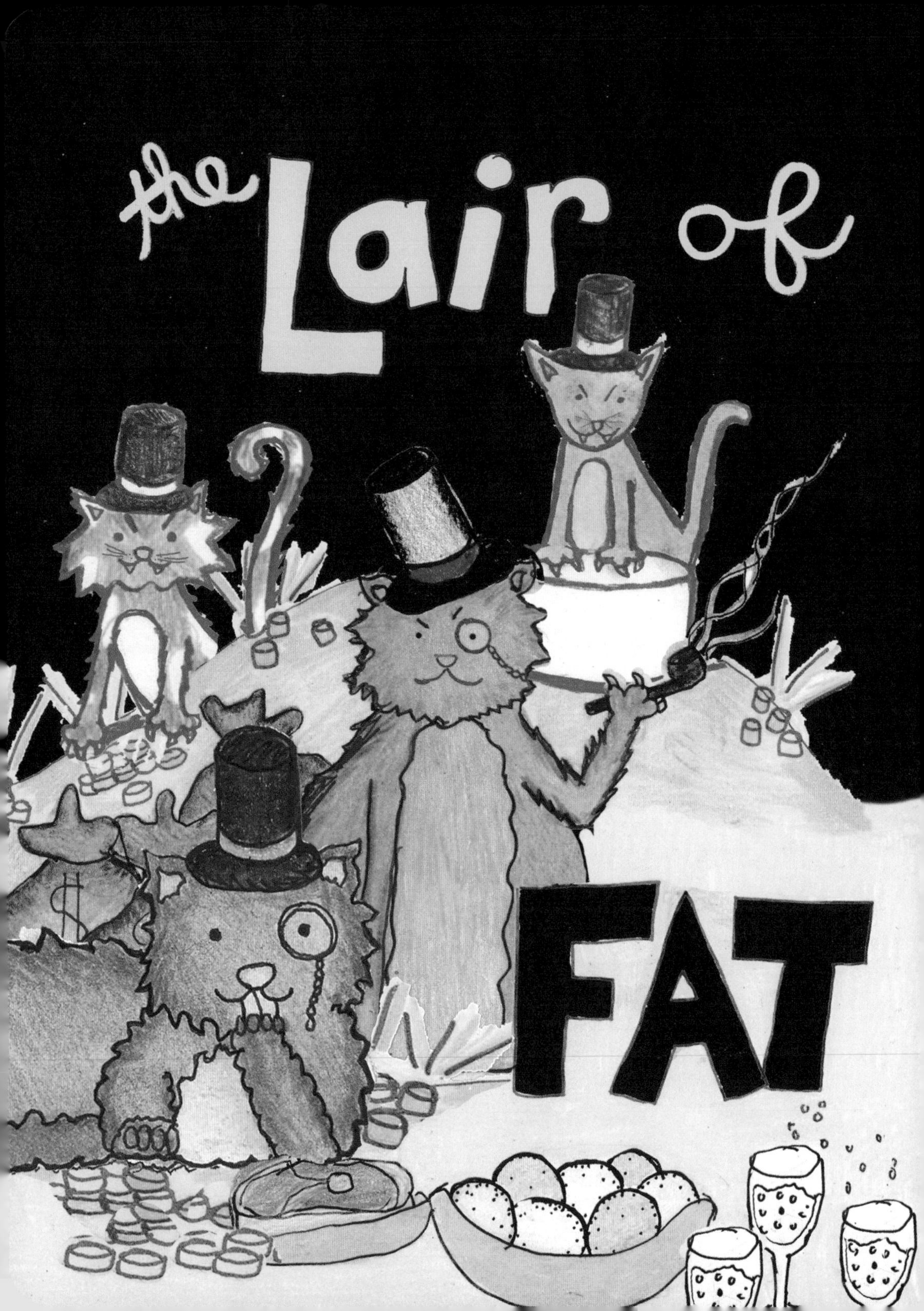
the Lair of
FAT

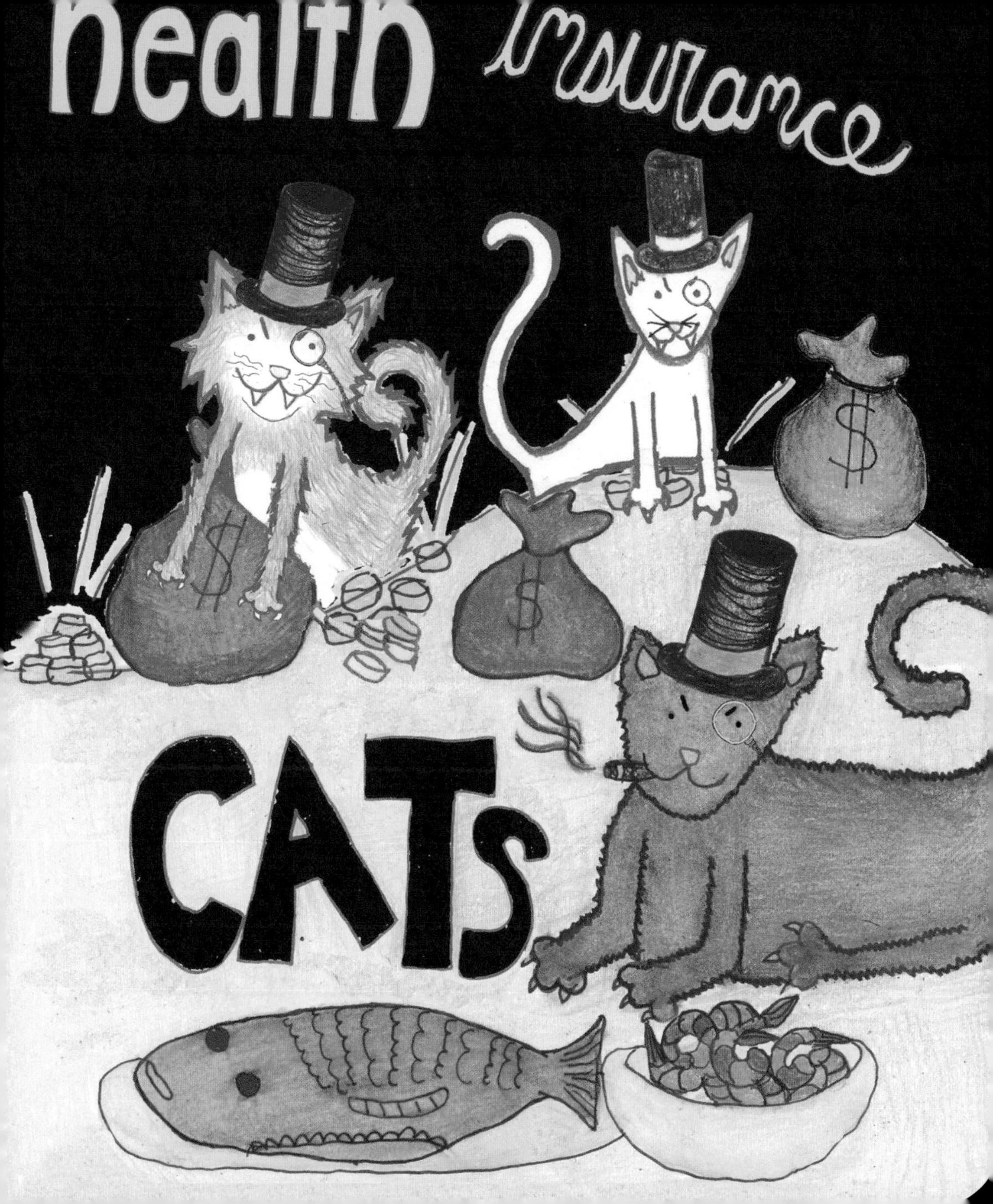
Health insurance
CATS

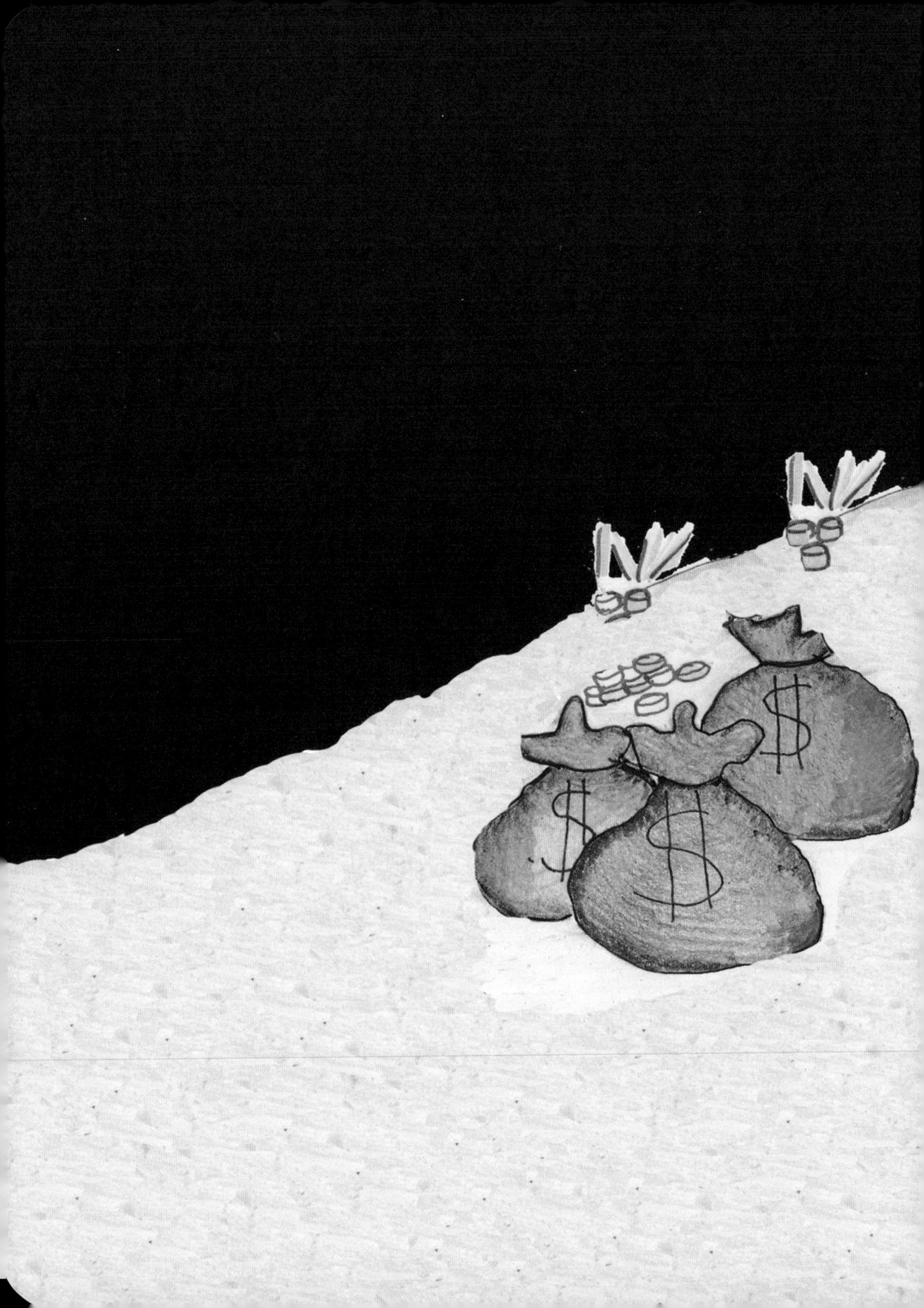

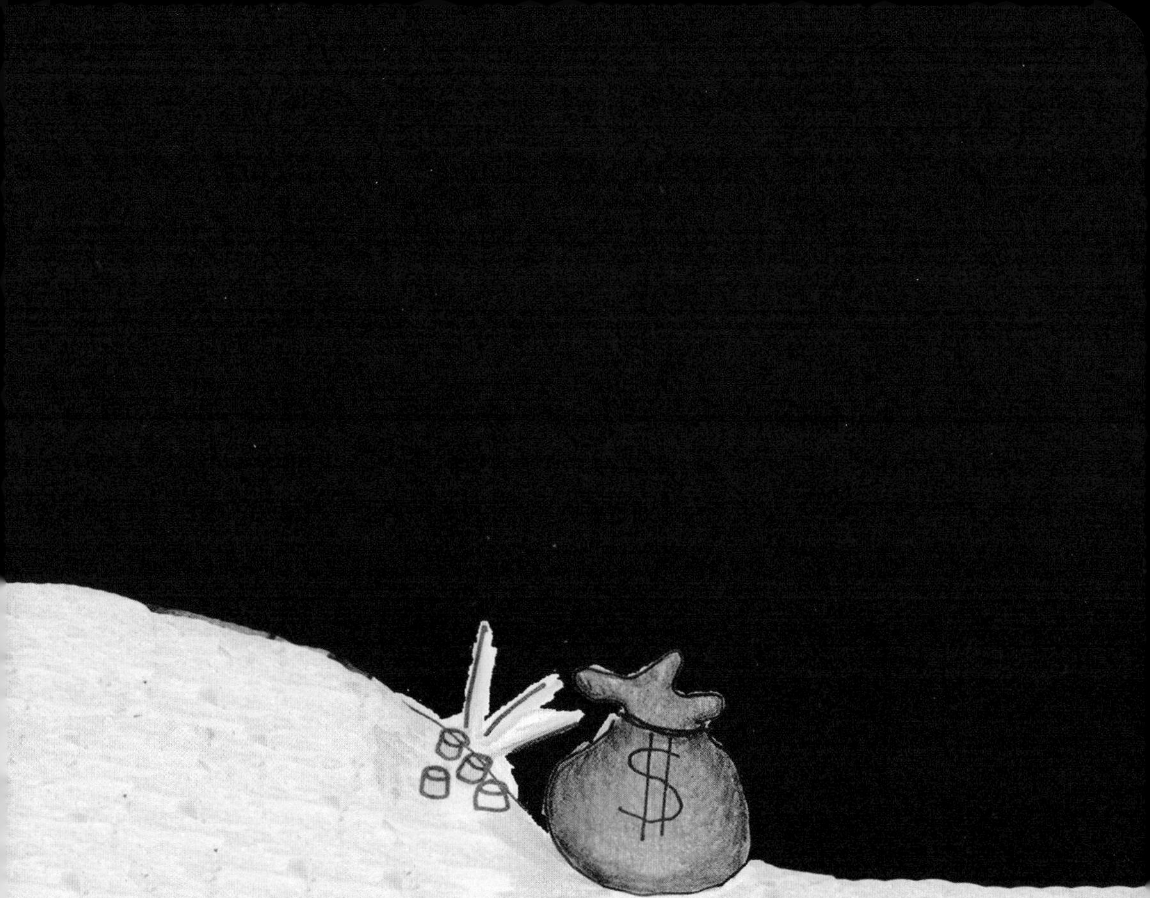
$

chapter three:

The Lair

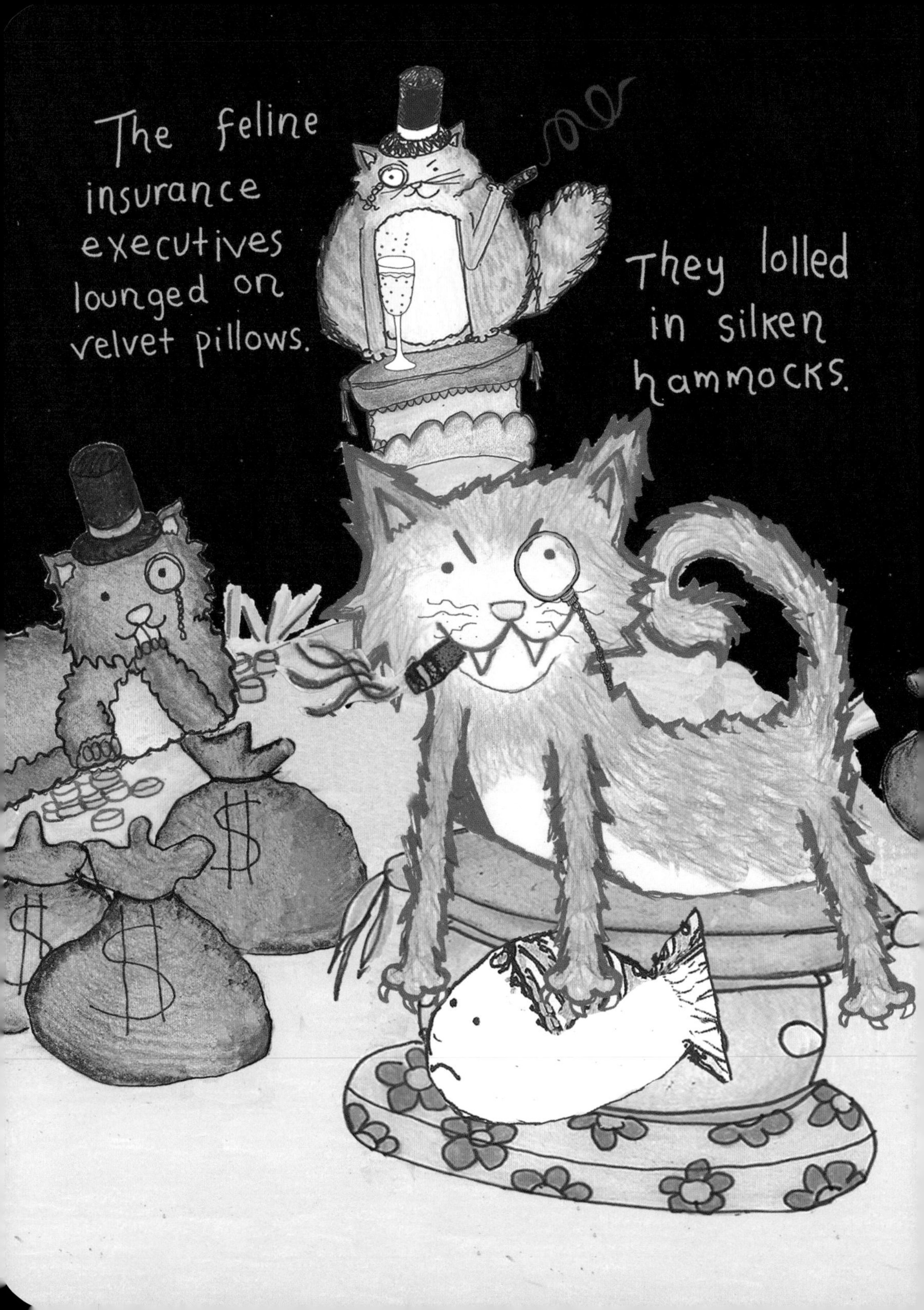
The feline insurance executives lounged on velvet pillows.
They lolled in silken hammocks.

They feasted on bald eagle eggs and baby beluga whale.

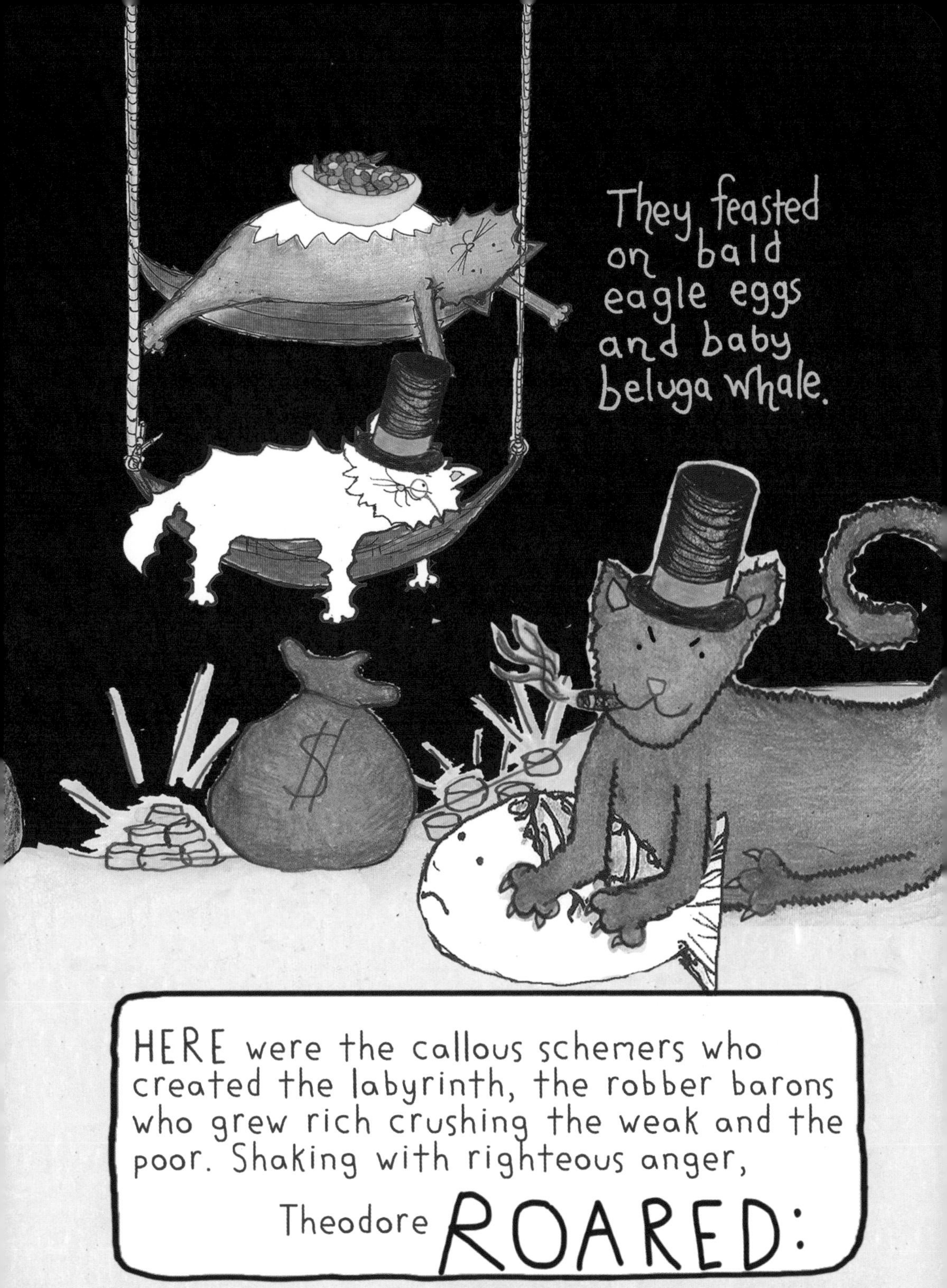

HERE were the callous schemers who created the labyrinth, the robber barons who grew rich crushing the weak and the poor. Shaking with righteous anger,

Theodore **ROARED:**

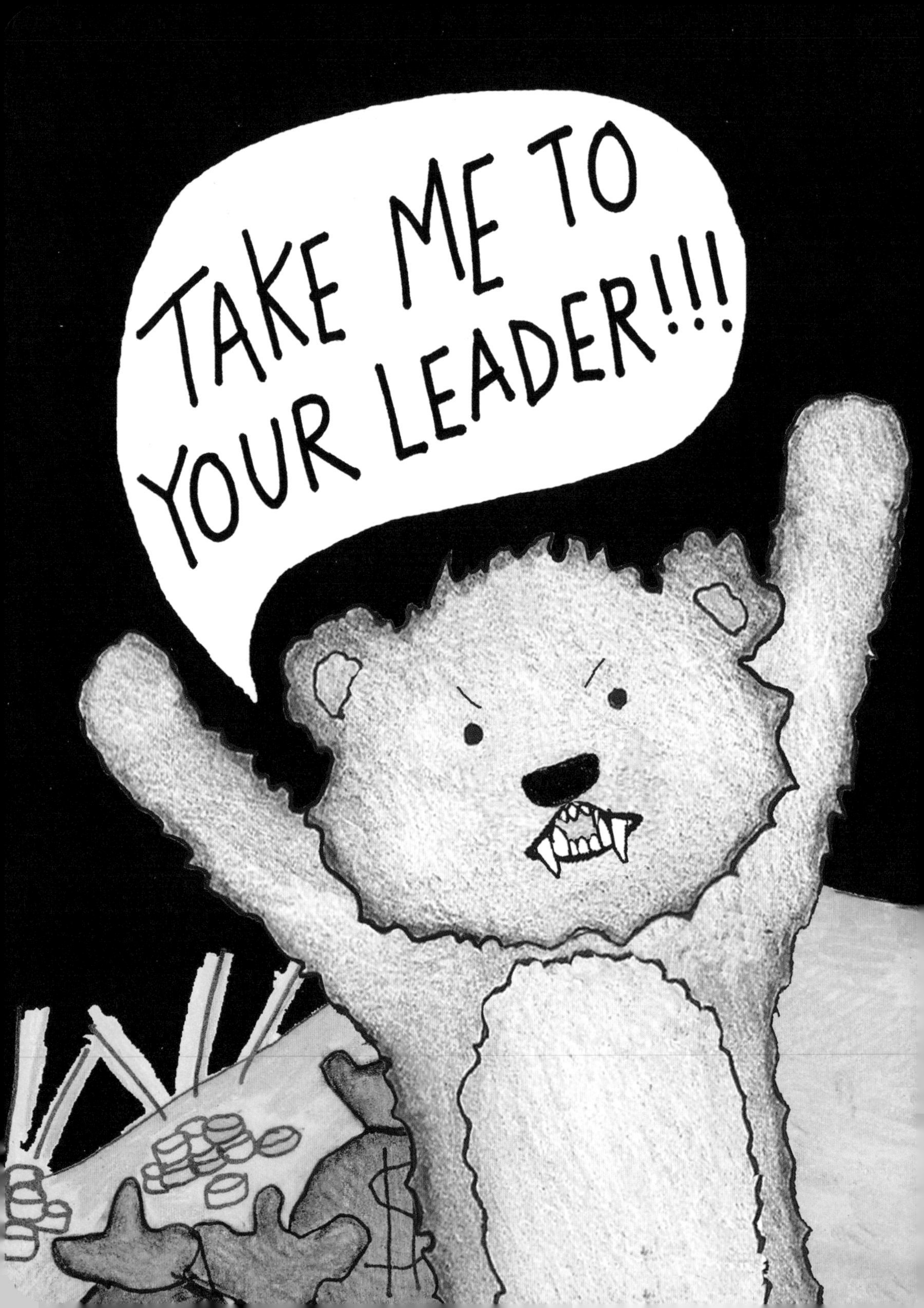
TAKE ME TO YOUR LEADER!!!

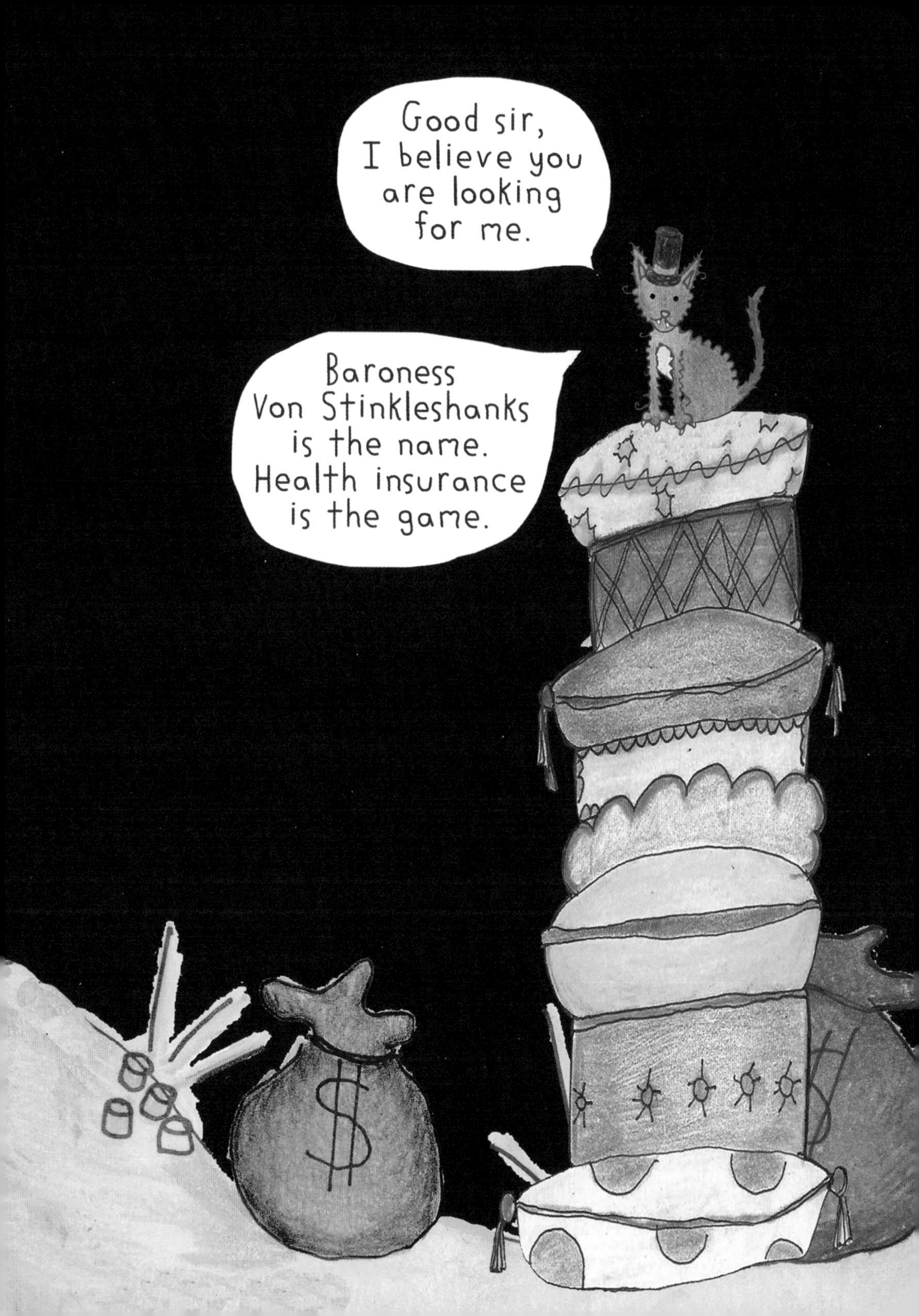
Good sir, I believe you are looking for me.
Baroness Von Stinkleshanks is the name. Health insurance is the game.

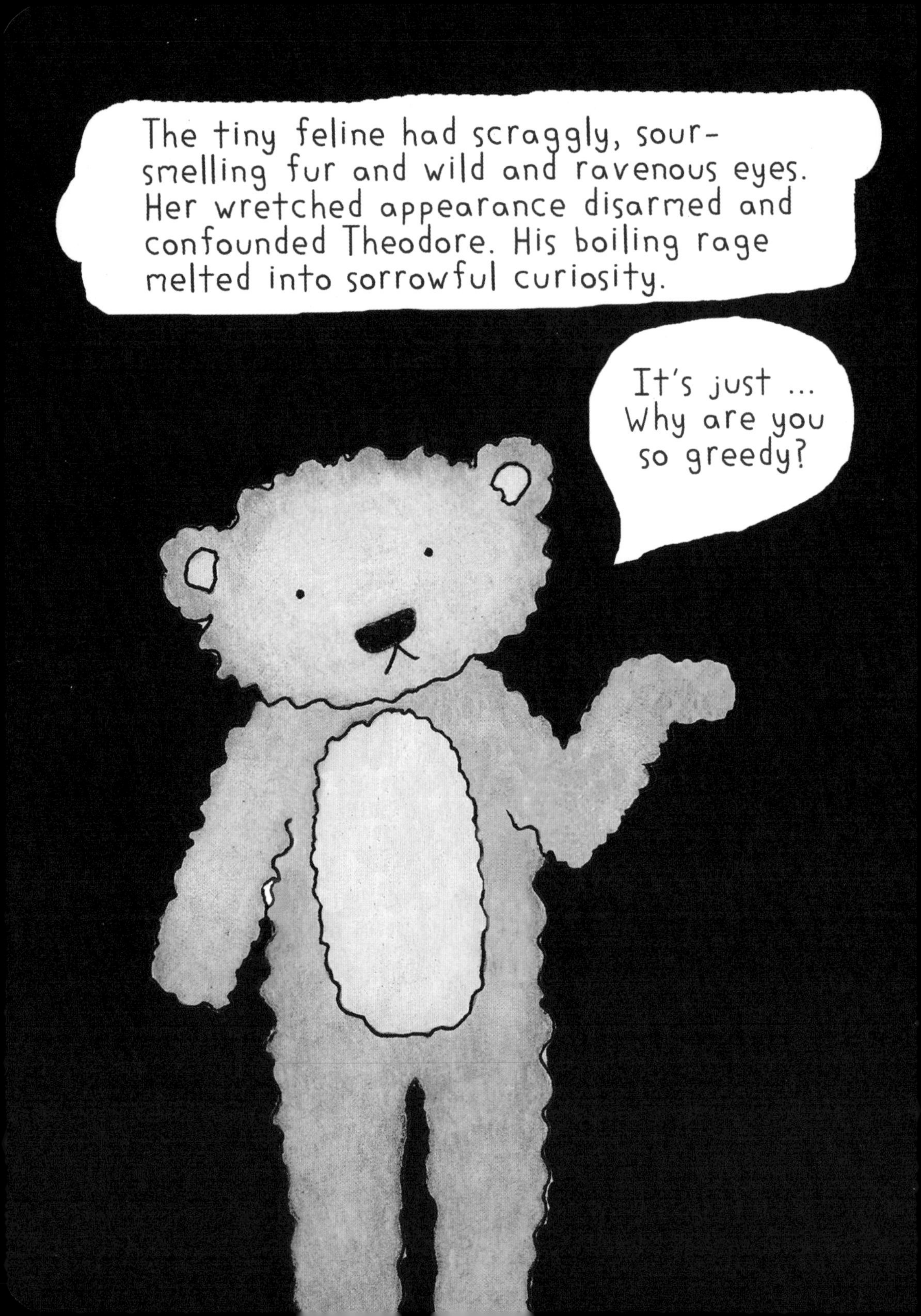
The tiny feline had scraggly, sour-smelling fur and wild and ravenous eyes. Her wretched appearance disarmed and confounded Theodore. His boiling rage melted into sorrowful curiosity.
It's just ... Why are you so greedy?

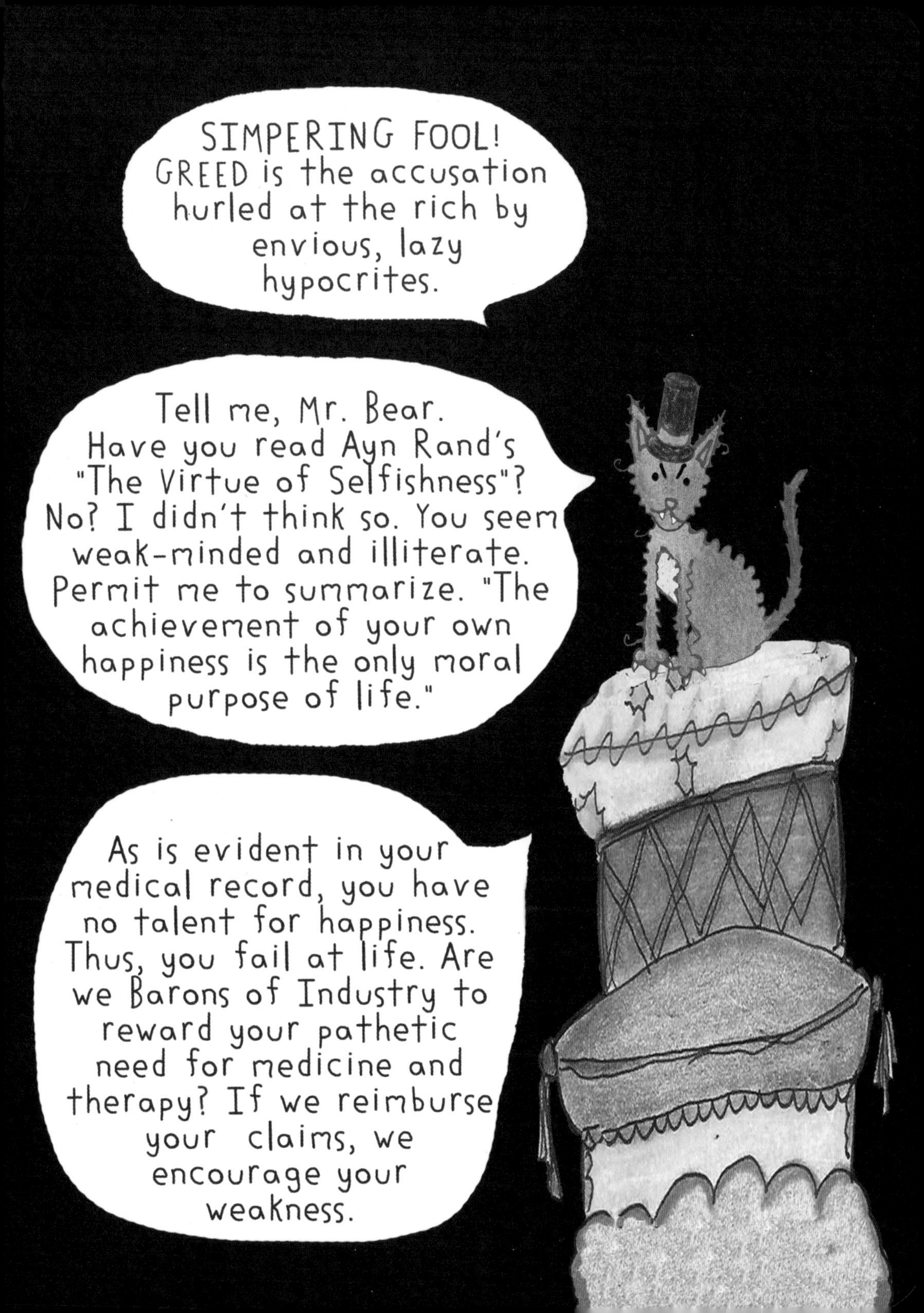
SIMPERING FOOL! GREED is the accusation hurled at the rich by envious, lazy hypocrites.
Tell me, Mr. Bear. Have you read Ayn Rand's "The Virtue of Selfishness"? No? I didn't think so. You seem weak-minded and illiterate. Permit me to summarize. "The achievement of your own happiness is the only moral purpose of life."
As is evident in your medical record, you have no talent for happiness. Thus, you fail at life. Are we Barons of Industry to reward your pathetic need for medicine and therapy? If we reimburse your claims, we encourage your weakness.

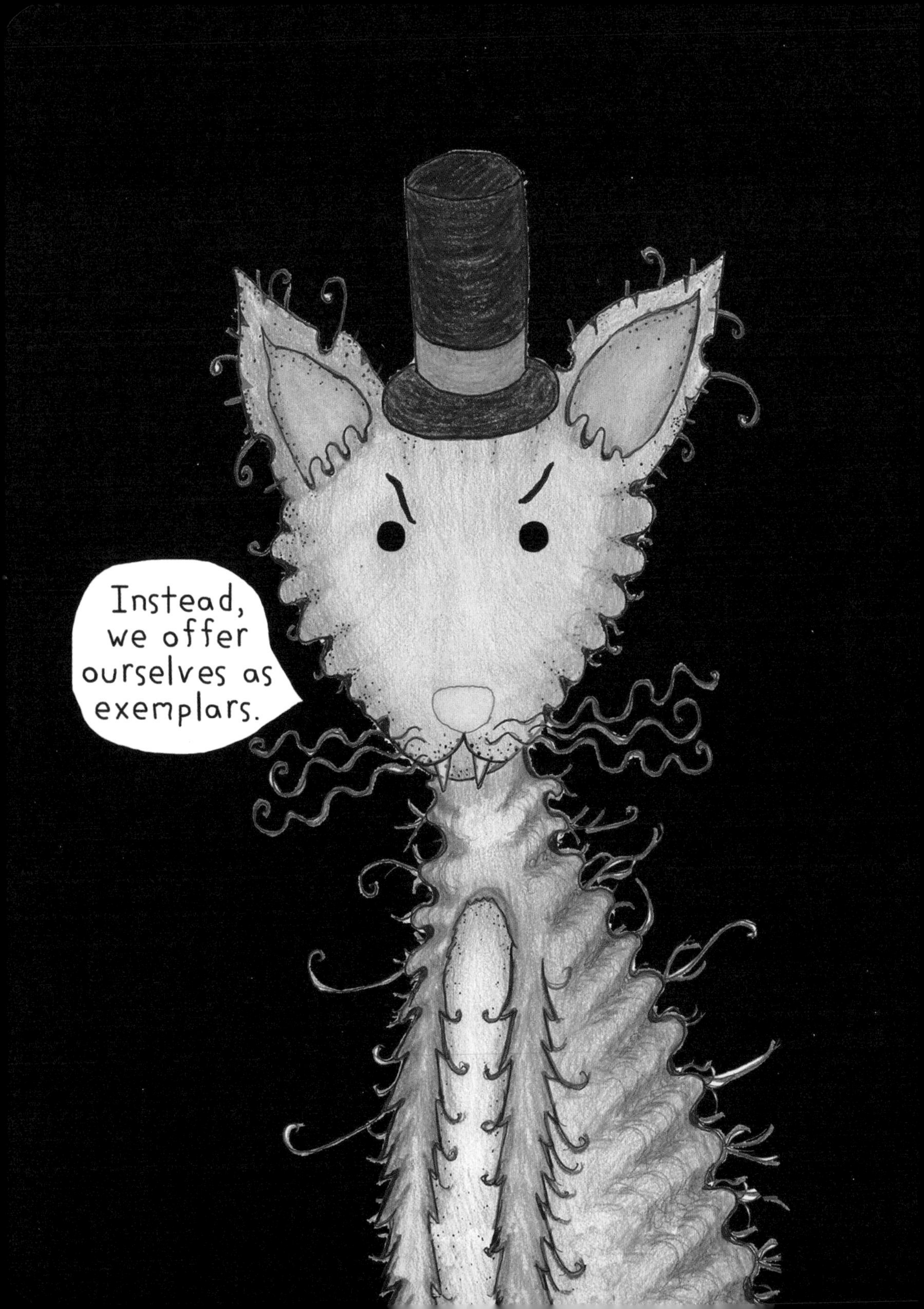
Instead, we offer ourselves as exemplars.

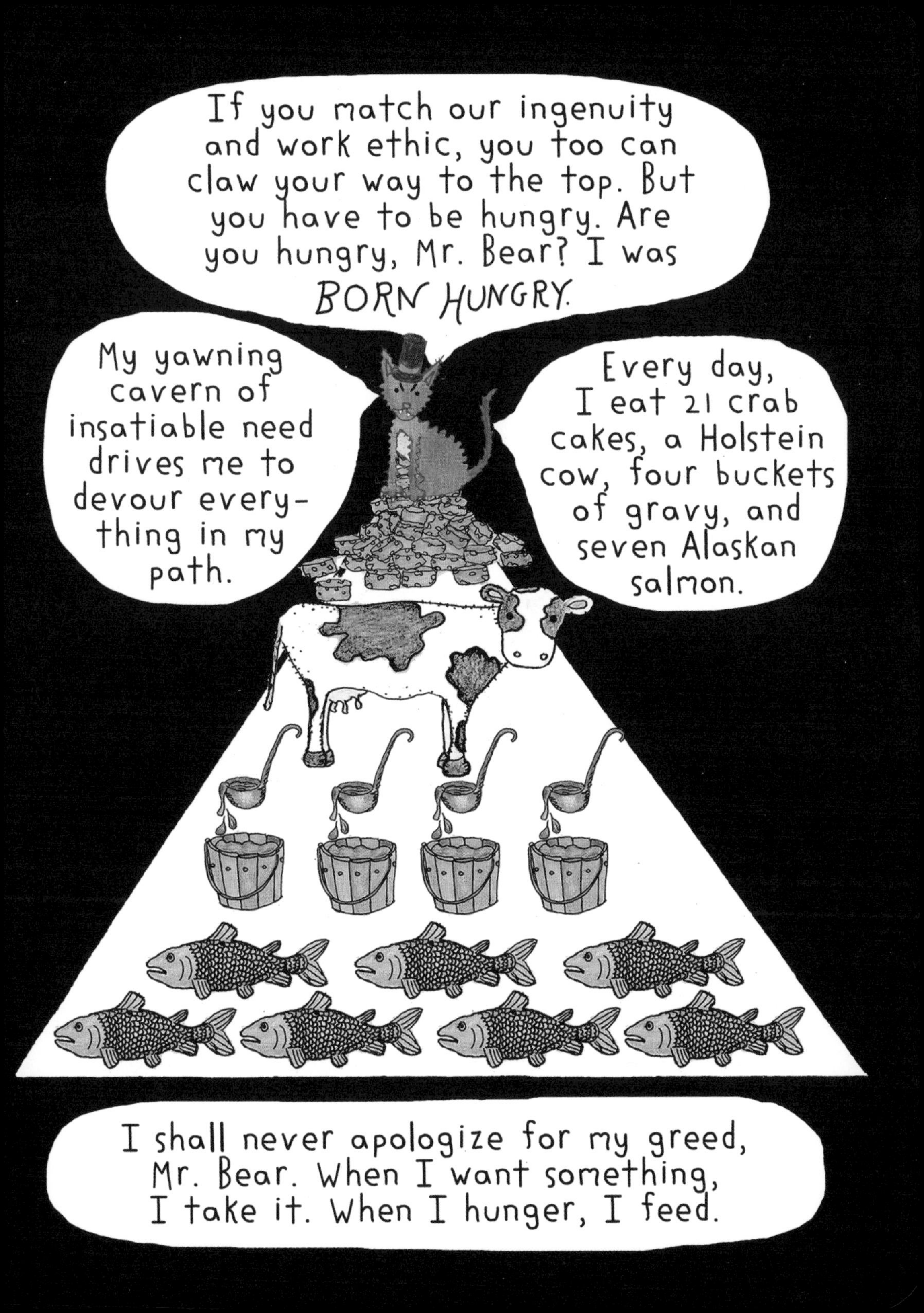
If you match our ingenuity and work ethic, you too can claw your way to the top. But you have to be hungry. Are you hungry, Mr. Bear? I was BORN HUNGRY.
My yawning cavern of insatiable need drives me to devour everything in my path.
Every day, I eat 21 crab cakes, a Holstein cow, four buckets of gravy, and seven Alaskan salmon.
I shall never apologize for my greed, Mr. Bear. When I want something, I take it. When I hunger, I feed.

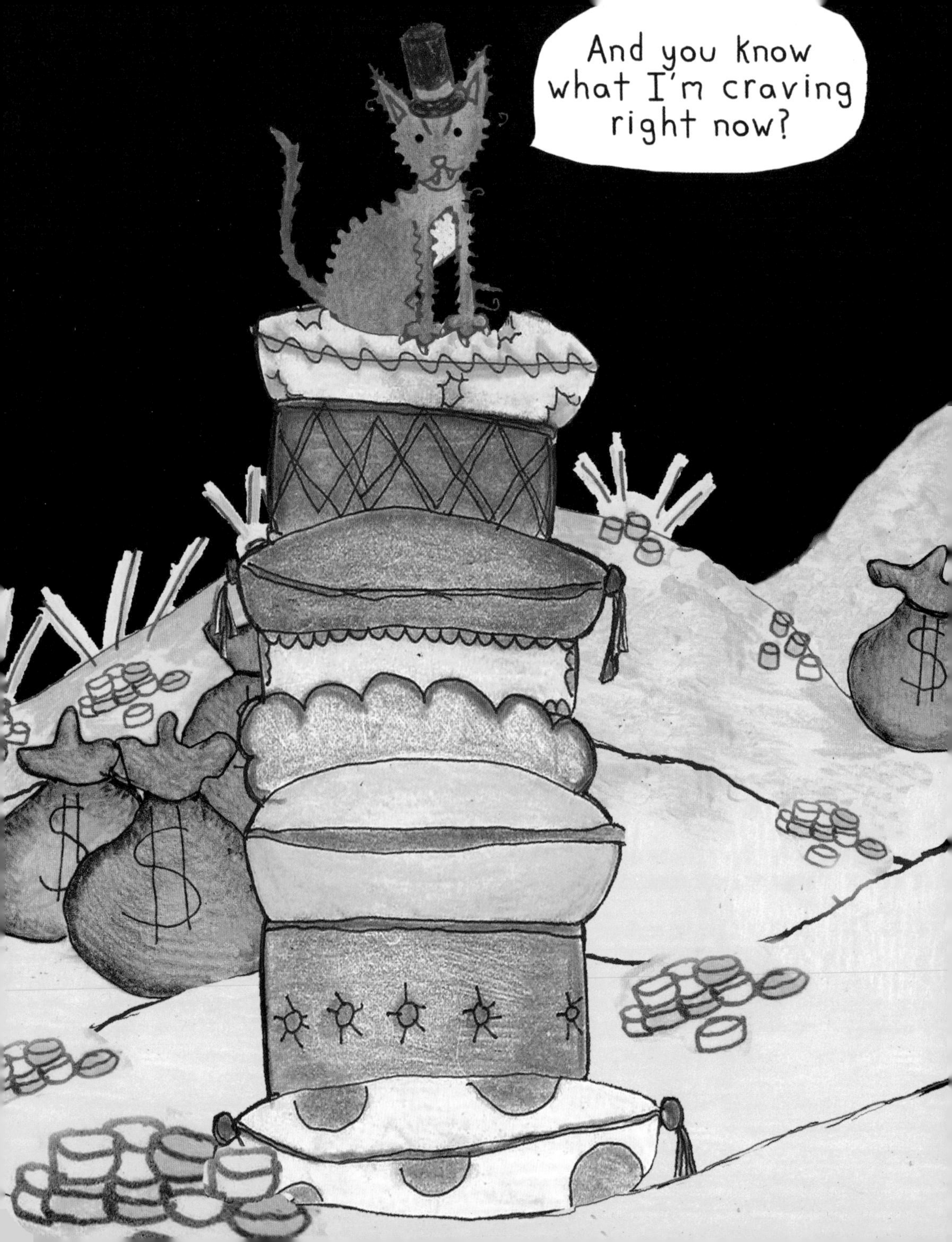
And you know what I'm craving right now?

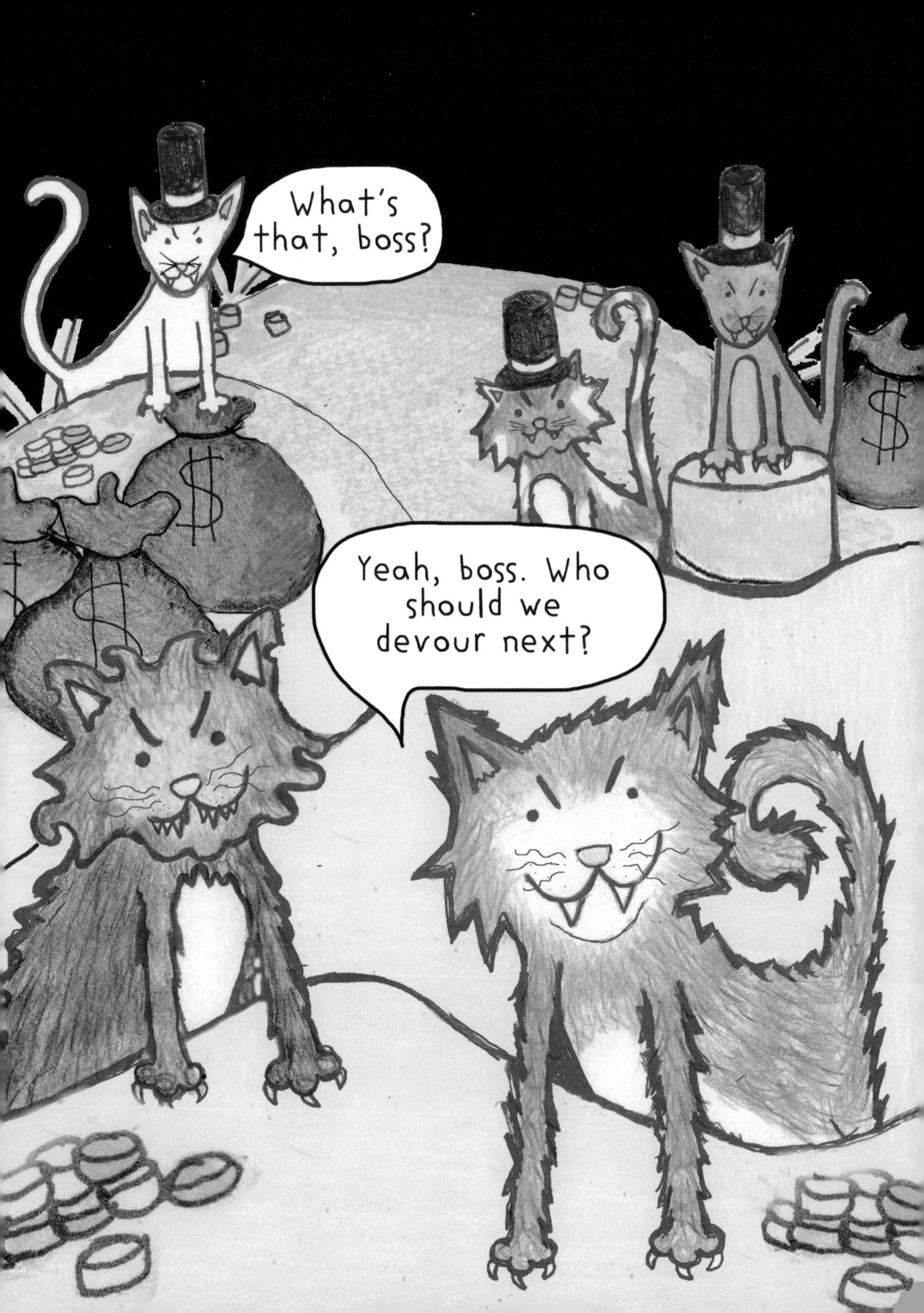
What's that, boss?
Yeah, boss. Who should we devour next?

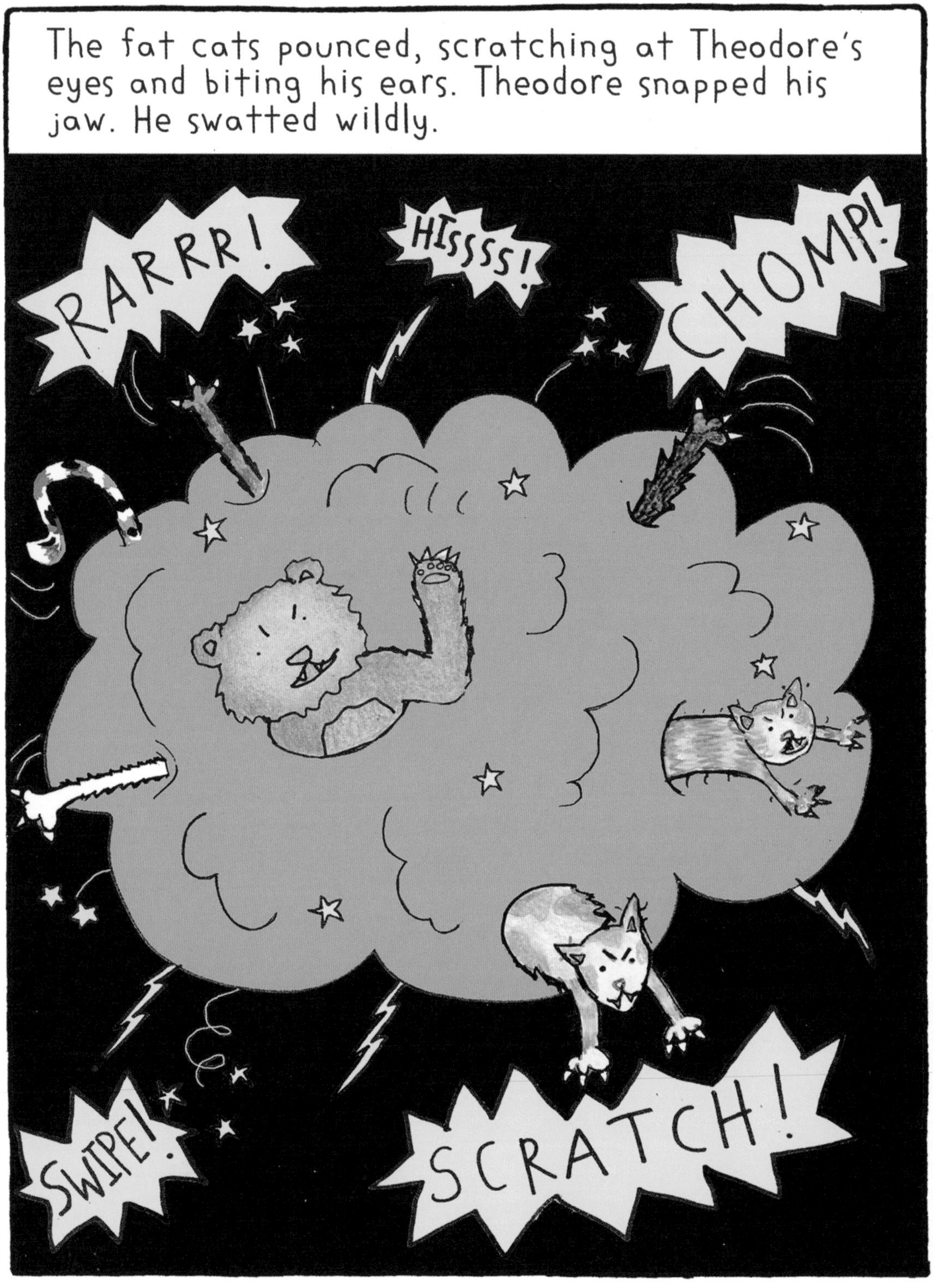
The fat cats pounced, scratching at Theodore's eyes and biting his ears. Theodore snapped his jaw. He swatted wildly.
RARRR!
HISSSS!
CHOMP!
SWIPE!
SCRATCH!

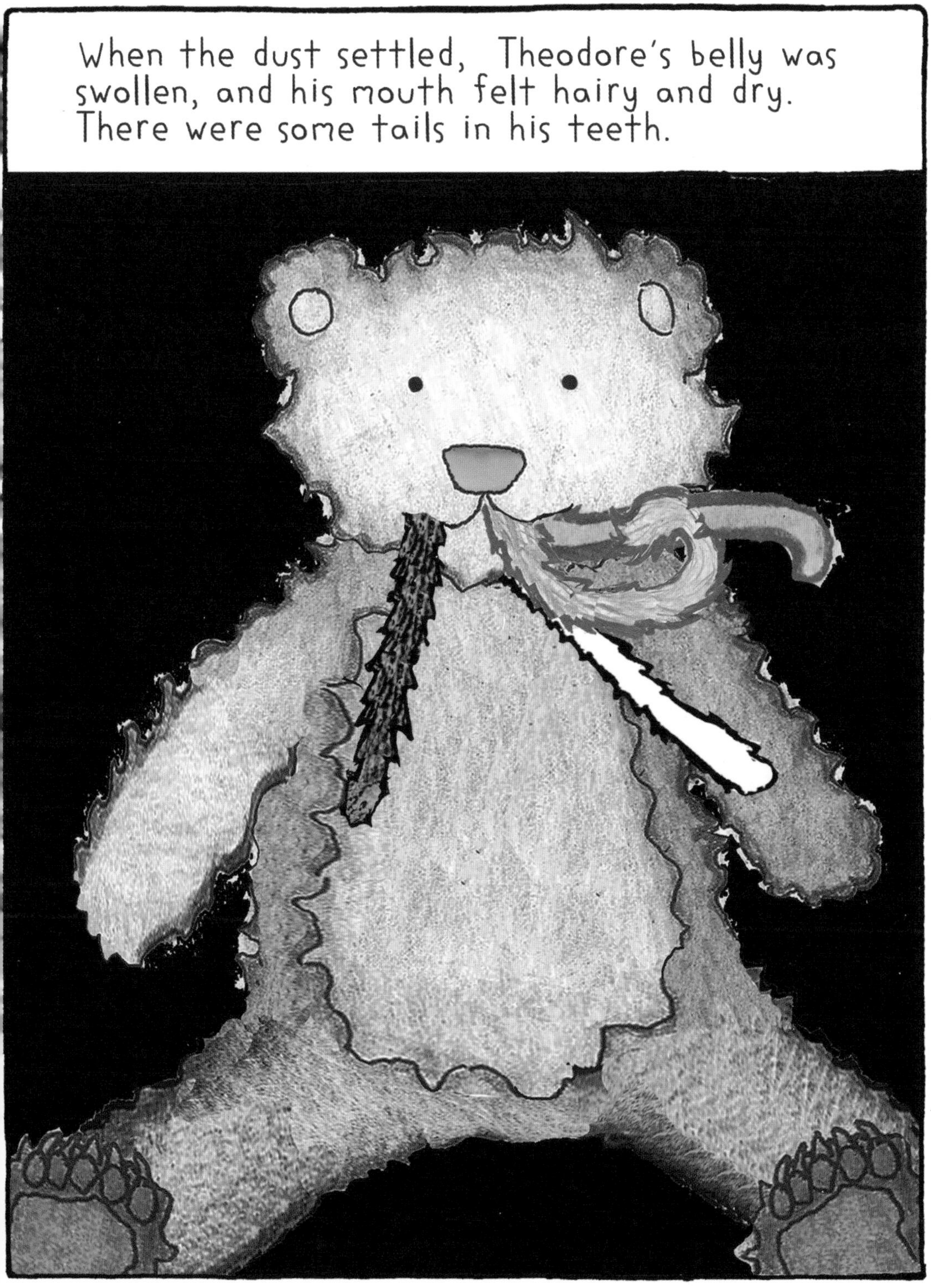
When the dust settled, Theodore's belly was swollen, and his mouth felt hairy and dry. There were some tails in his teeth.

Theodore made his way home, collapsed into bed, and pulled the covers over his head.

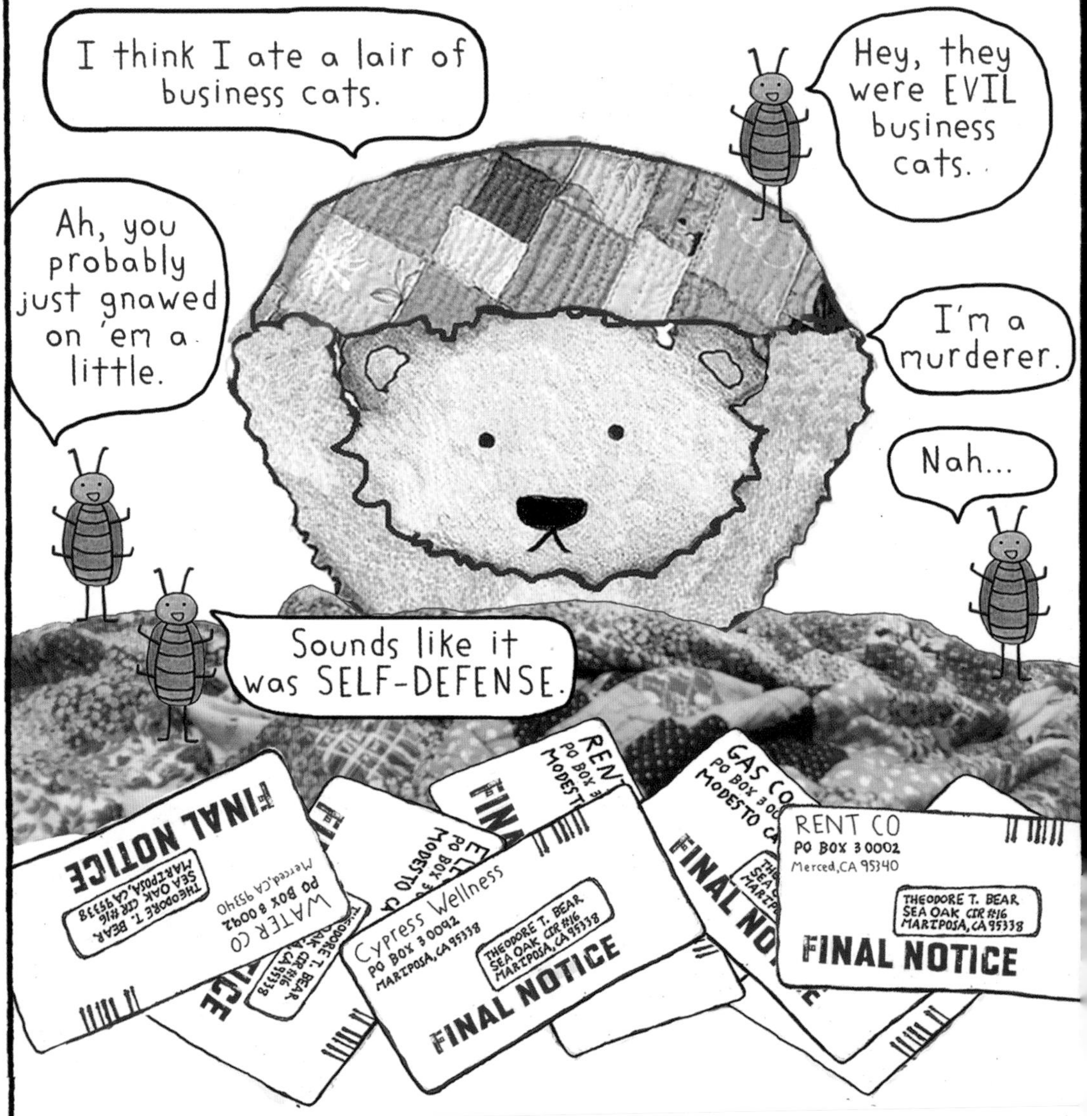

I think I ate a lair of business cats.
Hey, they were EVIL business cats.
Ah, you probably just gnawed on 'em a little.
I'm a murderer.
Nah...
Sounds like it was SELF-DEFENSE.
FINAL NOTICE
WATER CO
PO BOX 80042
Merced, CA 95340
THEODORE T. BEAR
SEA OAK CIR #16
MARIPOSA, CA 95338
Cypress Wellness
PO BOX 30092
MARIPOSA, CA 95338
THEODORE T. BEAR
SEA OAK CIR #16
MARIPOSA, CA 95338
FINAL NOTICE
RENT CO
PO BOX 30002
Merced, CA 95340
THEODORE T. BEAR
SEA OAK CIR #16
MARIPOSA, CA 95338
FINAL NOTICE

Theodore didn't bother calling in sick to work. The bills piled up. Eventually, there was a knock at the door.

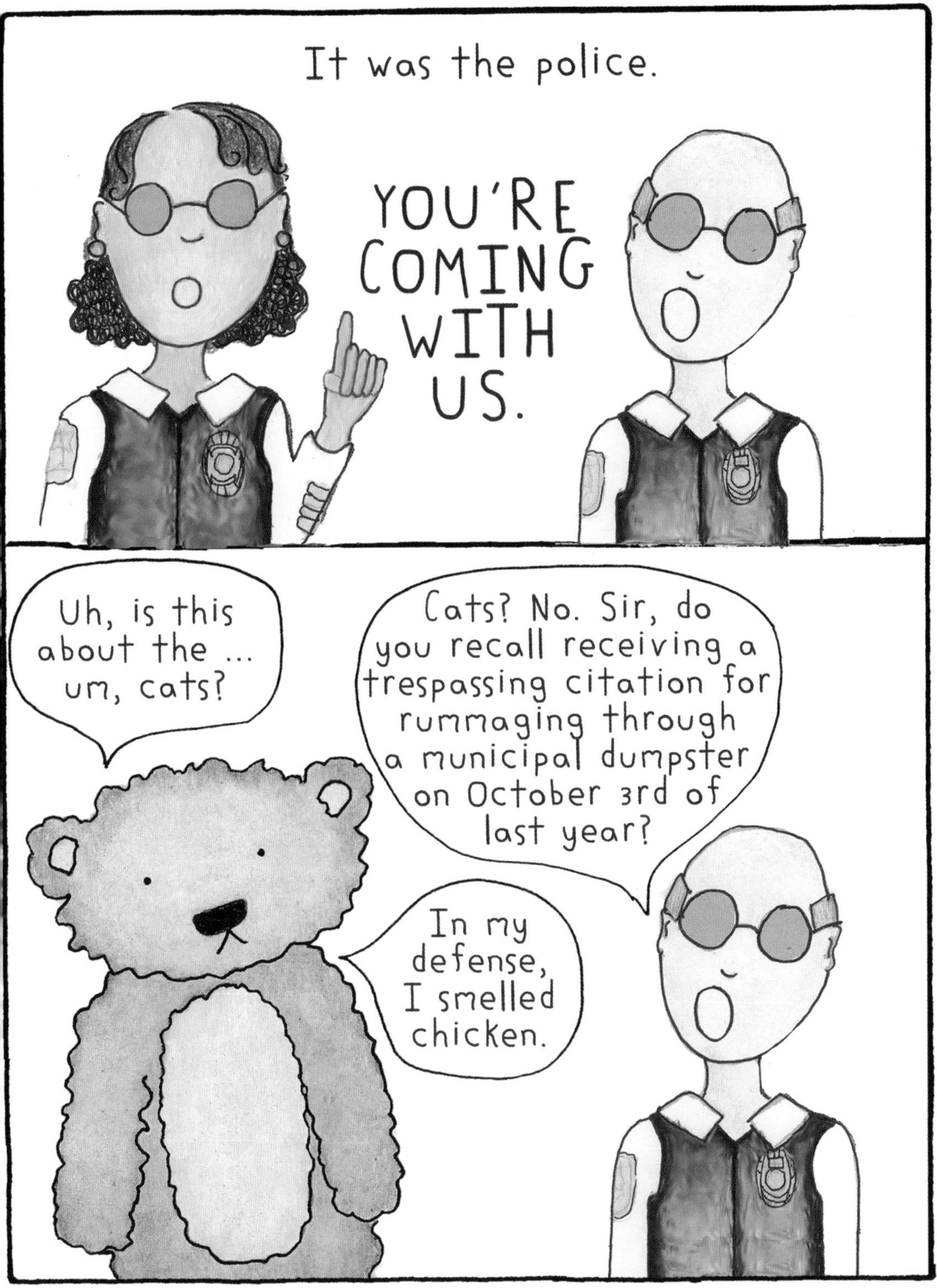
It was the police.
YOU'RE COMING WITH US.
Uh, is this about the ... um, cats?
Cats? No. Sir, do you recall receiving a trespassing citation for rummaging through a municipal dumpster on October 3rd of last year?
In my defense, I smelled chicken.

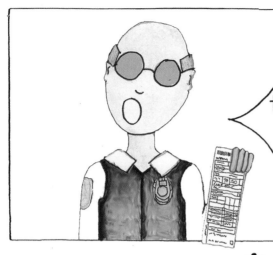

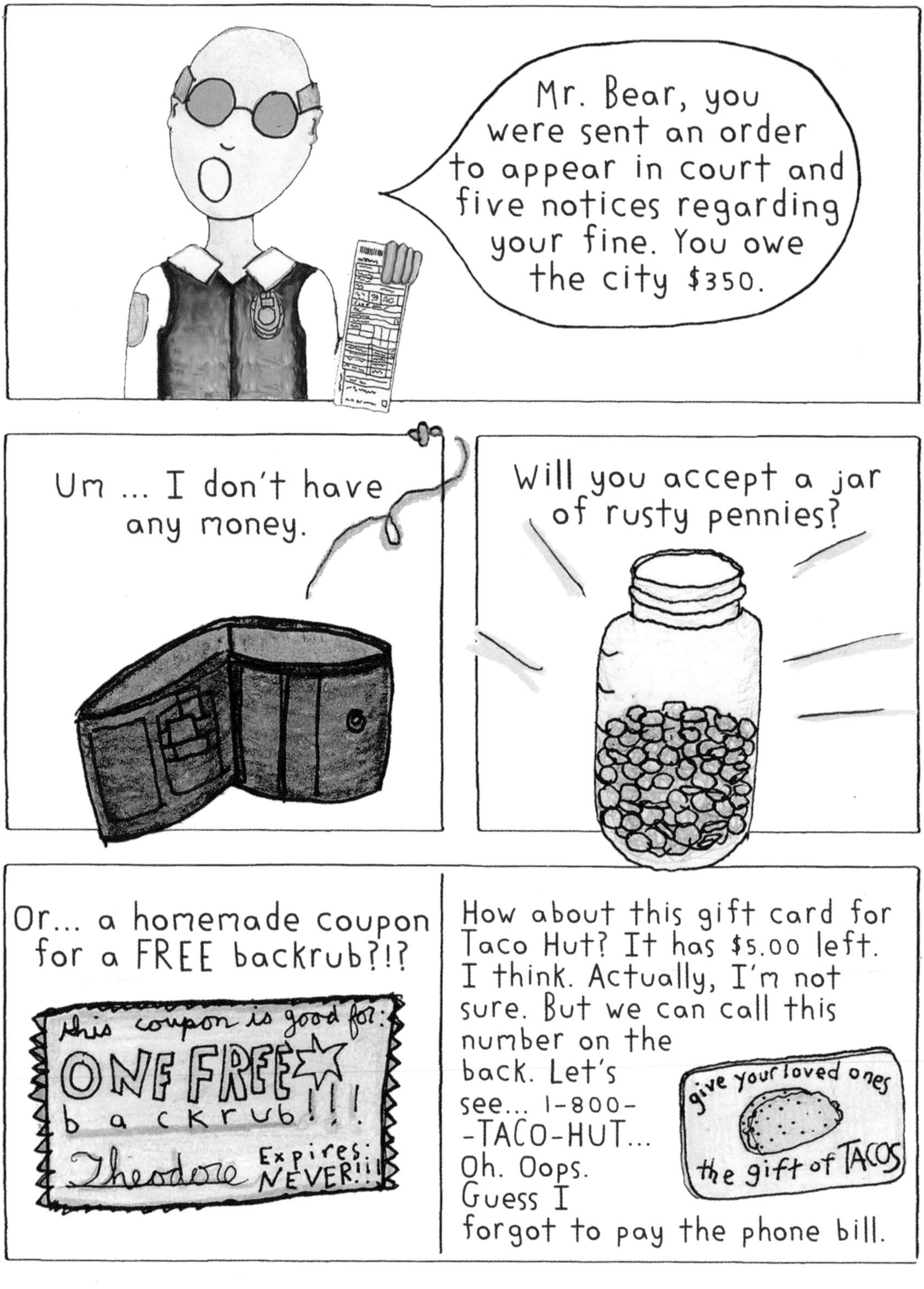

Mr. Bear, you were sent an order to appear in court and five notices regarding your fine. You owe the city $350.

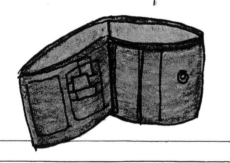

Um ... I don't have any money.

Will you accept a jar of rusty pennies?

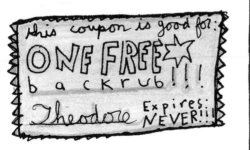

Or... a homemade coupon for a FREE backrub?!?

this coupon is good for: ONE FREE☆ b a c k r u b !!! Theodore Expires: NEVER!!!

How about this gift card for Taco Hut? It has $5.00 left. I think. Actually, I'm not sure. But we can call this number on the back. Let's see... 1-800-TACO-HUT... Oh. Oops. Guess I forgot to pay the phone bill.

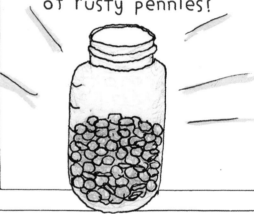

give your loved ones the gift of TACOS

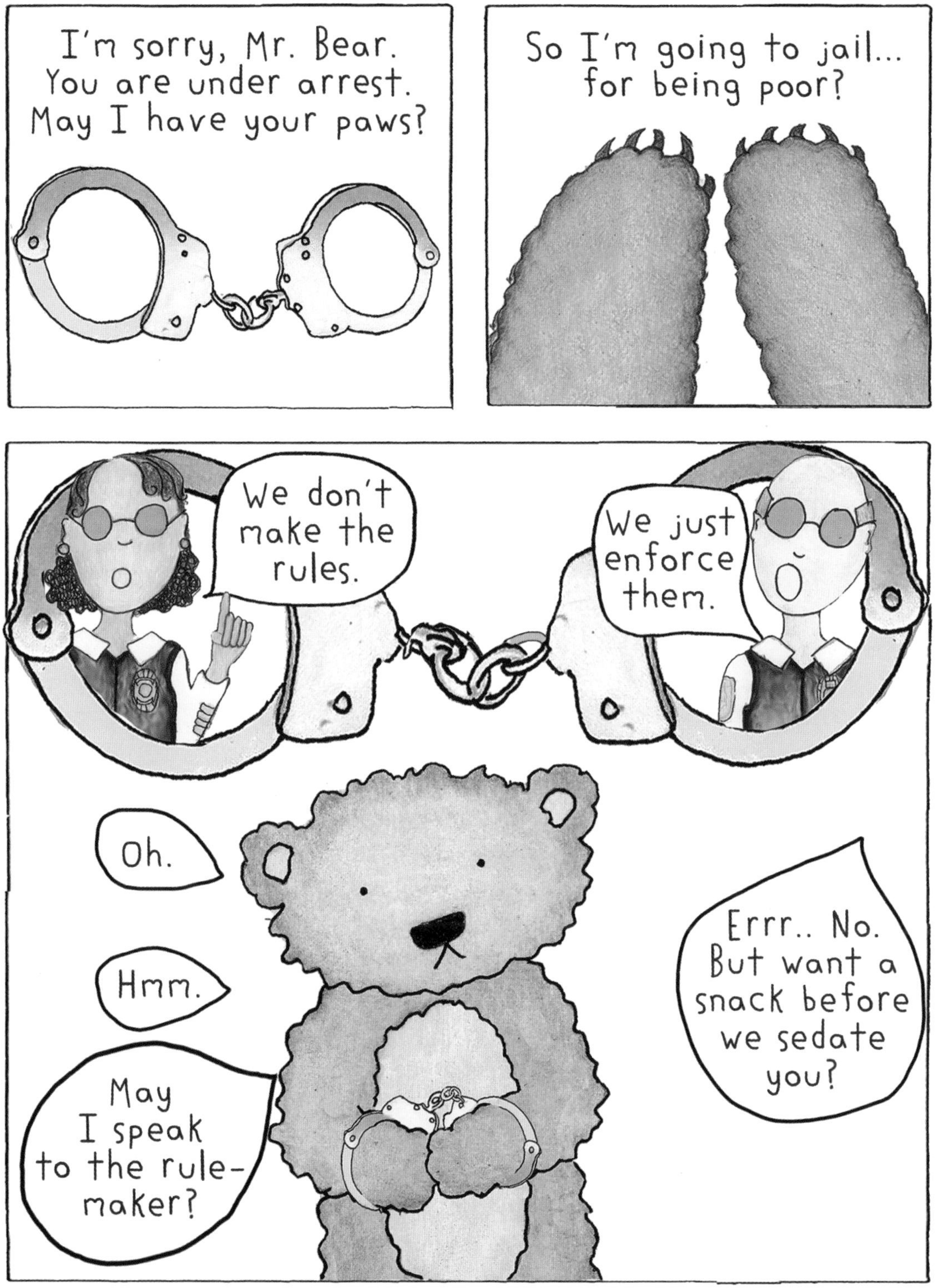
I'm sorry, Mr. Bear. You are under arrest. May I have your paws?
So I'm going to jail... for being poor?
We don't make the rules.
We just enforce them.
Oh.
Hmm.
May I speak to the rule-maker?
Errr.. No. But want a snack before we sedate you?

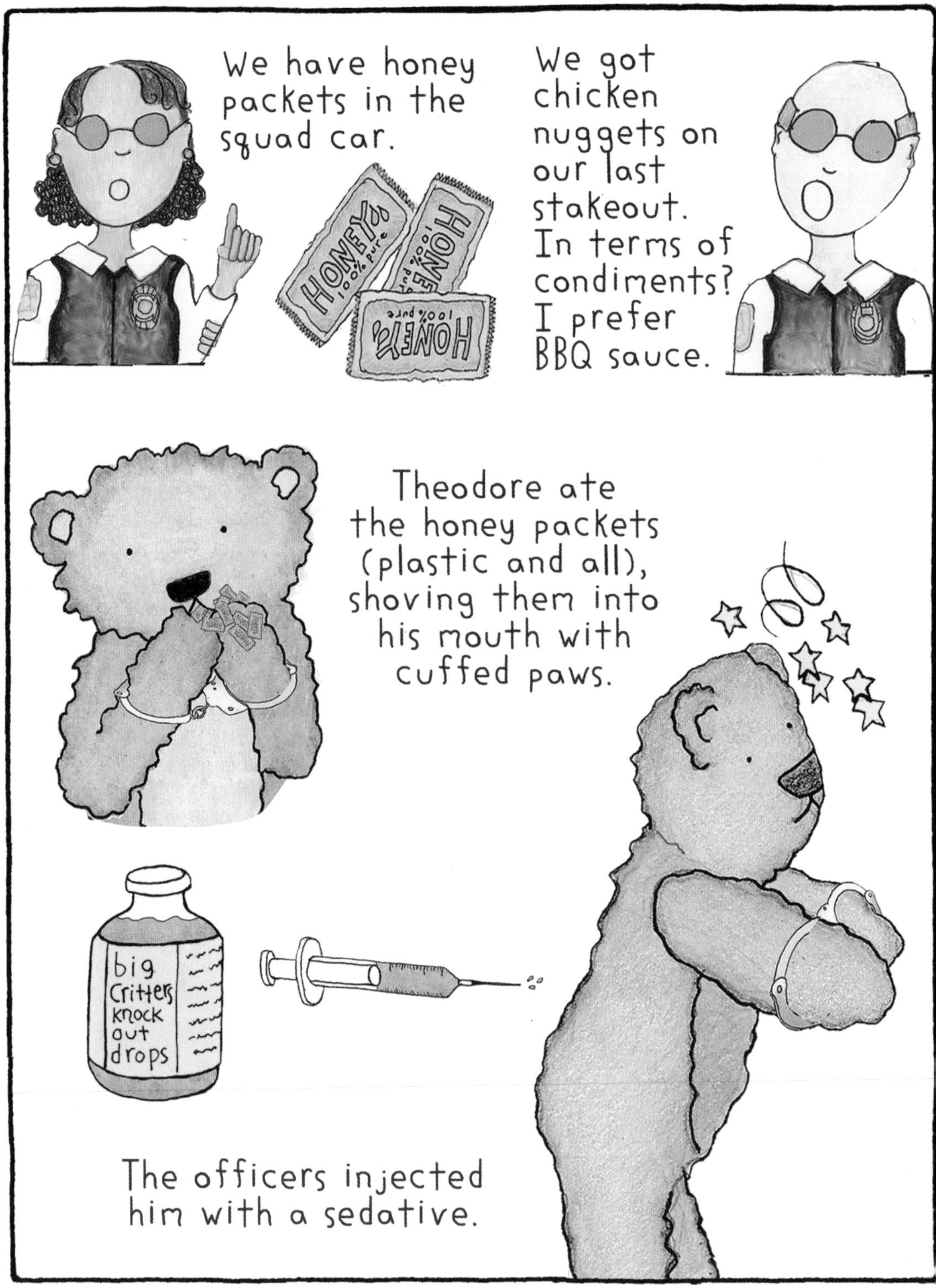
We have honey packets in the squad car.
HONEY 100% pure
We got chicken nuggets on our last stakeout. In terms of condiments? I prefer BBQ sauce.
Theodore ate the honey packets (plastic and all), shoving them into his mouth with cuffed paws.
big critters knock out drops
The officers injected him with a sedative.

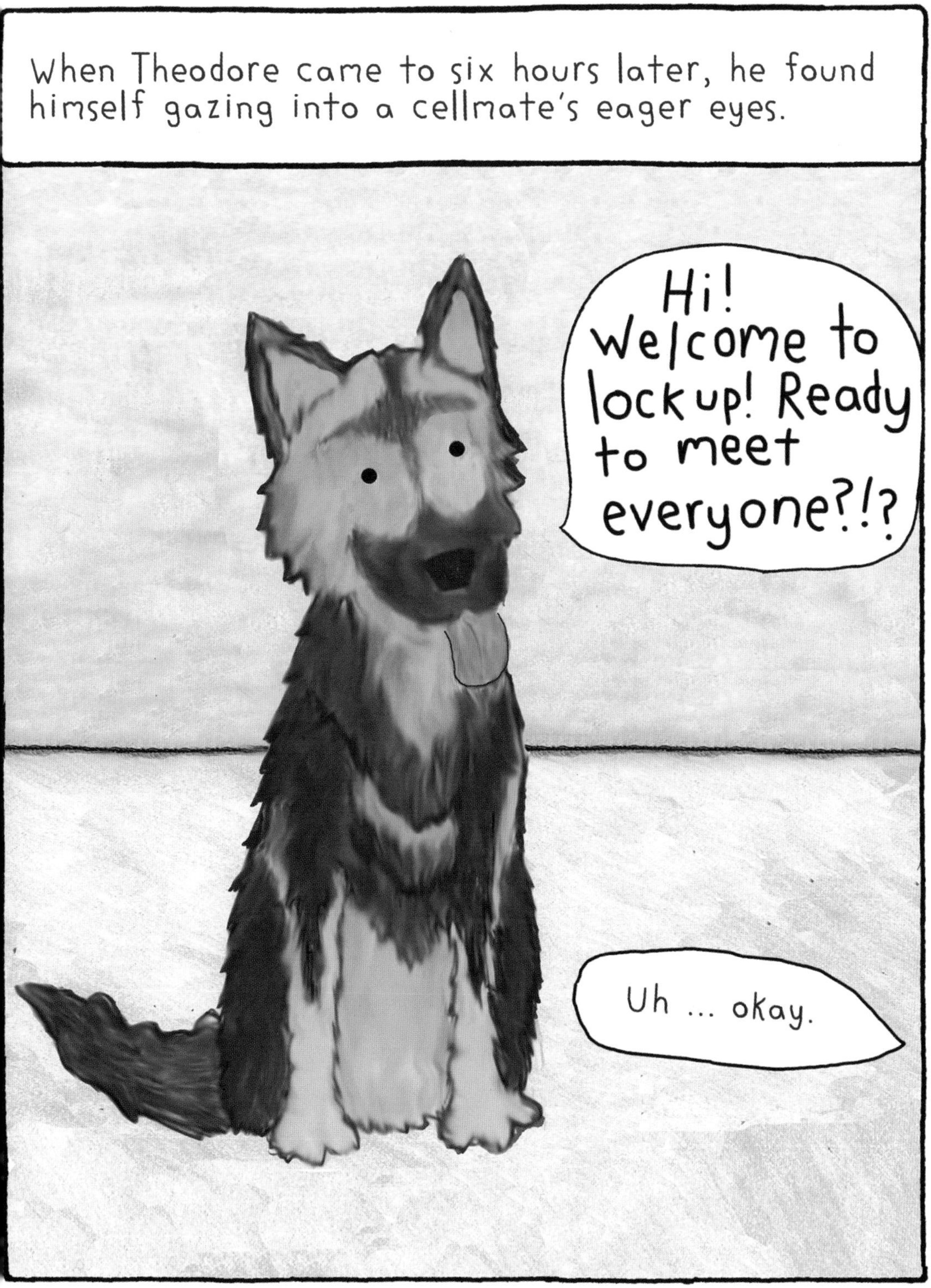
When Theodore came to six hours later, he found himself gazing into a cellmate's eager eyes.
Hi! Welcome to lockup! Ready to meet everyone?!?
Uh ... okay.

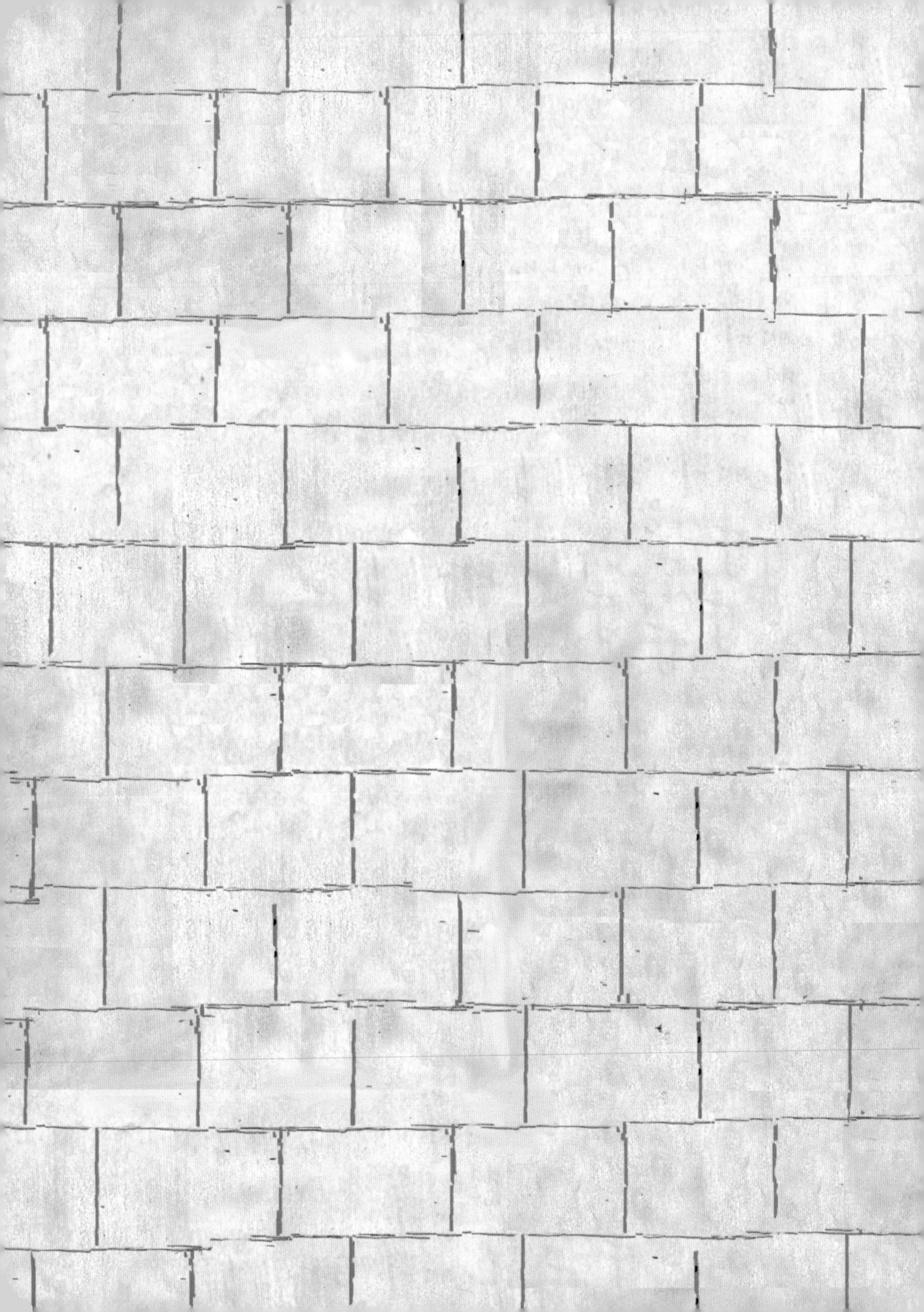

chapter four:
Crime & Punishment

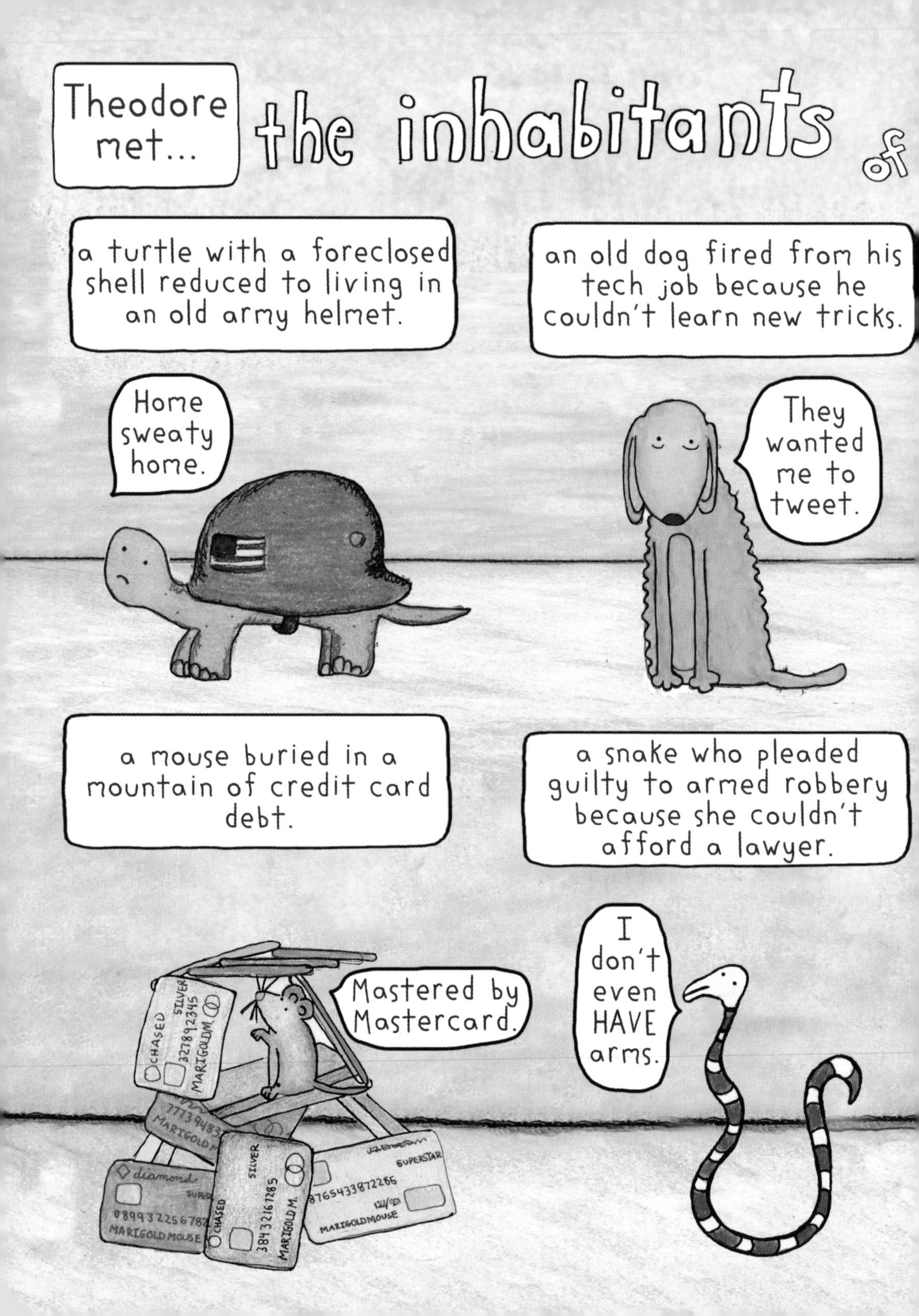

Theodore met...
the inhabitants of
a turtle with a foreclosed shell reduced to living in an old army helmet.
Home sweaty home.
an old dog fired from his tech job because he couldn't learn new tricks.
They wanted me to tweet.
a mouse buried in a mountain of credit card debt.
Mastered by Mastercard.
a snake who pleaded guilty to armed robbery because she couldn't afford a lawyer.
I don't even HAVE arms.

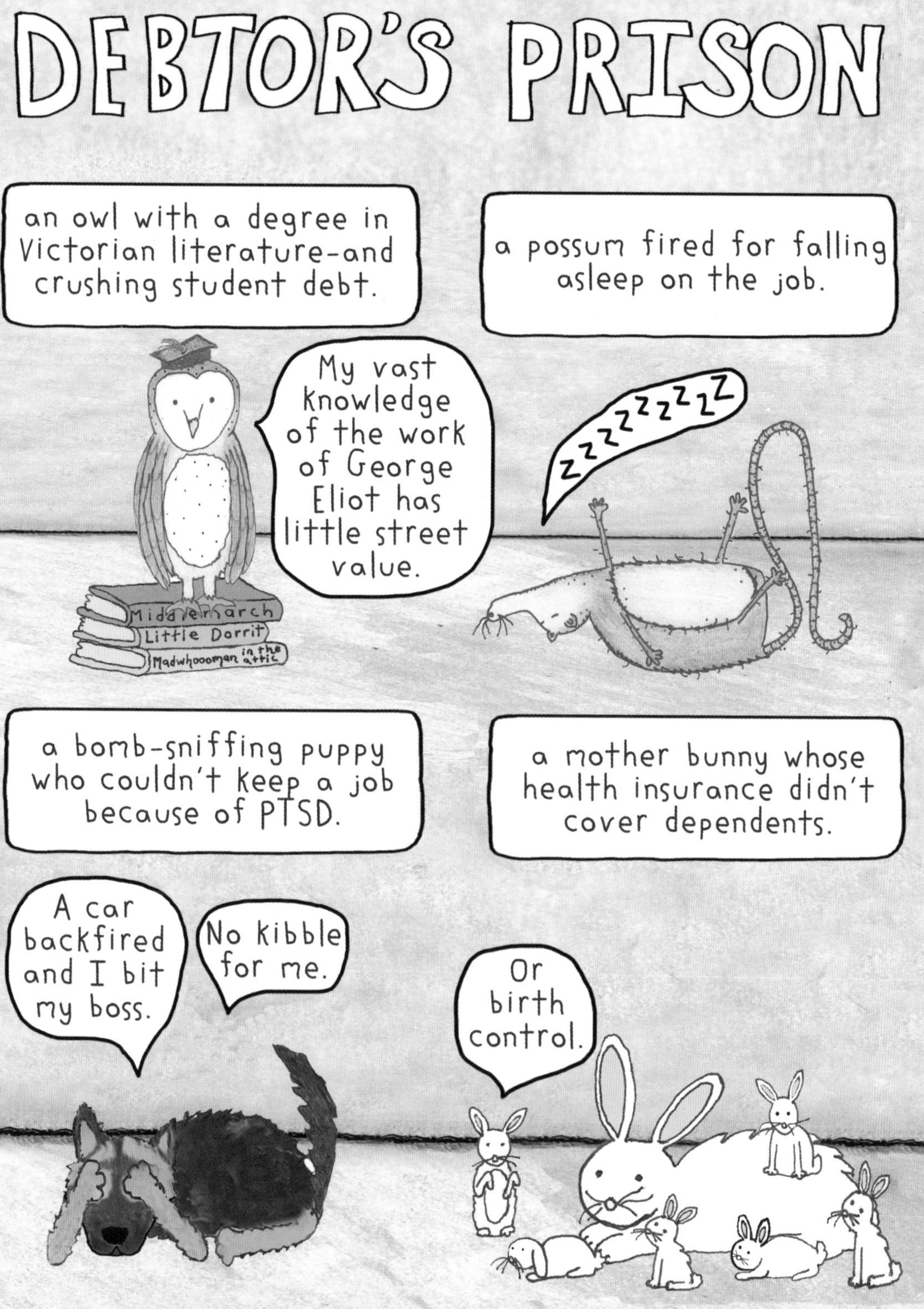

DEBTOR'S PRISON

an owl with a degree in Victorian literature-and crushing student debt.

a possum fired for falling asleep on the job.

My vast knowledge of the work of George Eliot has little street value.

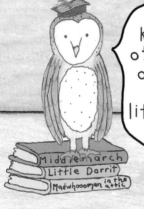

Middlemarch
Little Dorrit
Madwhoooman *in the attic*

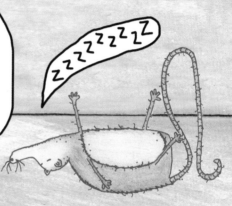
ZZZZZZZZZ

a bomb-sniffing puppy who couldn't keep a job because of PTSD.

a mother bunny whose health insurance didn't cover dependents.

A car backfired and I bit my boss.

No kibble for me.

Or birth control.

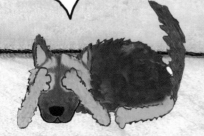

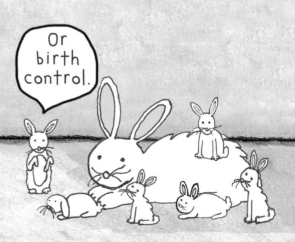

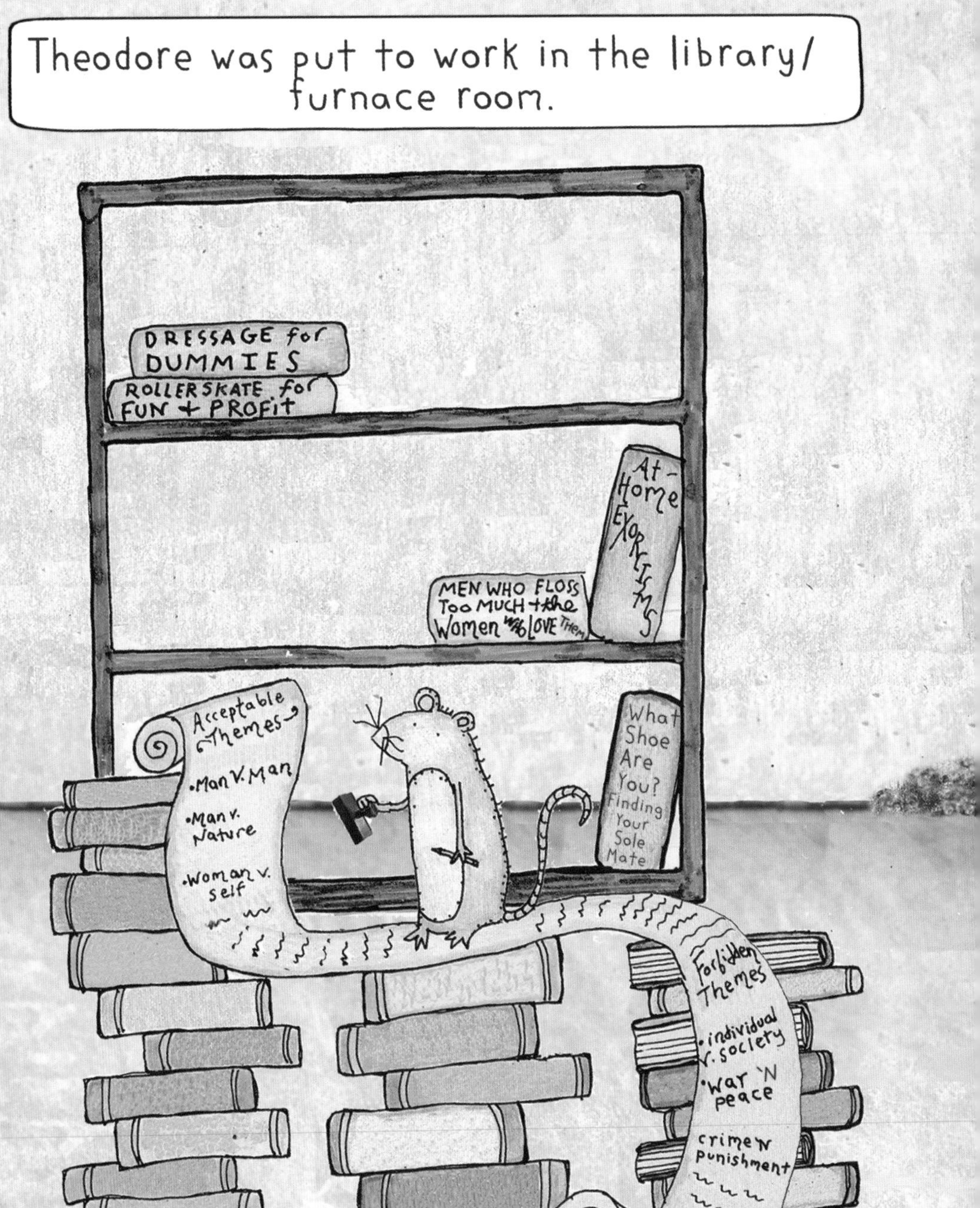
Theodore was put to work in the library/ furnace room.
DRESSAGE for DUMMIES
ROLLERSKATE for FUN + PROFIT
At-Home EXORCISMS
MEN WHO FLOSS Too MUCH + the Women WHO LOVE THEM
What Shoe Are You? Finding Your Sole Mate
Acceptable Themes
•Man V. Man
•Man v. Nature
•Woman v. self
Forbidden Themes
•individual v. society
•War 'N peace
crime 'N punishment

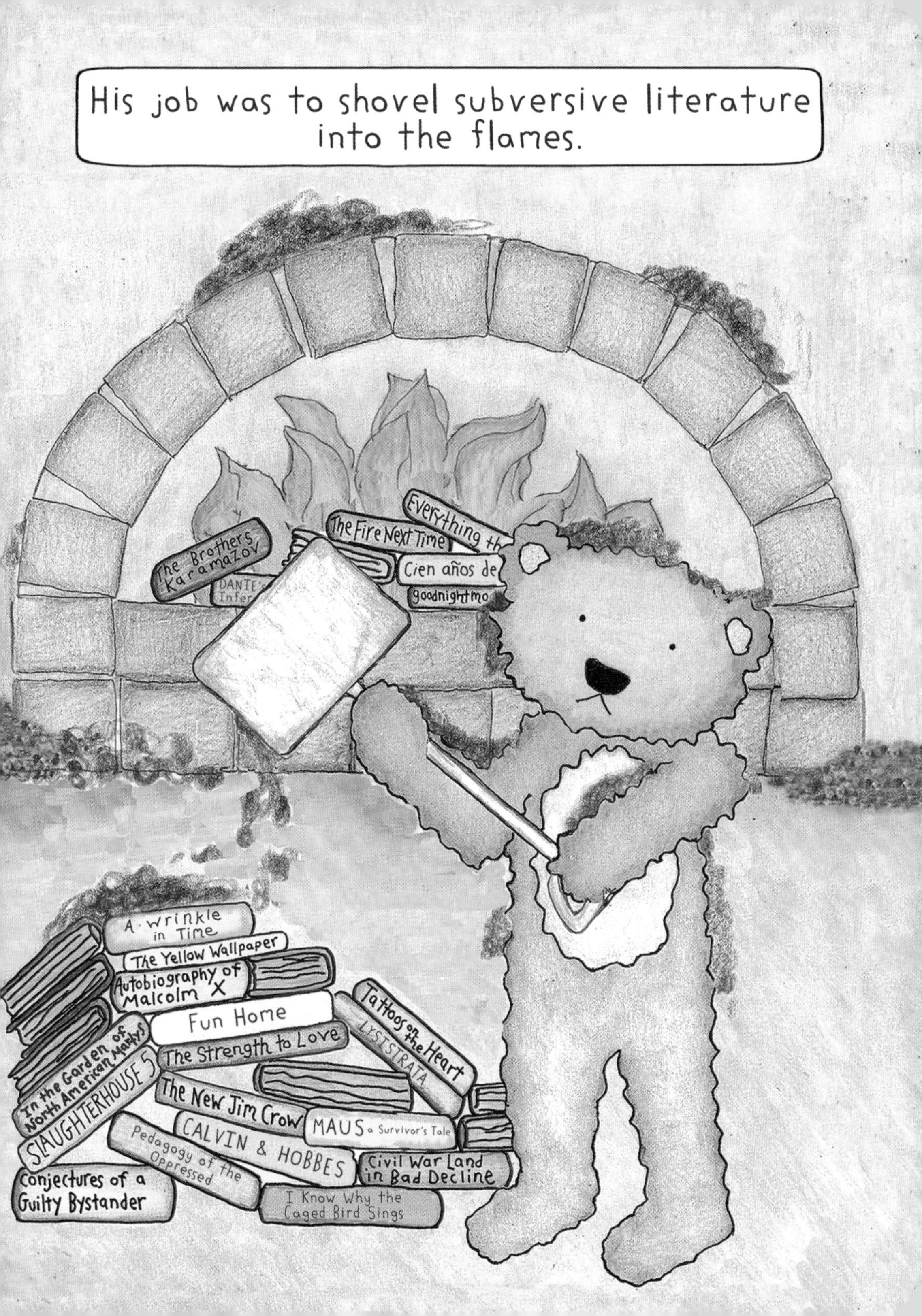
His job was to shovel subversive literature into the flames.
The Brothers Karamazov
The Fire Next Time
Everything th
Cien años de
goodnightmo
A Wrinkle in Time
The Yellow Wallpaper
Autobiography of Malcolm X
Fun Home
The Strength to Love
Tattoos on the Heart
LYSISTRATA
In the Garden of North American Martyrs
SLAUGHTERHOUSE 5
The New Jim Crow
MAUS a Survivor's Tale
CALVIN & HOBBES
Pedagogy of the Oppressed
Civil War Land in Bad Decline
Conjectures of a Guilty Bystander
I Know Why the Caged Bird Sings

Theodore paged through the books before casting them into the fire.

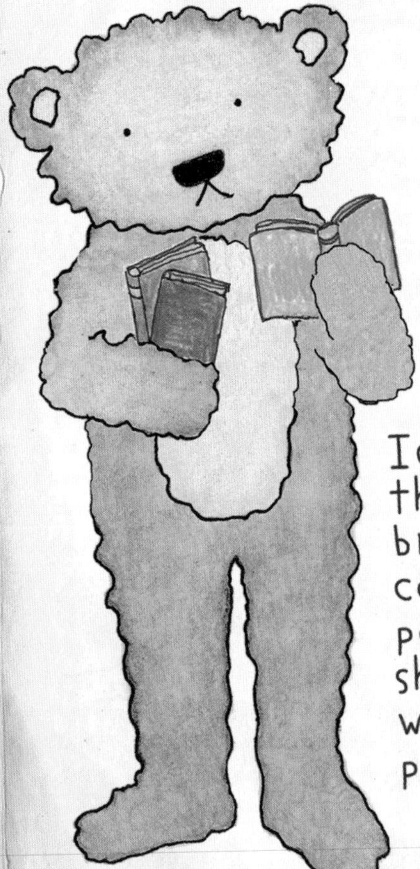

Ideas swirled through his brain. He copied down passages and shared them with fellow prisoners.

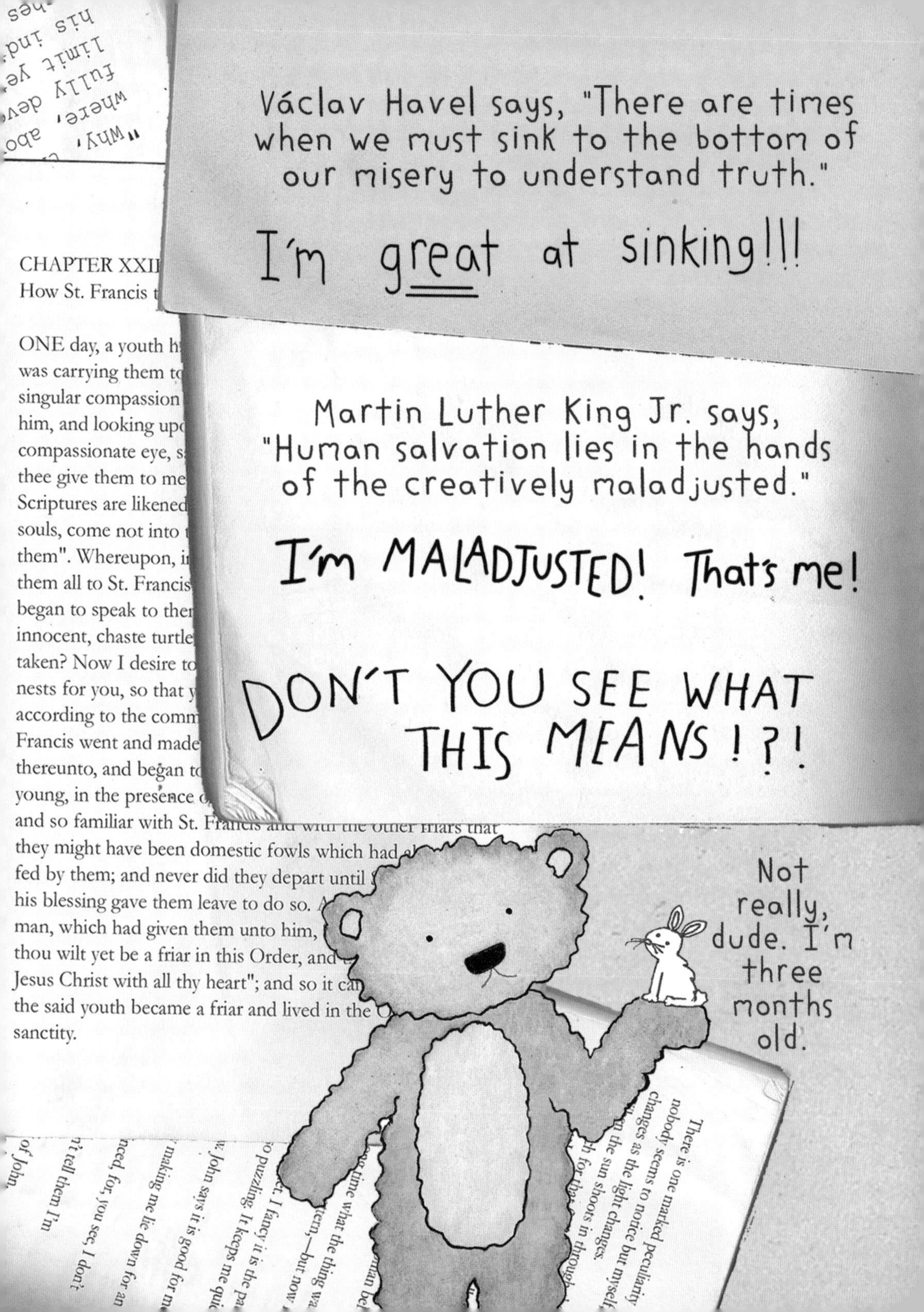
Václav Havel says, "There are times when we must sink to the bottom of our misery to understand truth."
I'm great at sinking!!!
Martin Luther King Jr. says, "Human salvation lies in the hands of the creatively maladjusted."
I'm MALADJUSTED! That's me!
DON'T YOU SEE WHAT THIS MEANS!?!
Not really, dude. I'm three months old.
CHAPTER XXII
How St. Francis
ONE day, a youth
was carrying them to
singular compassion
him, and looking upo
compassionate eye,
thee give them to me
Scriptures are likened
souls, come not into
them". Whereupon, i
them all to St. Francis
began to speak to the
innocent, chaste turtle
taken? Now I desire to
nests for you, so that
according to the comm
Francis went and made
thereunto, and began to
young, in the presence
and so familiar with St. Francis and with the other friars that
they might have been domestic fowls which had
fed by them; and never did they depart until
his blessing gave them leave to do so.
man, which had given them unto him,
thou wilt yet be a friar in this Order, and
Jesus Christ with all thy heart"; and so it ca
the said youth became a friar and lived in the
sanctity.

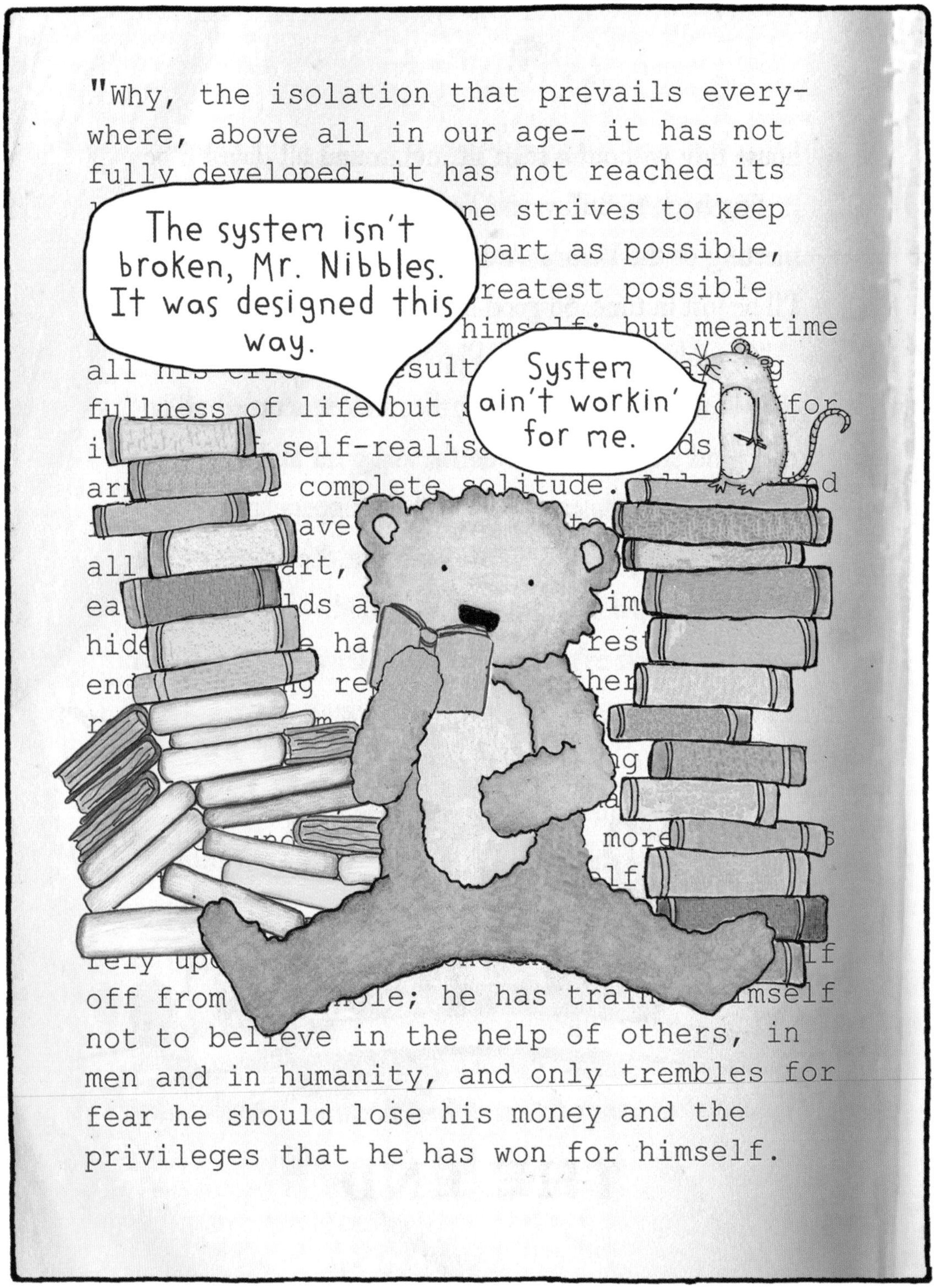
"Why, the isolation that prevails every-
where, above all in our age- it has not
fully developed, it has not reached its
The system isn't broken, Mr. Nibbles. It was designed this way.
System ain't workin' for me.
off from the whole; he has trained himself
not to believe in the help of others, in
men and in humanity, and only trembles for
fear he should lose his money and the
privileges that he has won for himself.

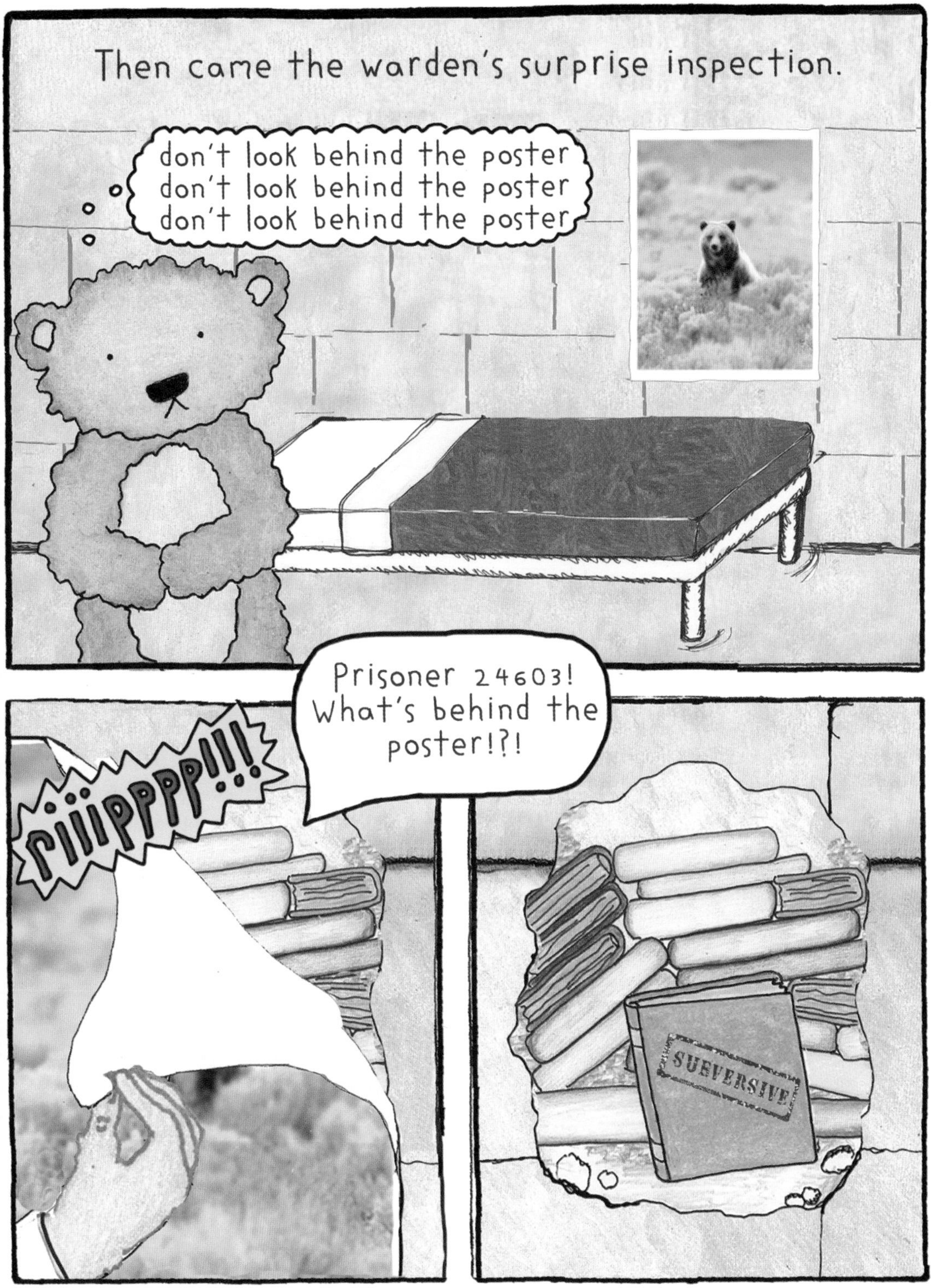
Then came the warden's surprise inspection.
don't look behind the poster
don't look behind the poster
don't look behind the poster
riiiPPPP!!!
Prisoner 24603! What's behind the poster!?!
SUBVERSIVE

Theodore was thrown into solitary confinement.
He sank into an ocean of doom.

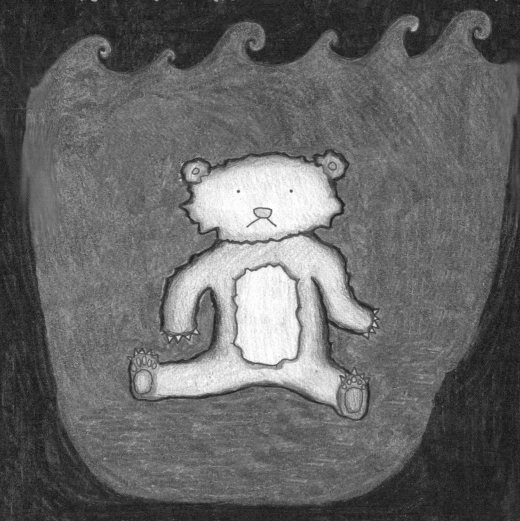

In his catatonic state, Theodore refused to eat or drink.
A shadow of himself, he grew thin and weak. An illness
spreading through the prison blossomed in his lungs.

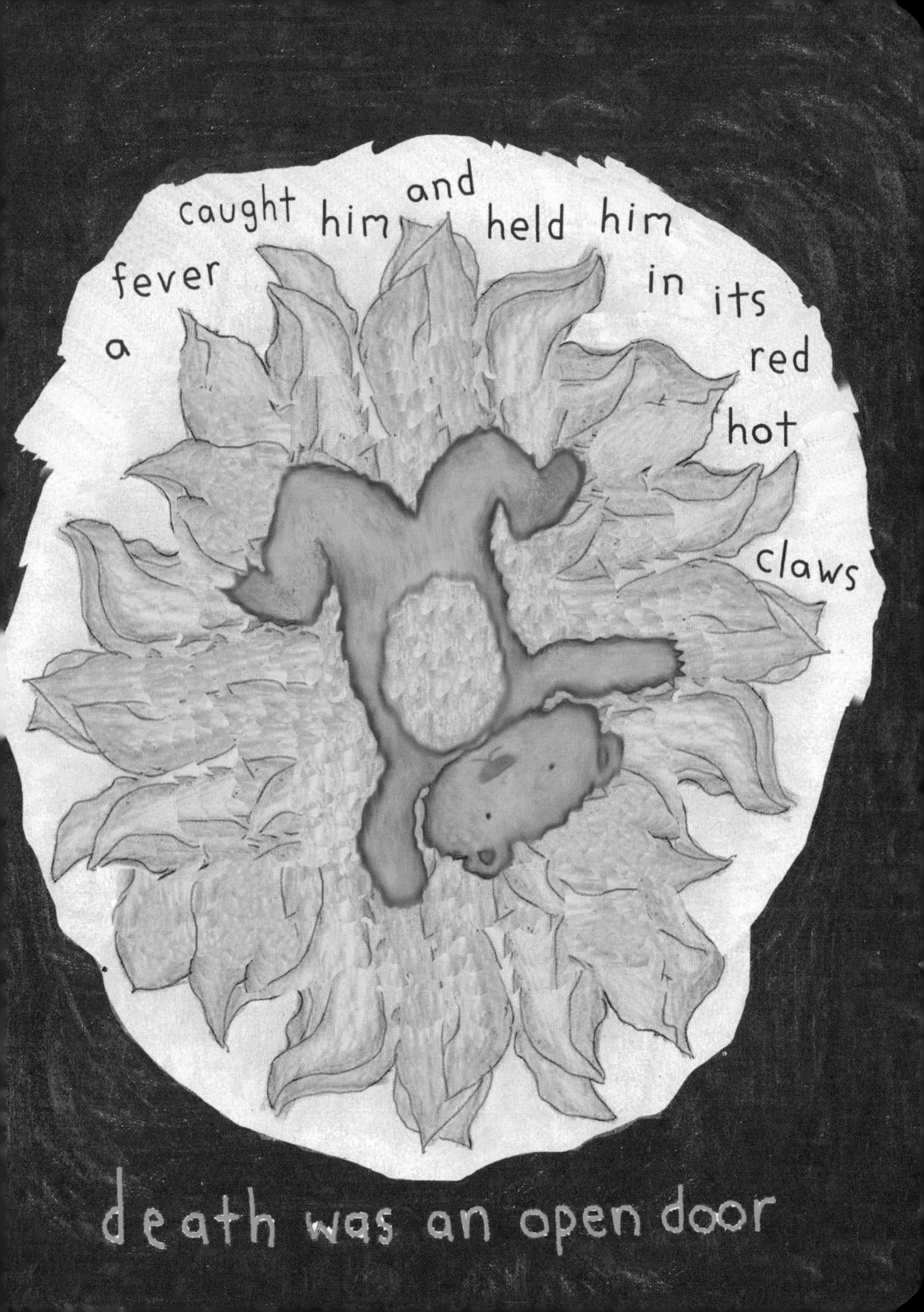
a fever caught him and held him in its red hot claws
death was an open door

And then...

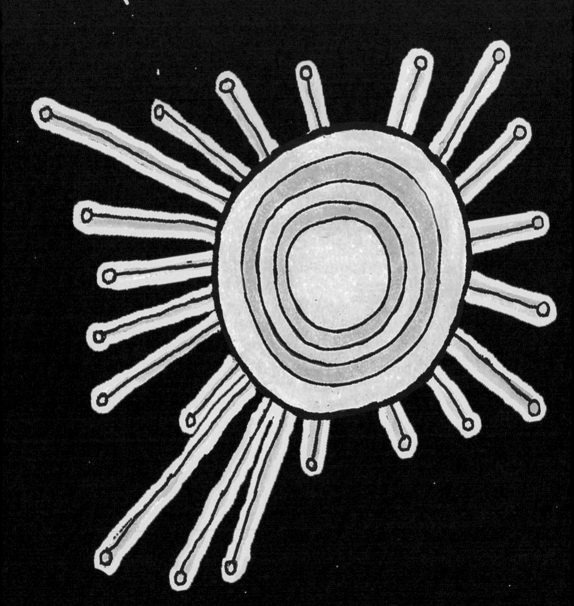

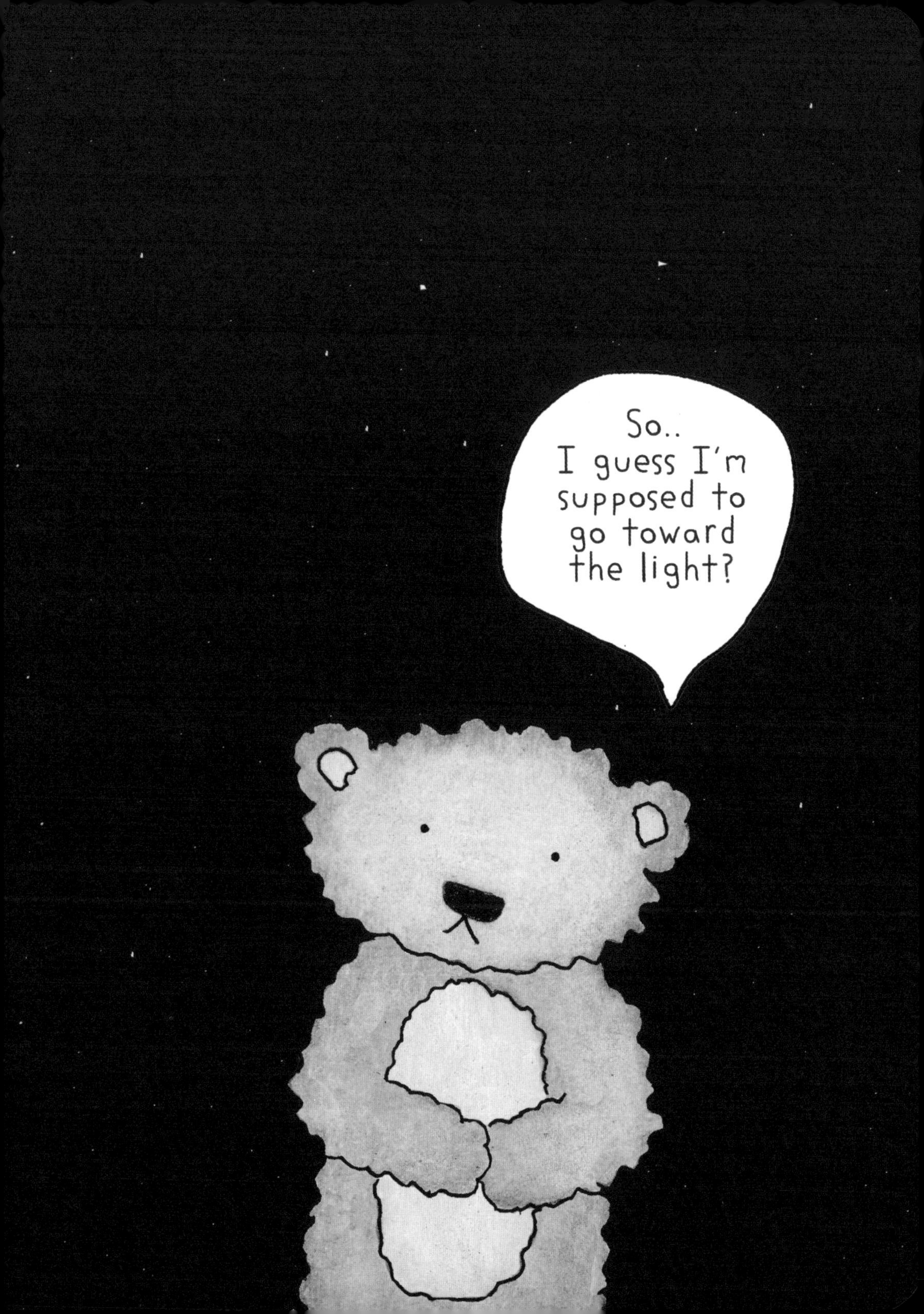
So.. I guess I'm supposed to go toward the light?

FEAR Not, THEODORE!

YOU ARE EXACTLY WHERE YOU ARE SUPPOSED TO BE

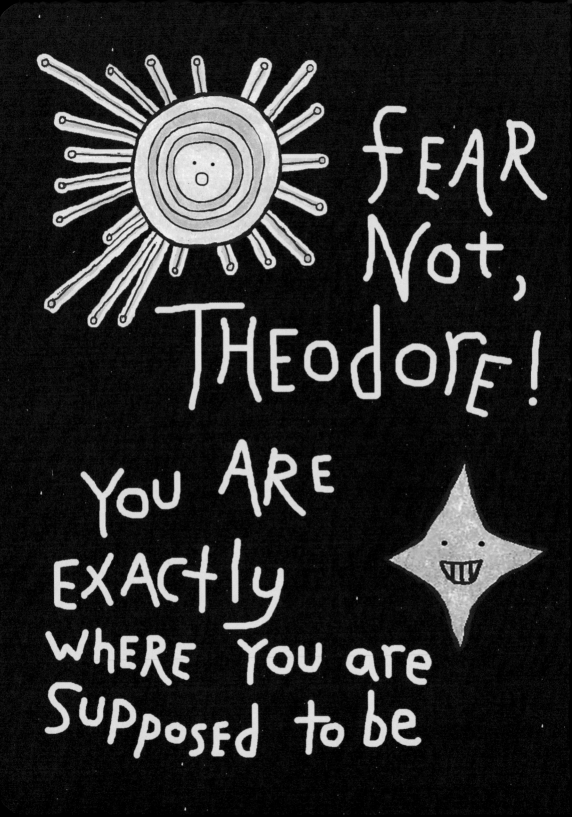

YOU MUST SAVE YOUR FELLOW debtors

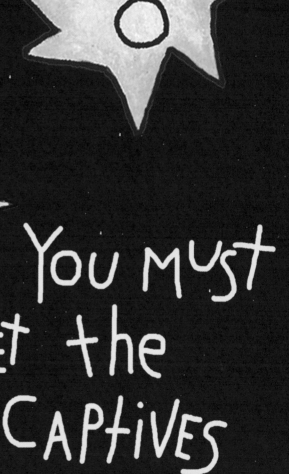

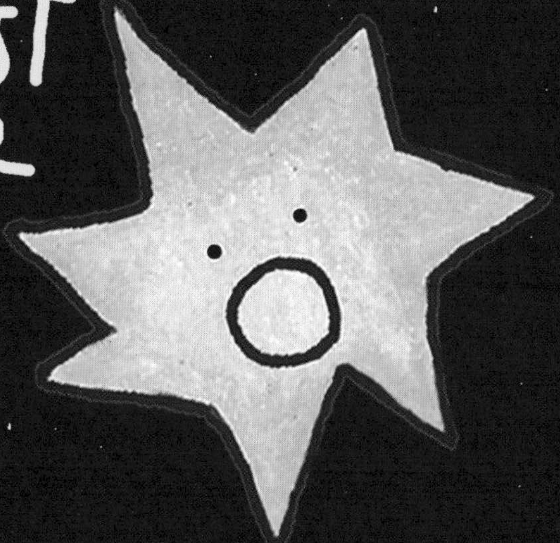

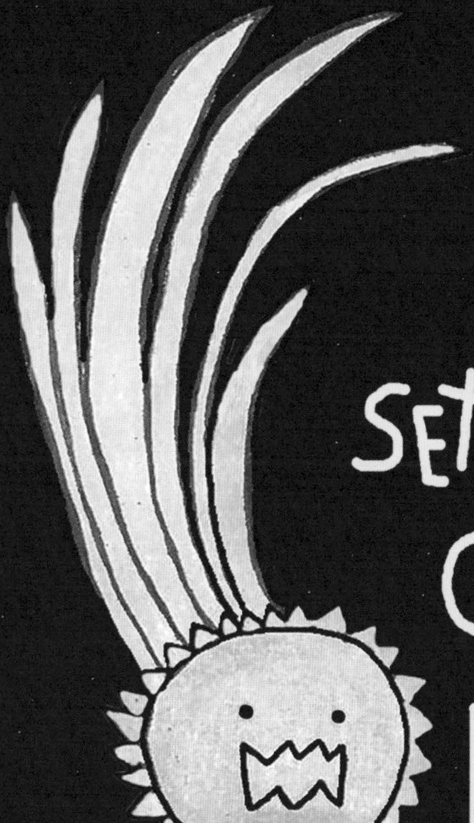

YOU MUST set the CAPTIVES FREE!

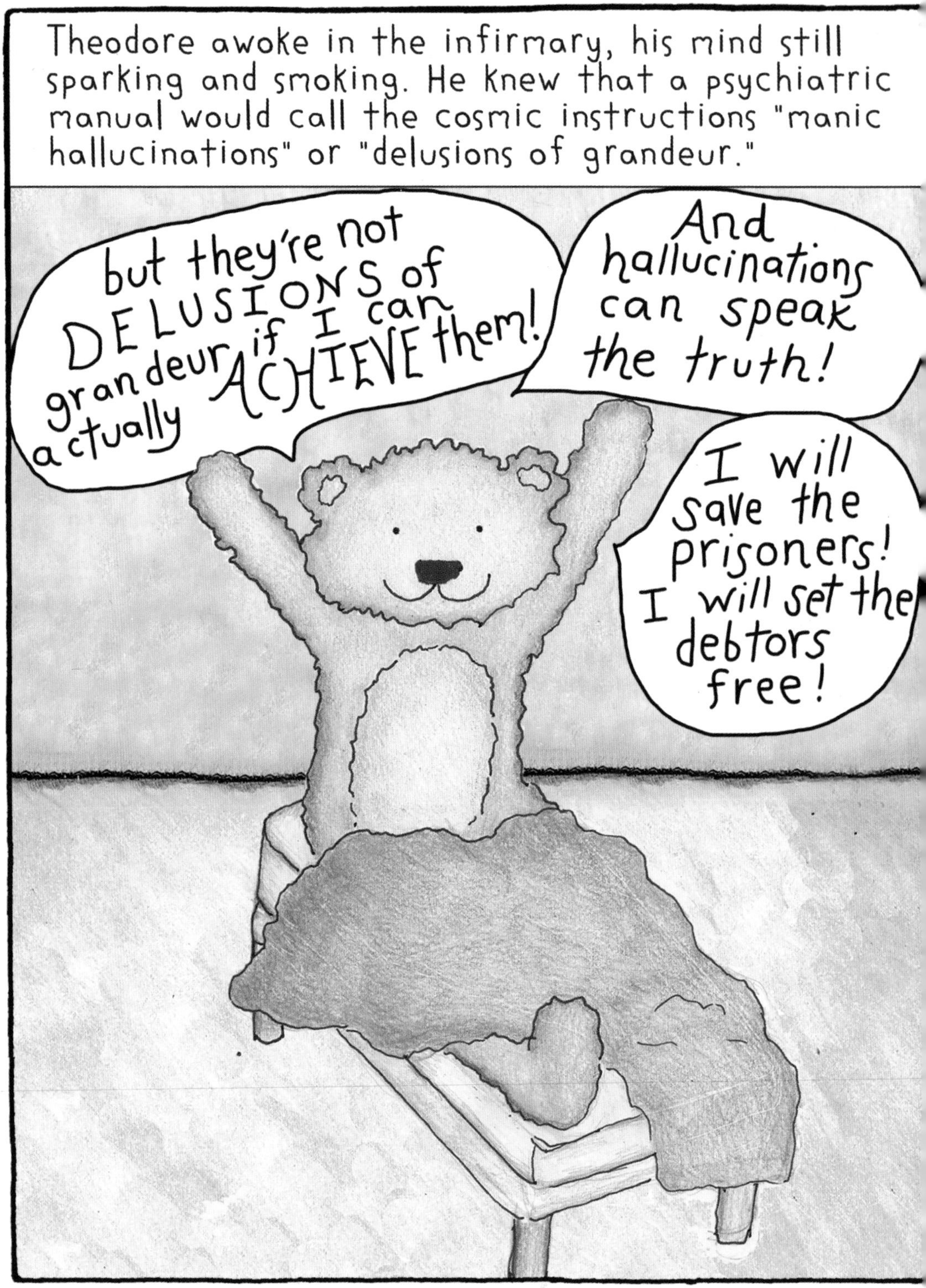
Theodore awoke in the infirmary, his mind still sparking and smoking. He knew that a psychiatric manual would call the cosmic instructions "manic hallucinations" or "delusions of grandeur."
but they're not DELUSIONS of grandeur if I can actually ACHIEVE them!
And hallucinations can speak the truth!
I will save the prisoners! I will set the debtors free!

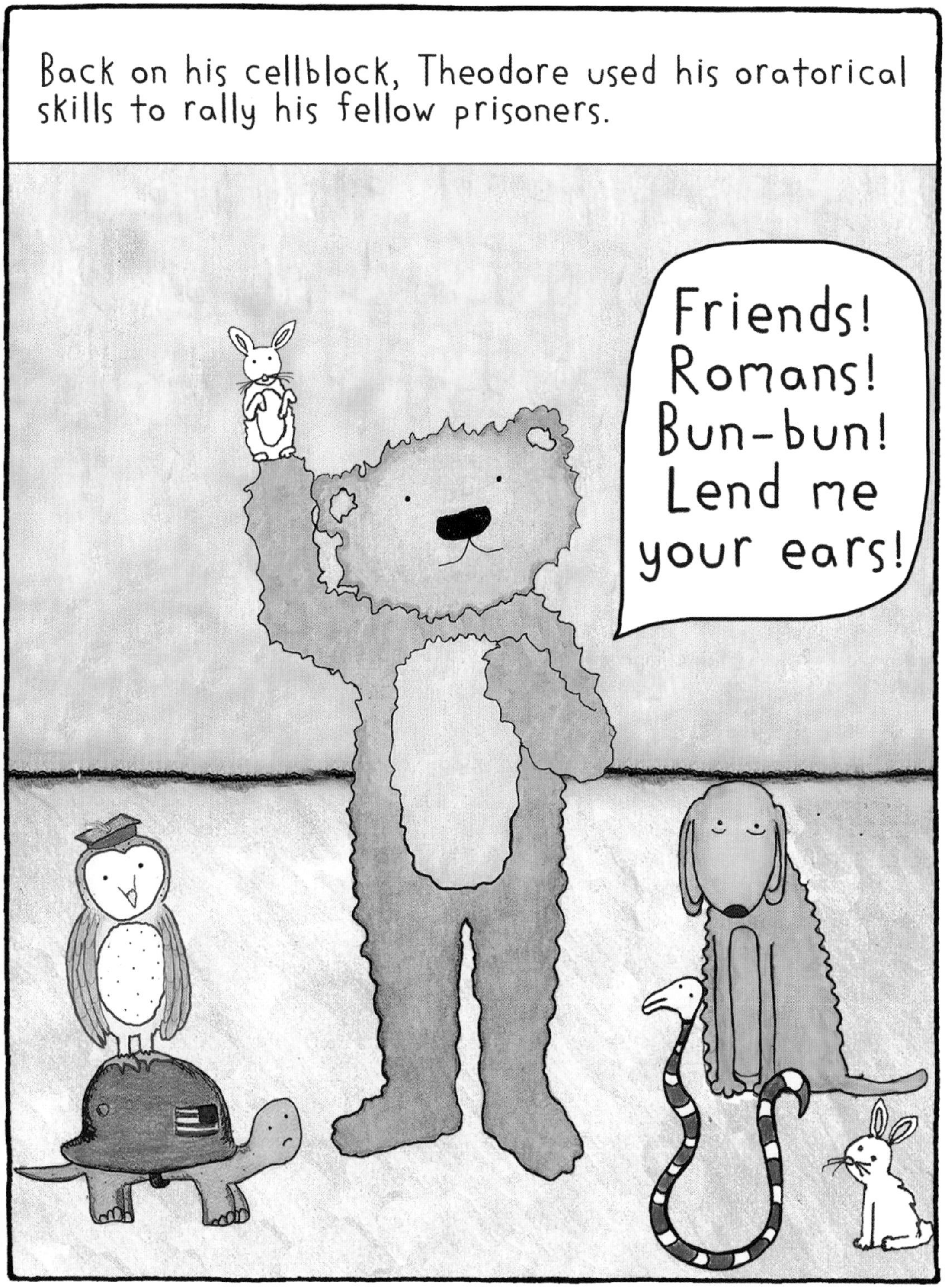
Back on his cellblock, Theodore used his oratorical skills to rally his fellow prisoners.
Friends! Romans! Bun-bun! Lend me your ears!

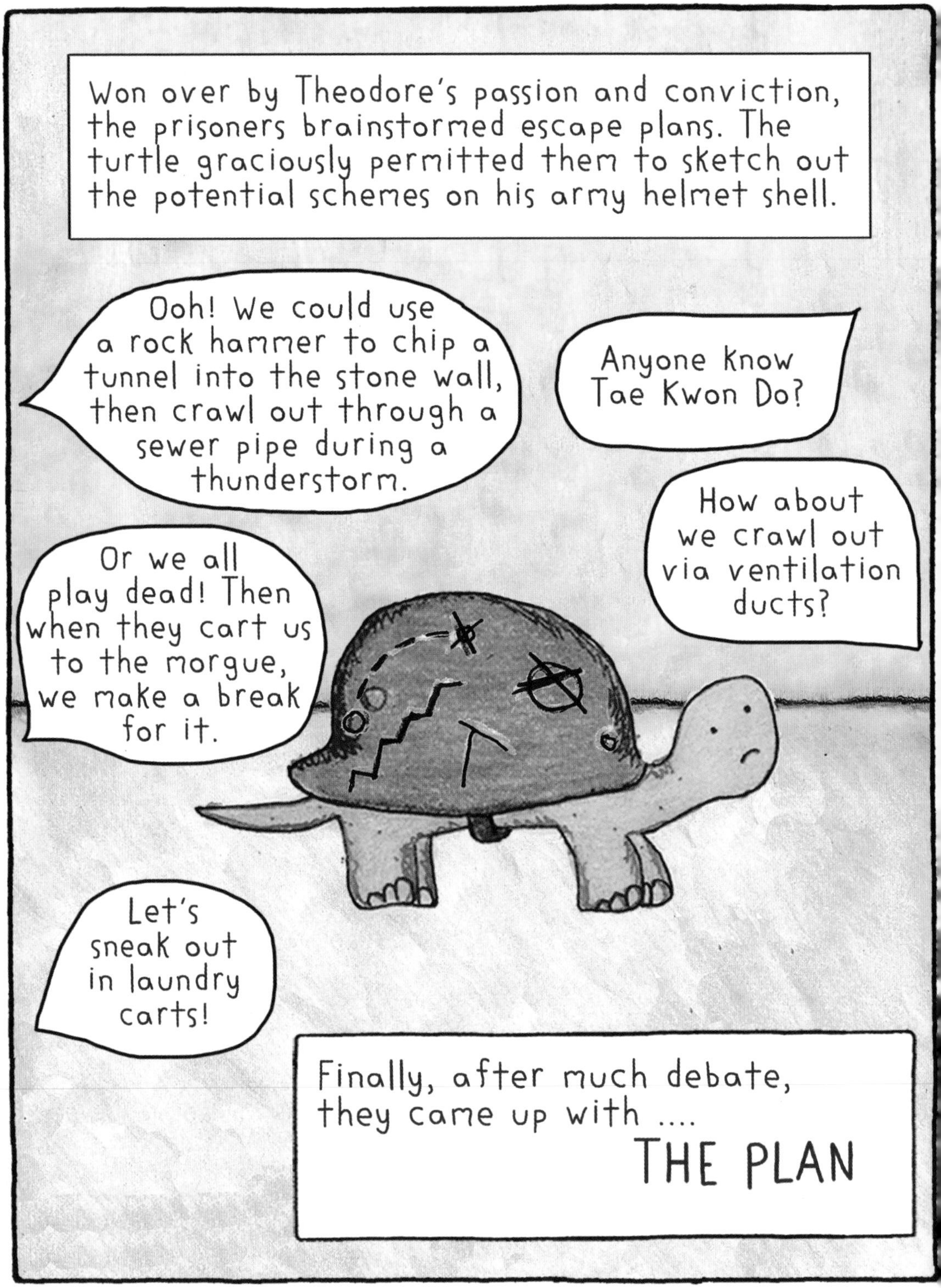
Won over by Theodore's passion and conviction, the prisoners brainstormed escape plans. The turtle graciously permitted them to sketch out the potential schemes on his army helmet shell.
Ooh! We could use a rock hammer to chip a tunnel into the stone wall, then crawl out through a sewer pipe during a thunderstorm.
Anyone know Tae Kwon Do?
Or we all play dead! Then when they cart us to the morgue, we make a break for it.
How about we crawl out via ventilation ducts?
Let's sneak out in laundry carts!
Finally, after much debate, they came up with ....
THE PLAN

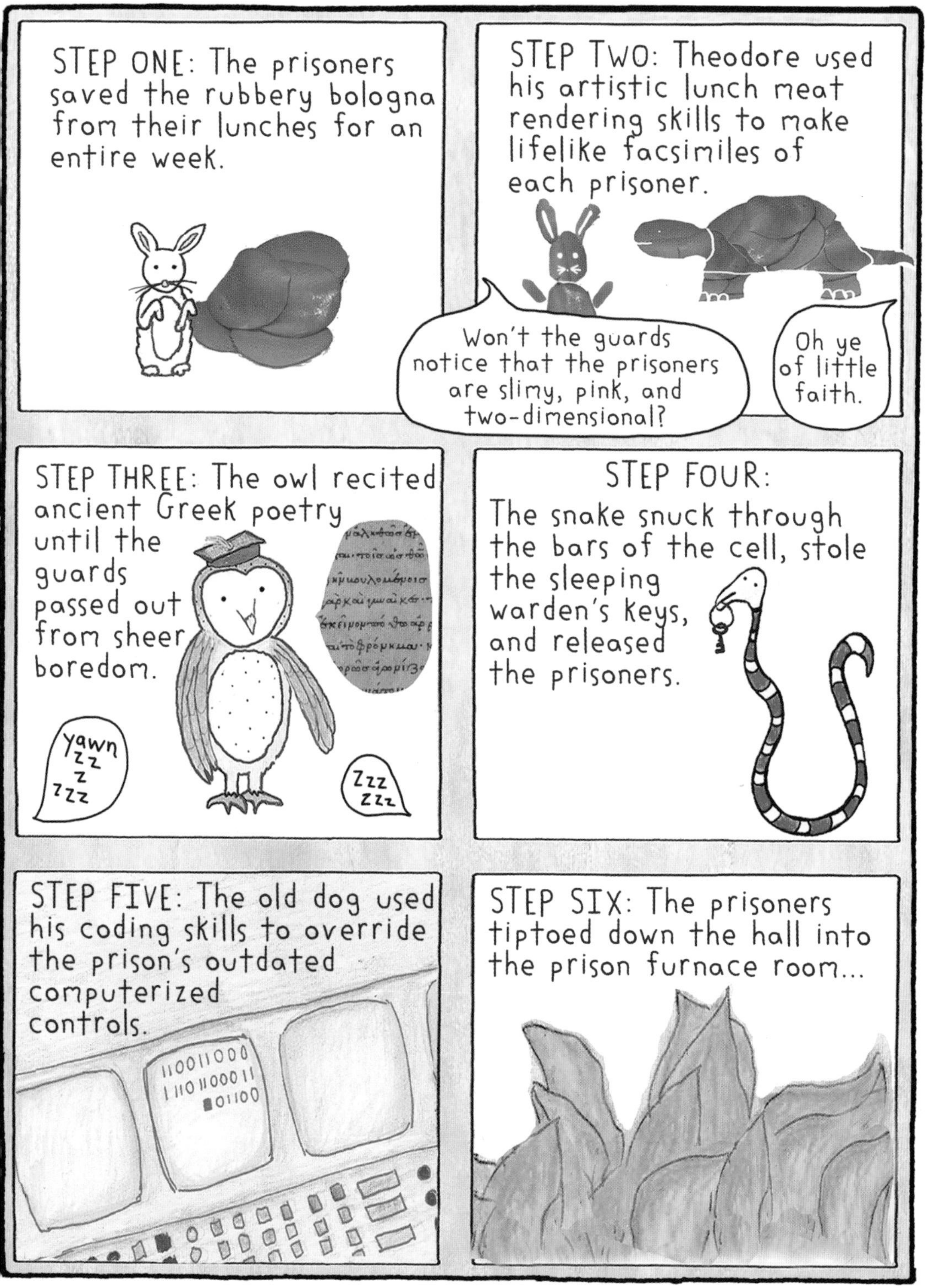
STEP ONE: The prisoners saved the rubbery bologna from their lunches for an entire week.
STEP TWO: Theodore used his artistic lunch meat rendering skills to make lifelike facsimiles of each prisoner.
Won't the guards notice that the prisoners are slimy, pink, and two-dimensional?
Oh ye of little faith.
STEP THREE: The owl recited ancient Greek poetry until the guards passed out from sheer boredom.
yawn zz z zzz
Zzz zzz
STEP FOUR: The snake snuck through the bars of the cell, stole the sleeping warden's keys, and released the prisoners.
STEP FIVE: The old dog used his coding skills to override the prison's outdated computerized controls.
STEP SIX: The prisoners tiptoed down the hall into the prison furnace room...

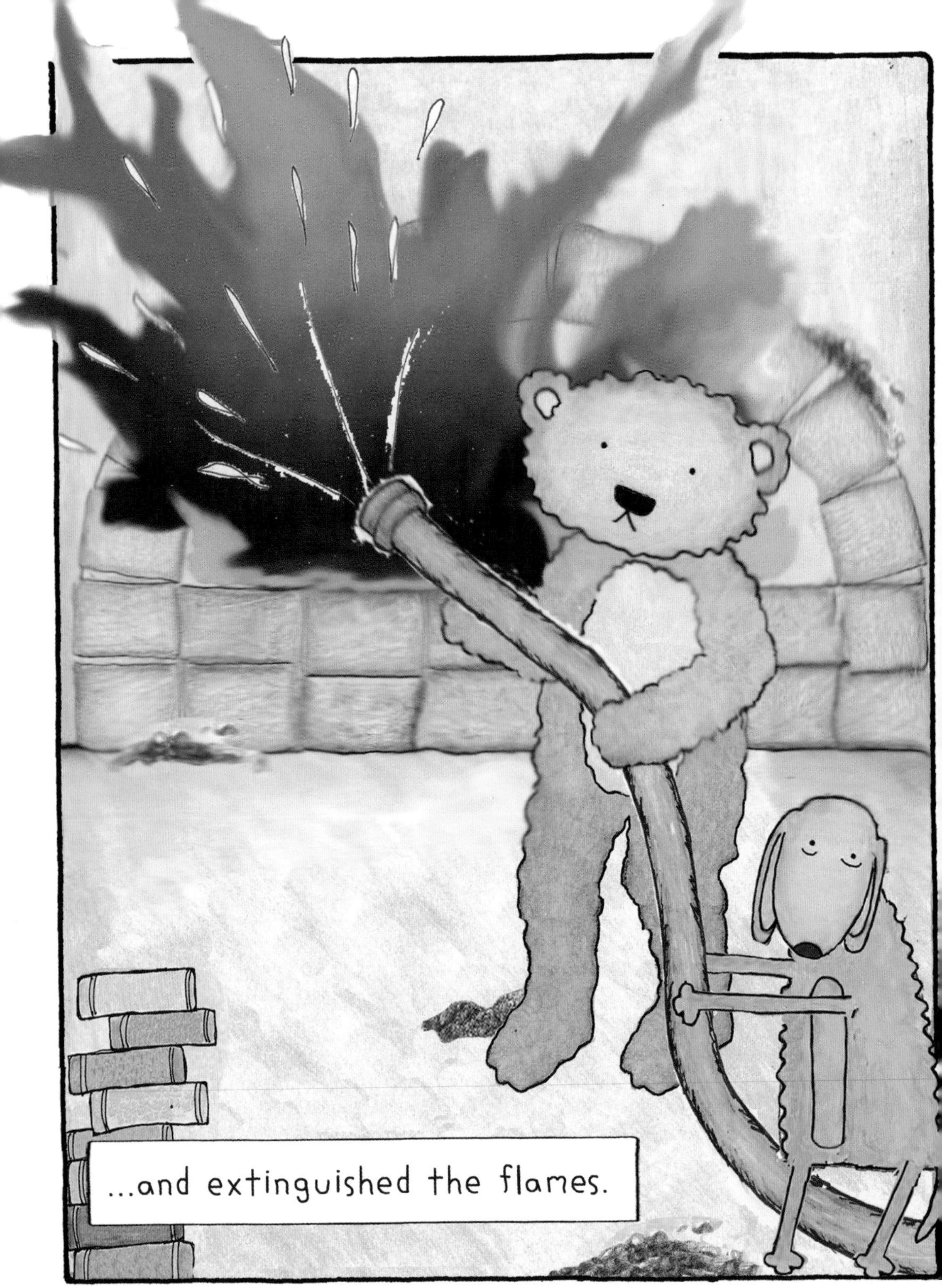
...and extinguished the flames.

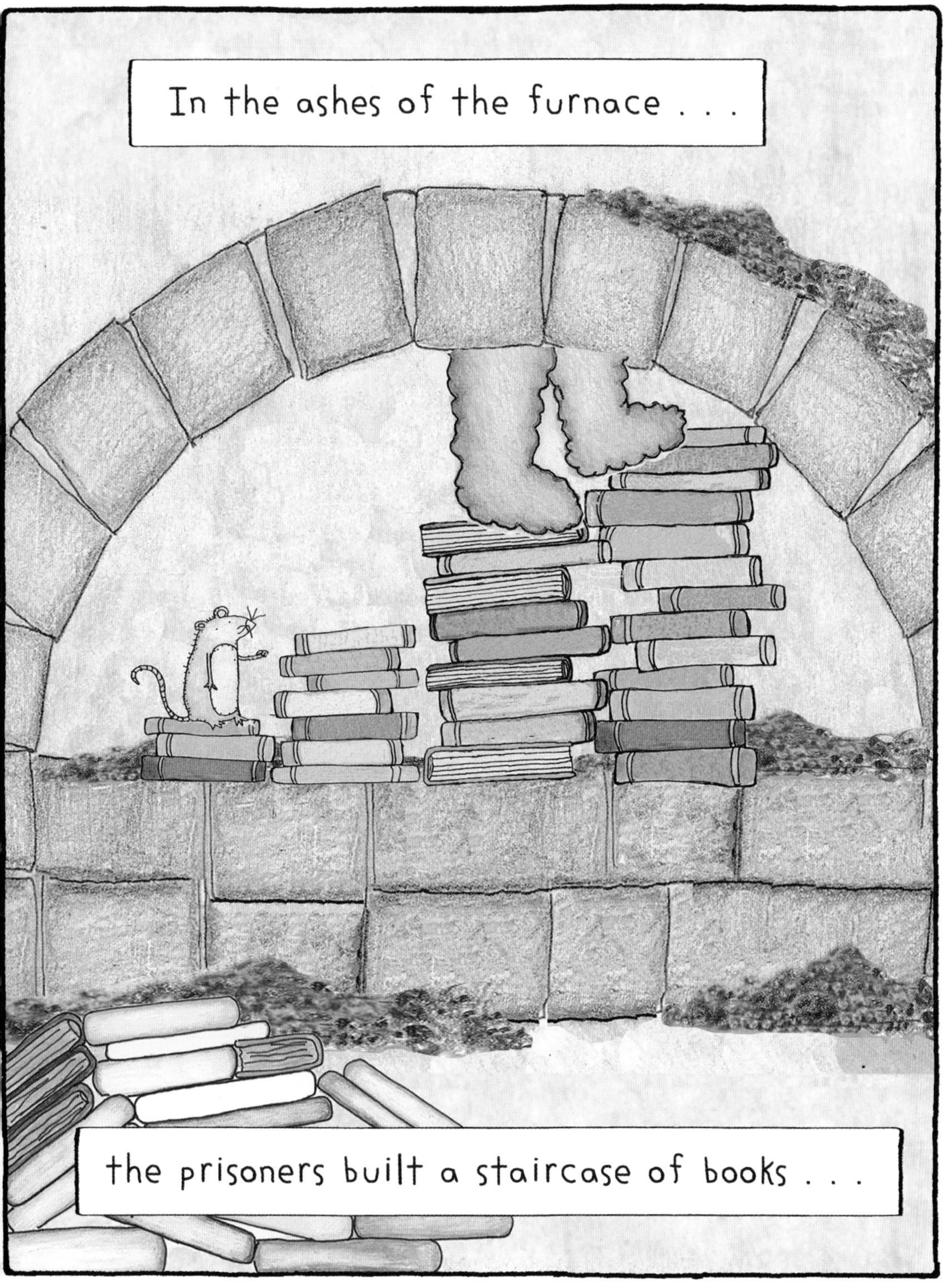
In the ashes of the furnace . . .
the prisoners built a staircase of books . . .

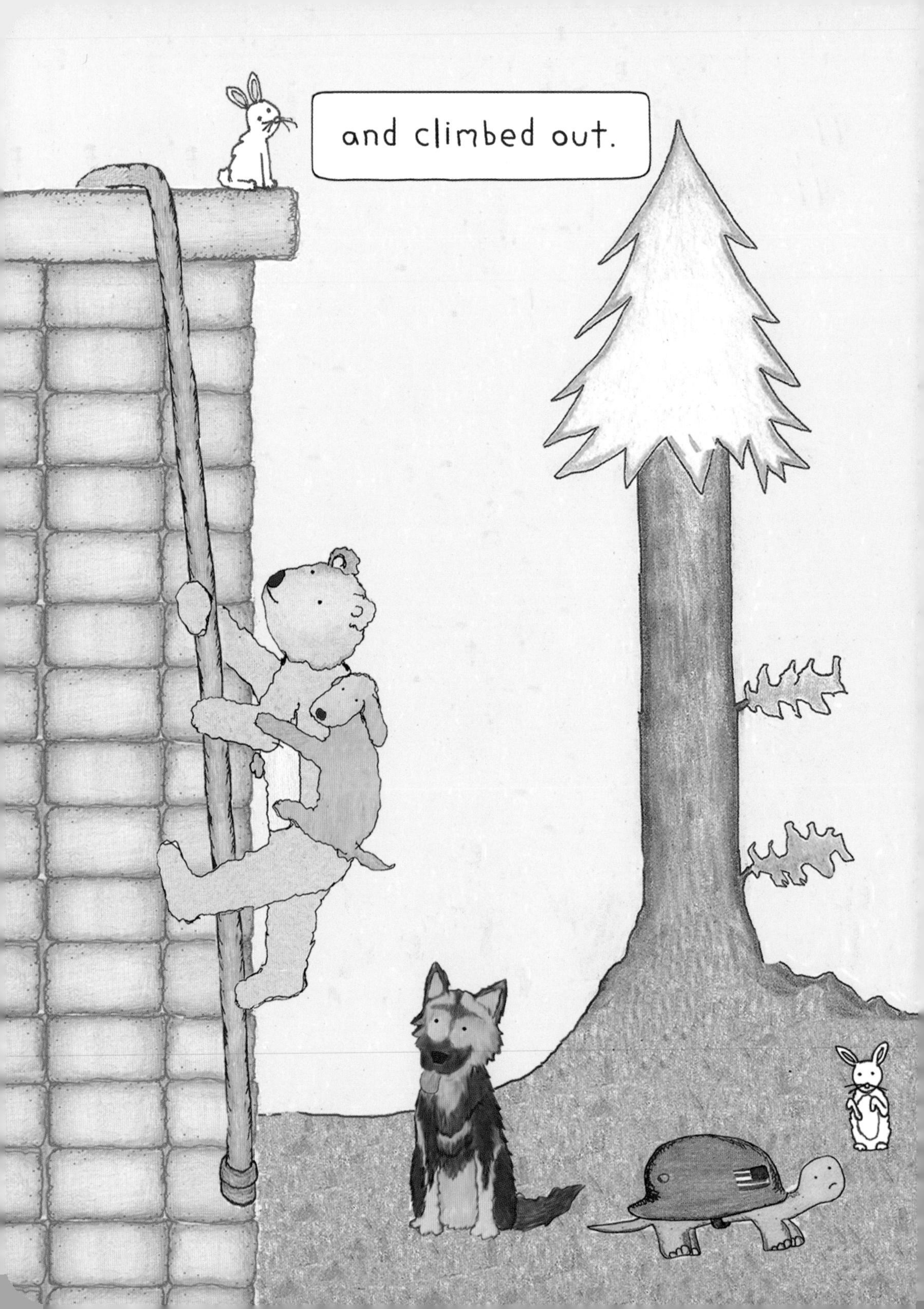
and climbed out.

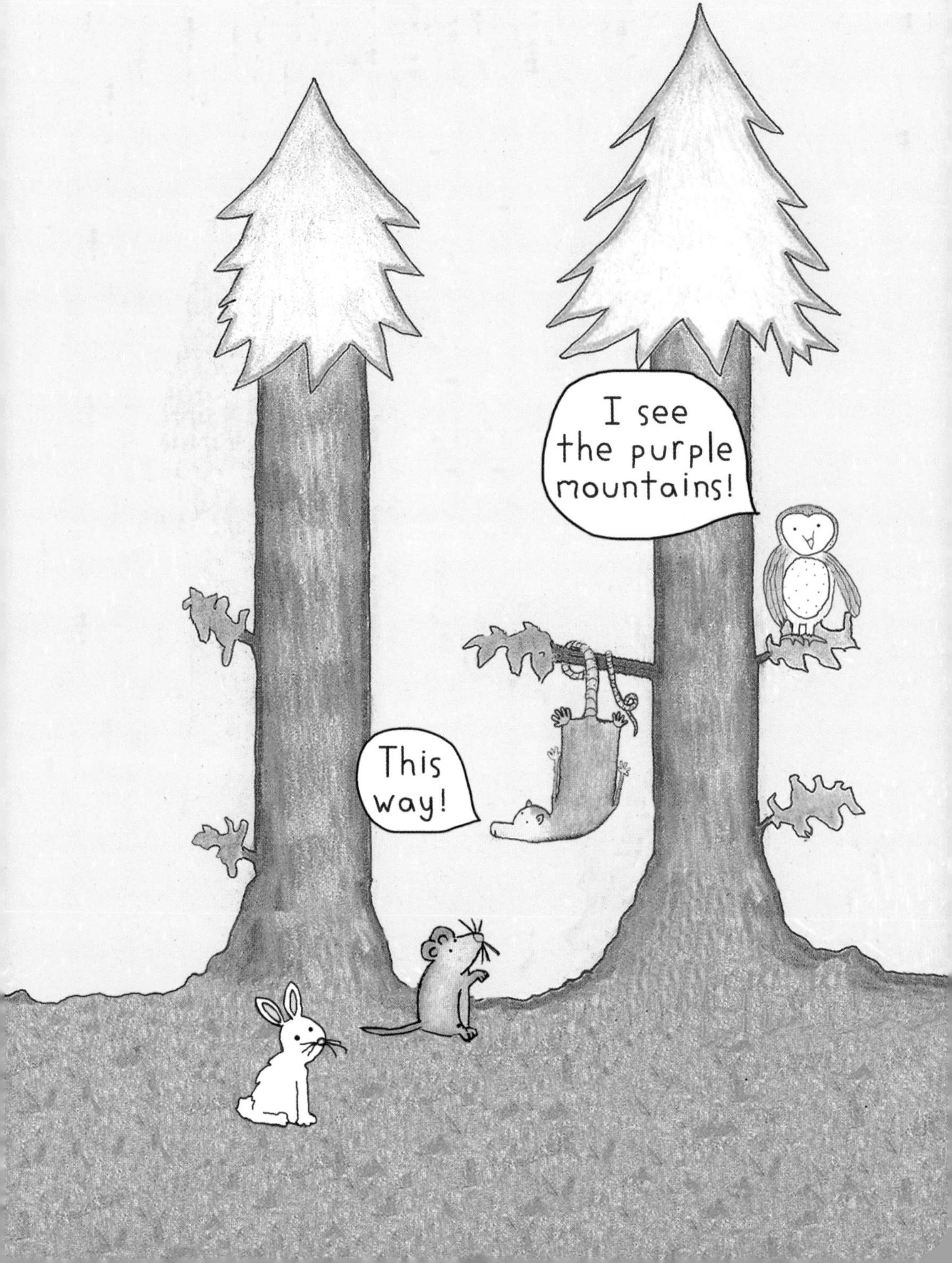
I see the purple mountains!
This way!

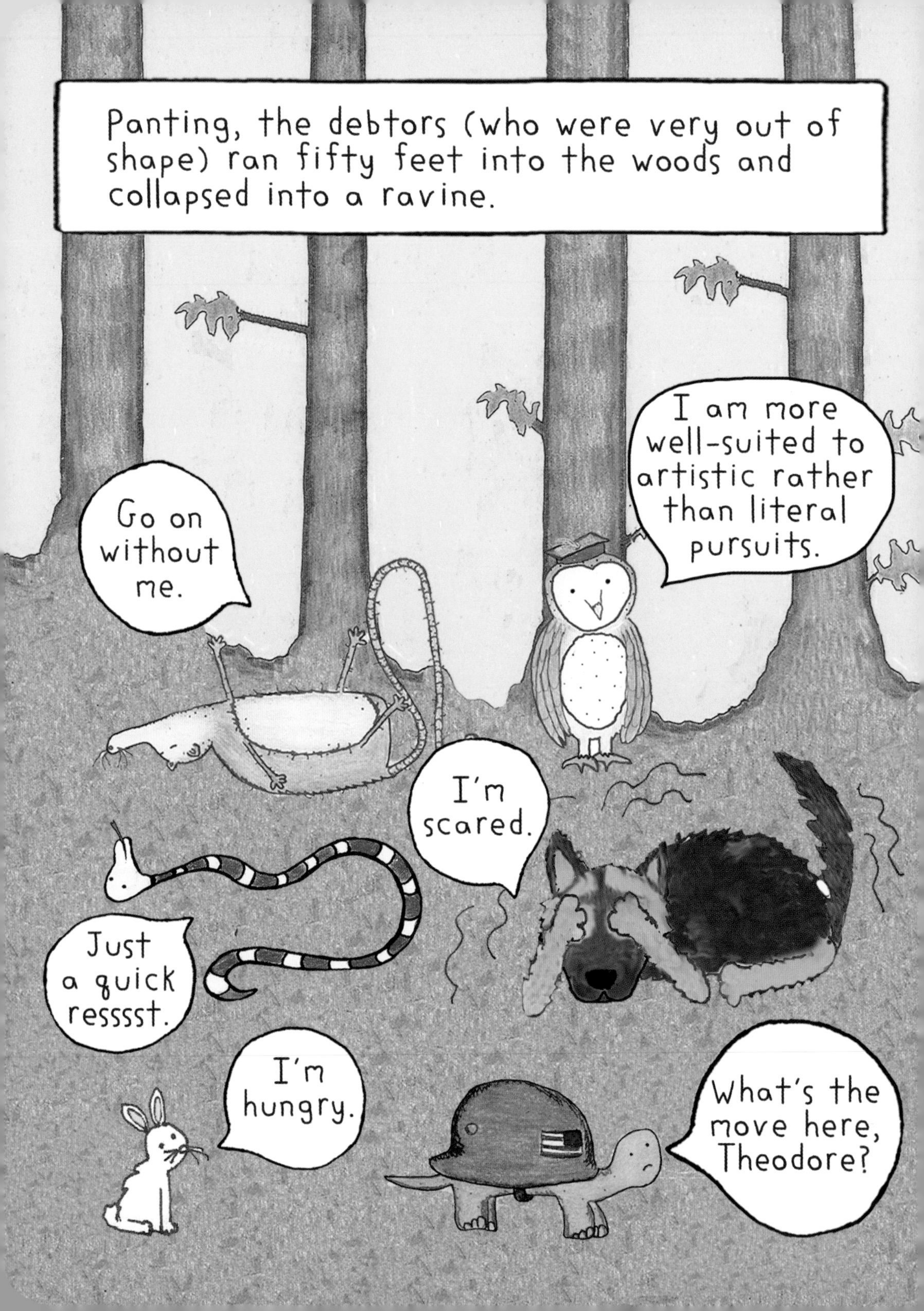
Panting, the debtors (who were very out of shape) ran fifty feet into the woods and collapsed into a ravine.
I am more well-suited to artistic rather than literal pursuits.
Go on without me.
I'm scared.
Just a quick resssst.
I'm hungry.
What's the move here, Theodore?

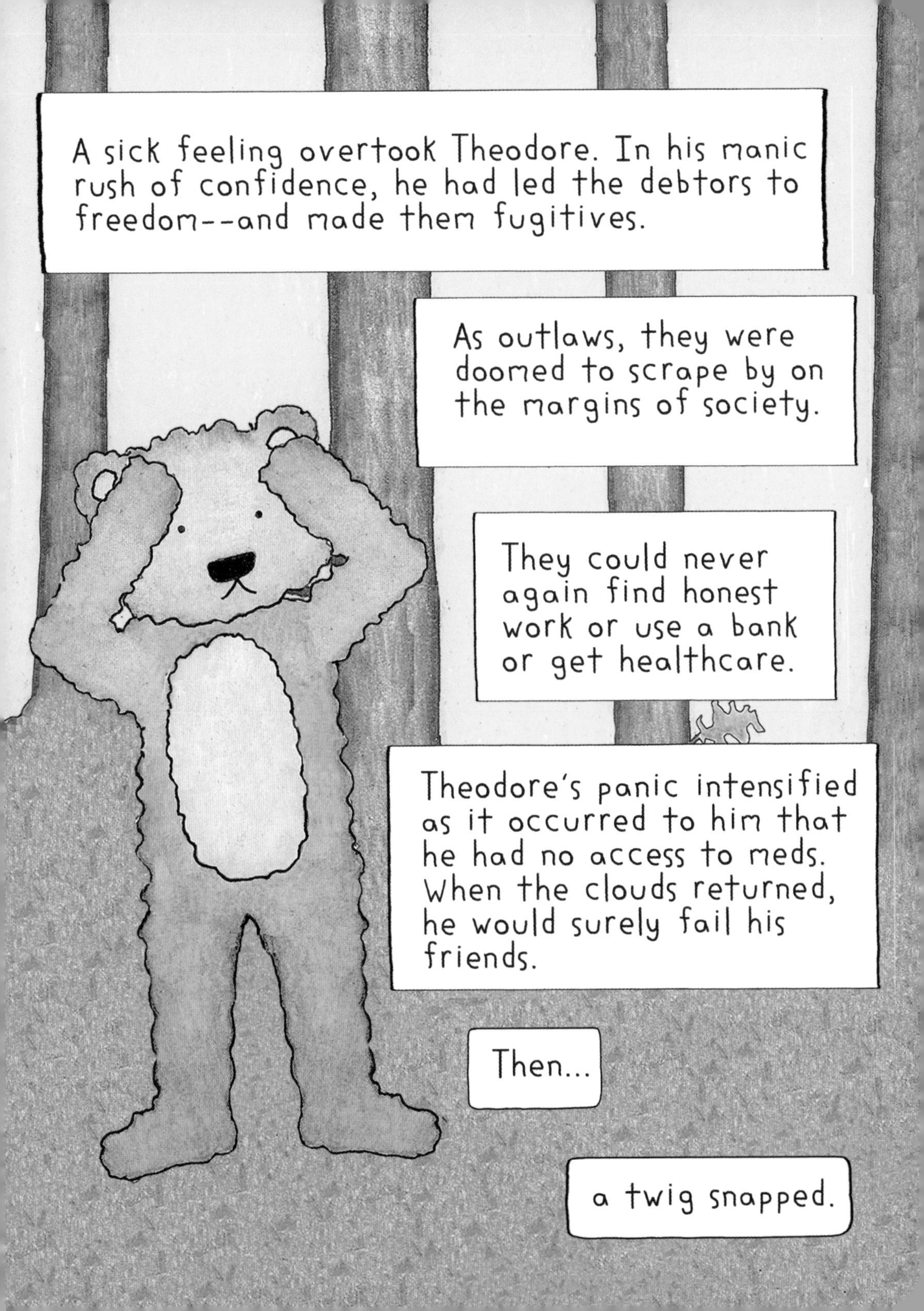
A sick feeling overtook Theodore. In his manic rush of confidence, he had led the debtors to freedom--and made them fugitives.
As outlaws, they were doomed to scrape by on the margins of society.
They could never again find honest work or use a bank or get healthcare.
Theodore's panic intensified as it occurred to him that he had no access to meds. When the clouds returned, he would surely fail his friends.
Then...
a twig snapped.

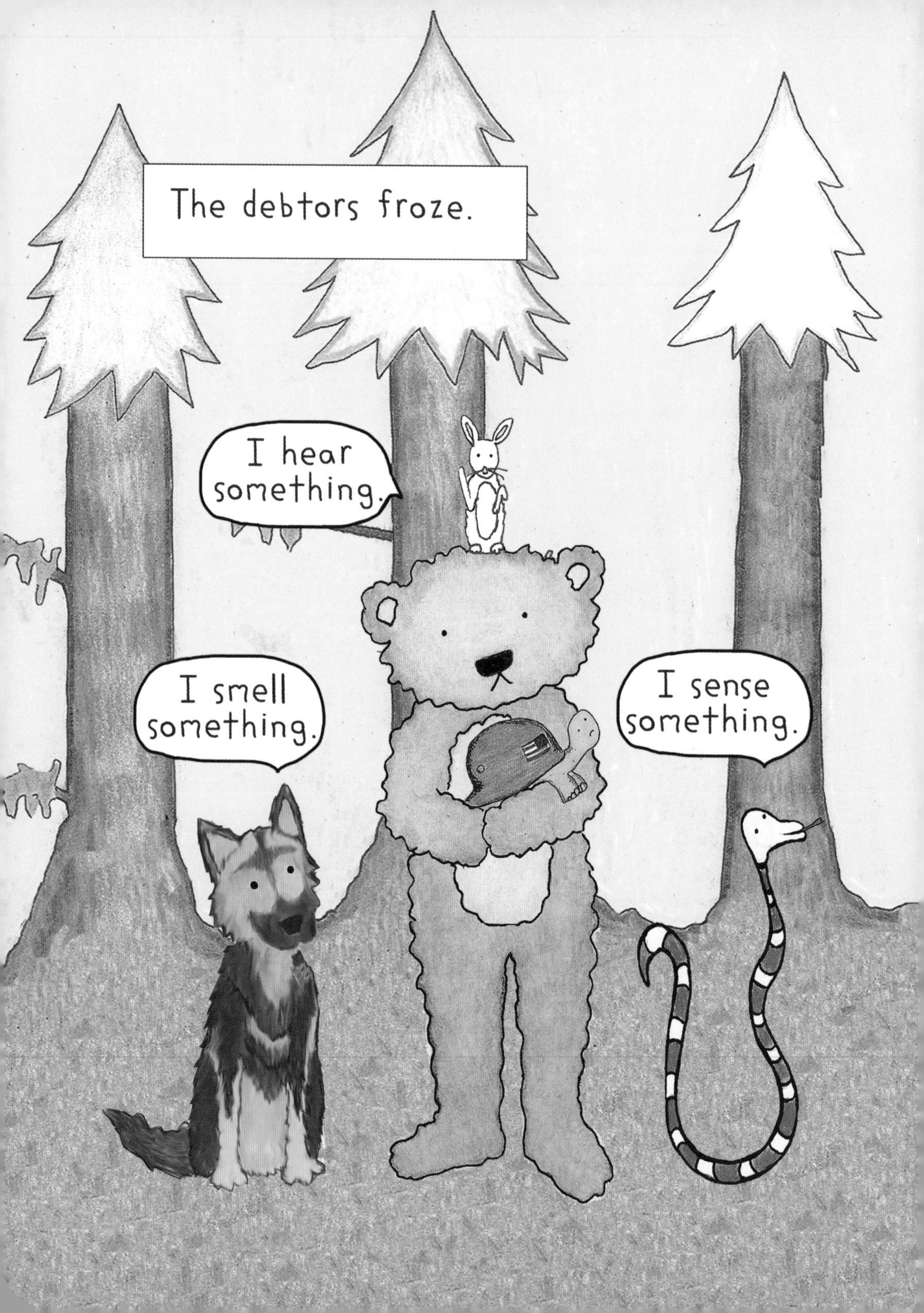
The debtors froze.
I hear something.
I smell something.
I sense something.

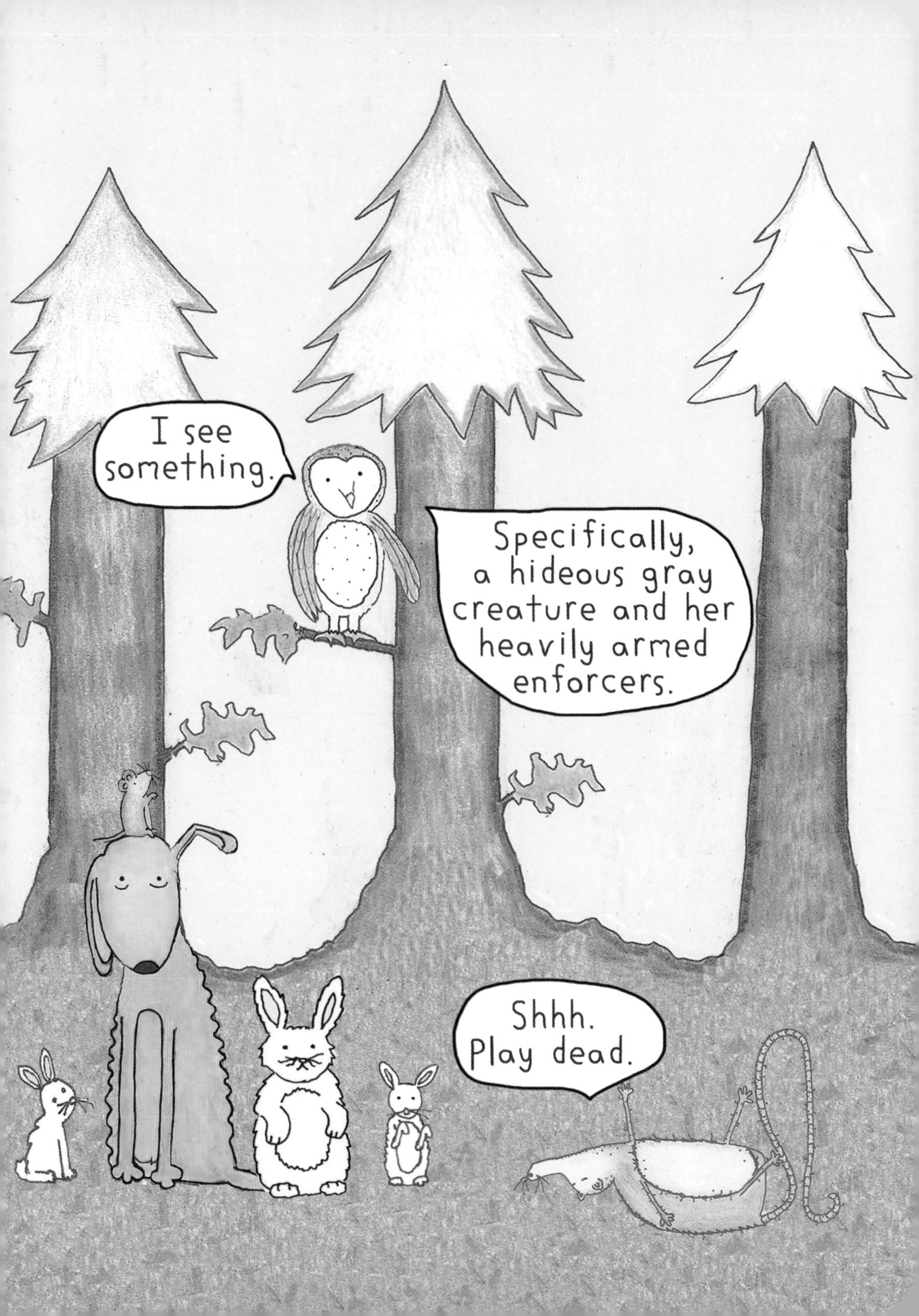
I see something.
Specifically, a hideous gray creature and her heavily armed enforcers.
Shhh. Play dead.

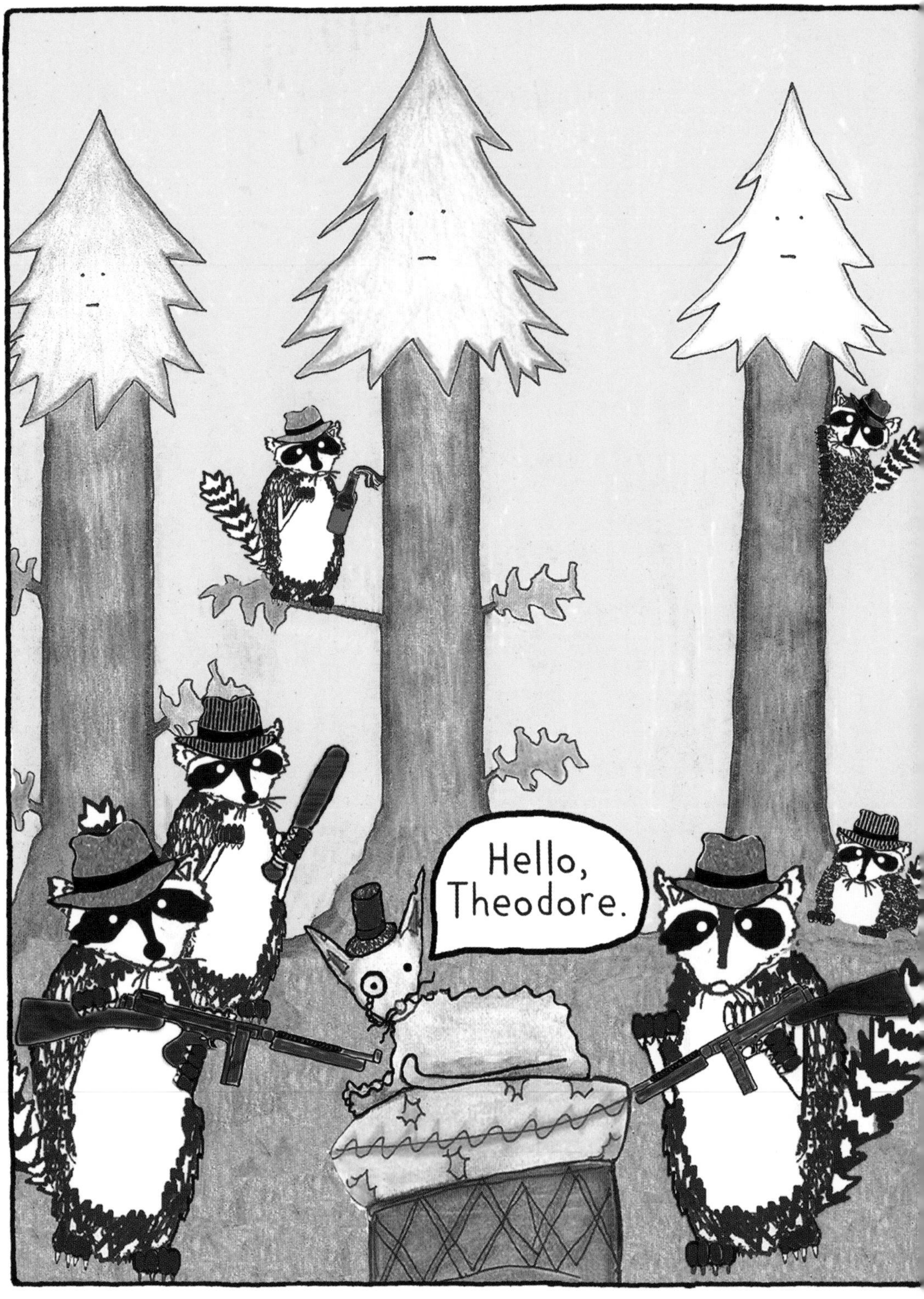
Hello, Theodore.

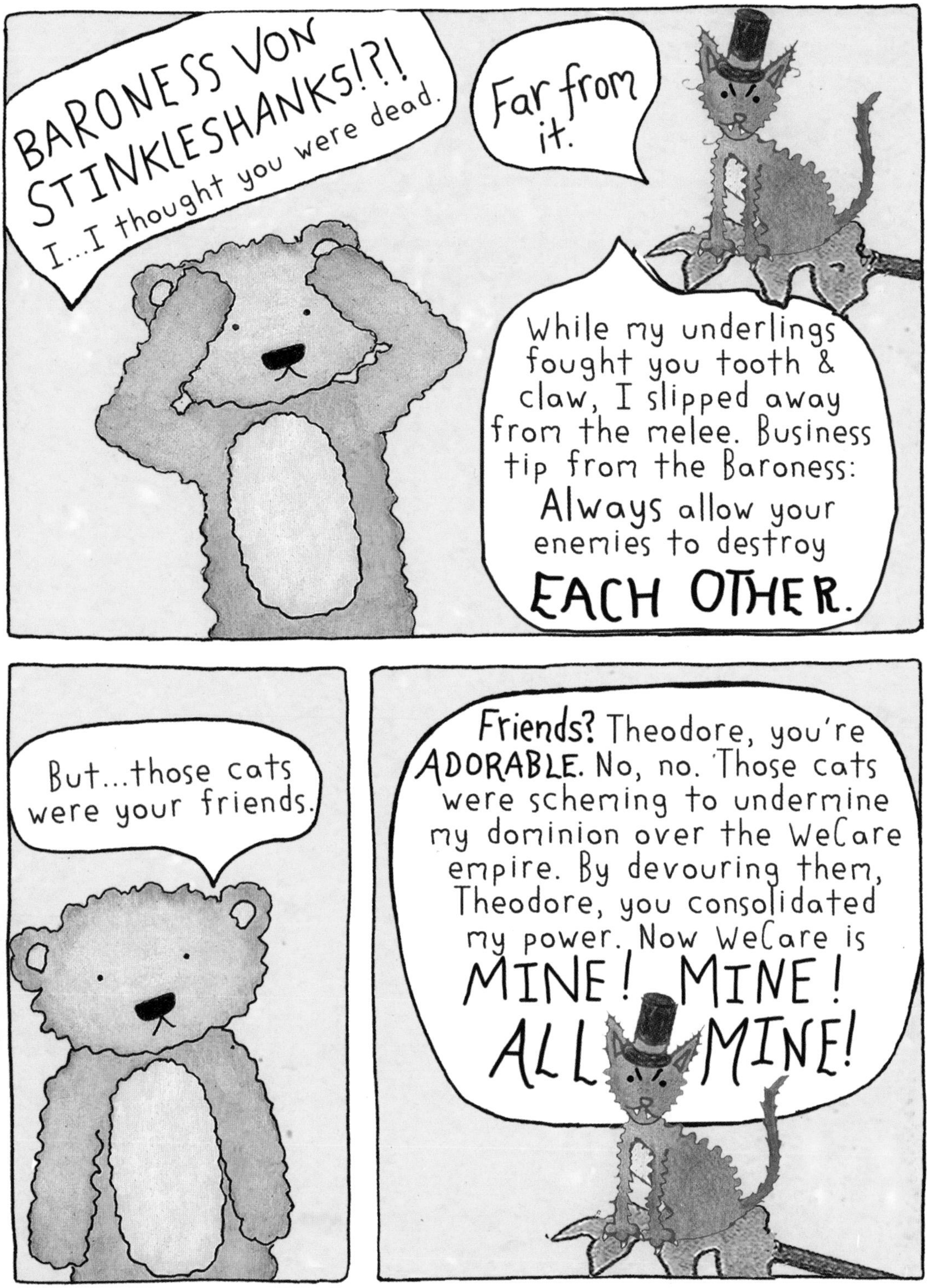

BARONESS VON STINKLESHANKS!?!! I...I thought you were dead.
Far from it.
While my underlings fought you tooth & claw, I slipped away from the melee. Business tip from the Baroness: Always allow your enemies to destroy EACH OTHER.
But...those cats were your friends.
Friends? Theodore, you're ADORABLE. No, no. Those cats were scheming to undermine my dominion over the WeCare empire. By devouring them, Theodore, you consolidated my power. Now WeCare is MINE! MINE! ALL MINE!

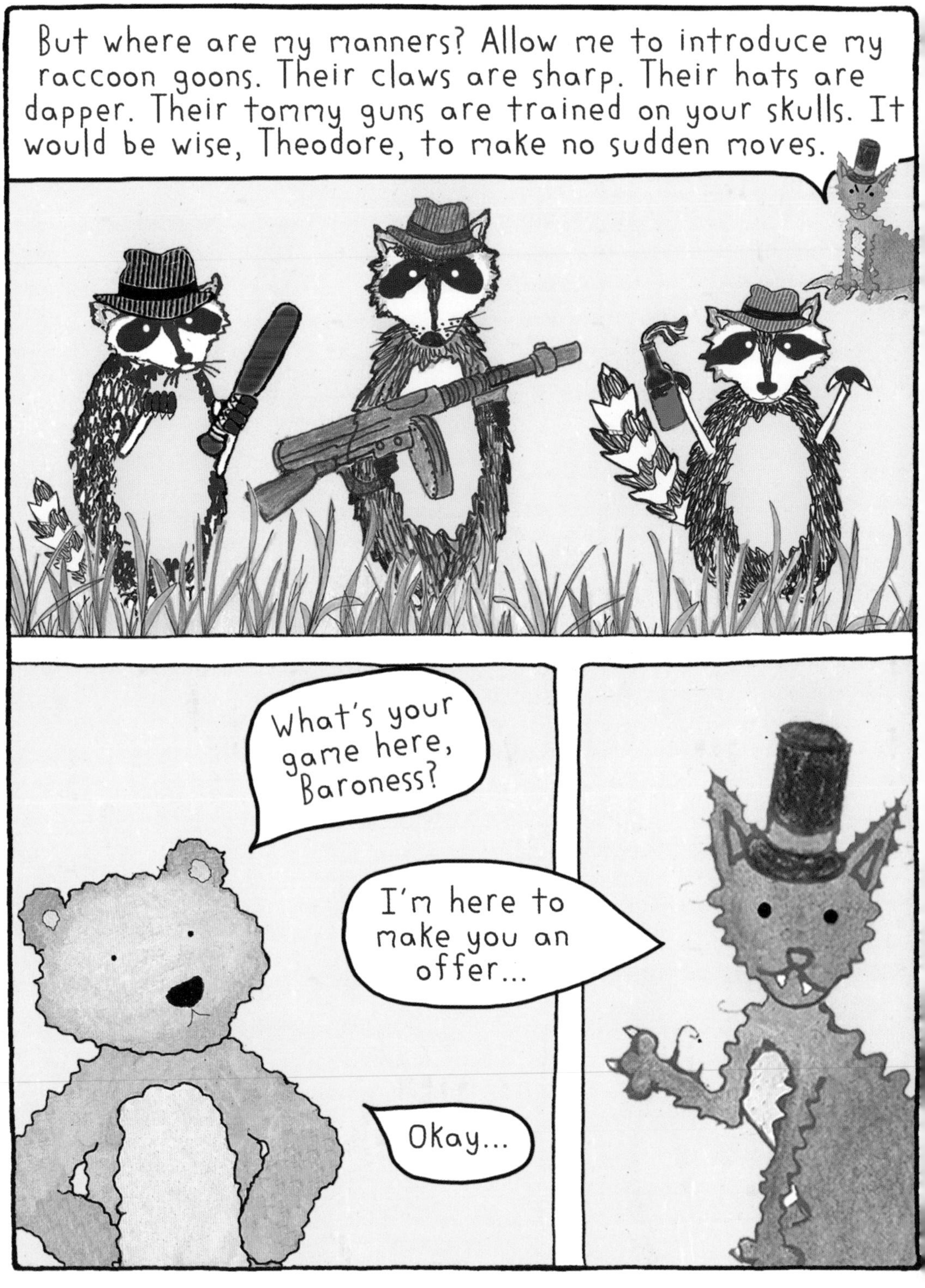
But where are my manners? Allow me to introduce my raccoon goons. Their claws are sharp. Their hats are dapper. Their tommy guns are trained on your skulls. It would be wise, Theodore, to make no sudden moves.
What's your game here, Baroness?
I'm here to make you an offer...
Okay...

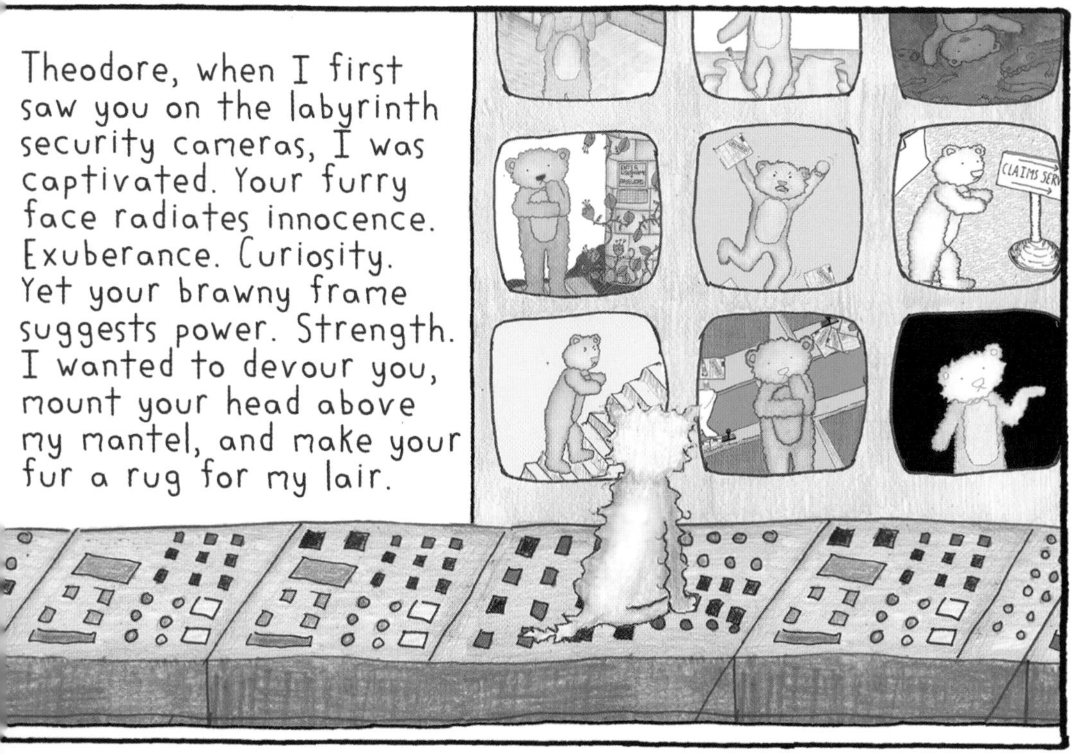
Theodore, when I first saw you on the labyrinth security cameras, I was captivated. Your furry face radiates innocence. Exuberance. Curiosity. Yet your brawny frame suggests power. Strength. I wanted to devour you, mount your head above my mantel, and make your fur a rug for my lair.
CLAIMS SERV

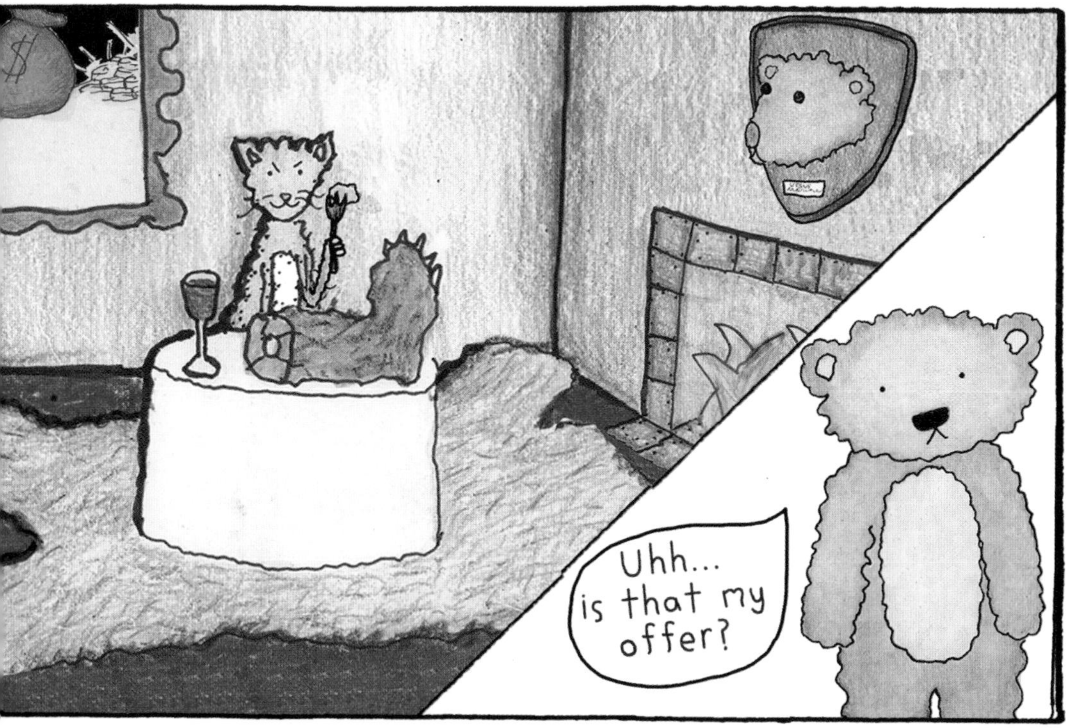
Uhh... is that my offer?

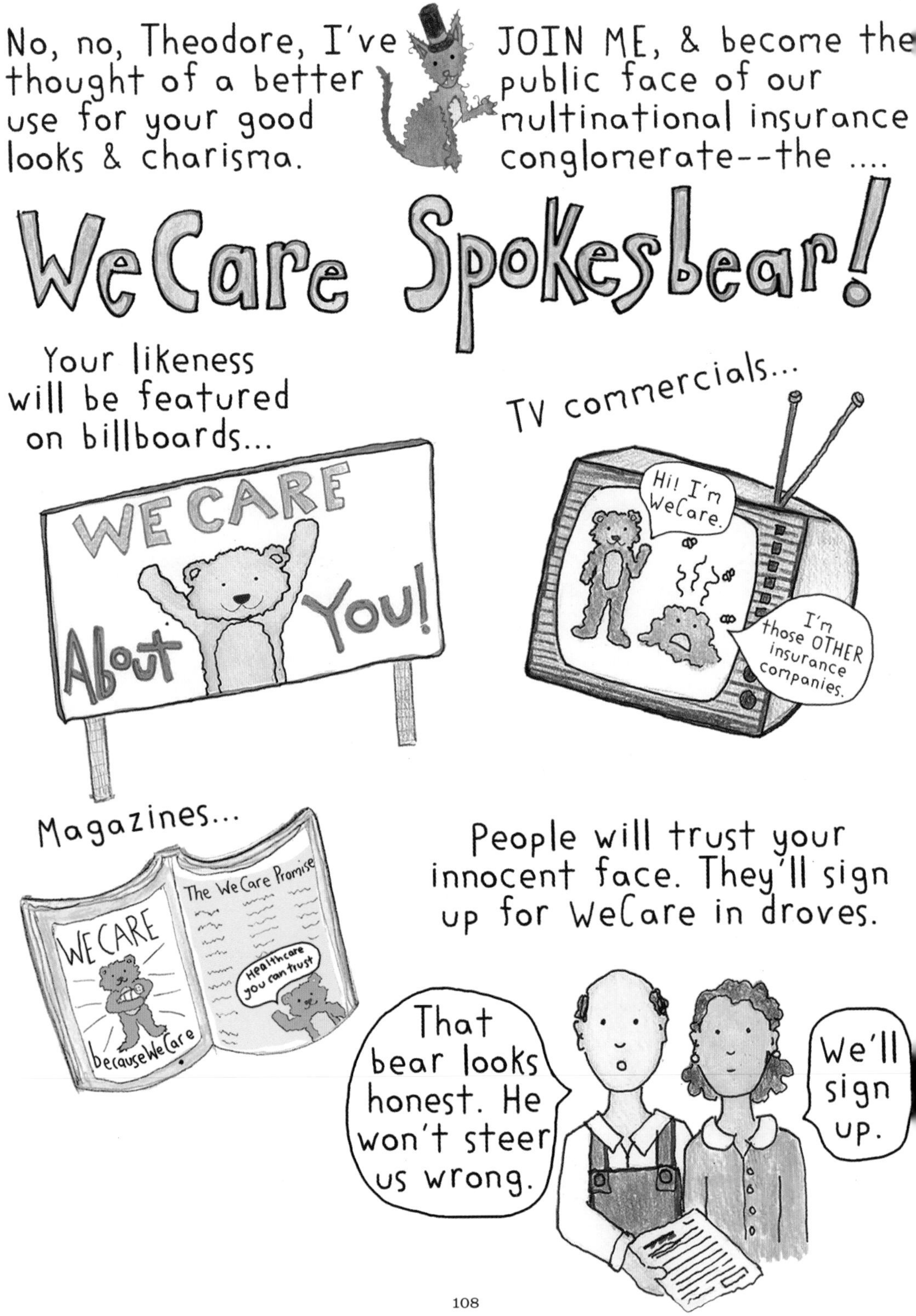
No, no, Theodore, I've thought of a better use for your good looks & charisma.
JOIN ME, & become the public face of our multinational insurance conglomerate--the ....
WeCare Spokesbear!
Your likeness will be featured on billboards...
WE CARE About YOU!
TV commercials...
Hi! I'm WeCare.
I'm those OTHER insurance companies.
Magazines...
WE CARE
because WeCare
The WeCare Promise
Healthcare you can trust
People will trust your innocent face. They'll sign up for WeCare in droves.
That bear looks honest. He won't steer us wrong.
We'll sign up.

You will, of course, be compensated. You'll have a swanky corporate apartment. Sumptuous meals. Bags of cash.

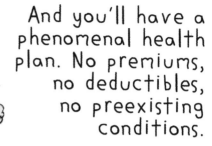

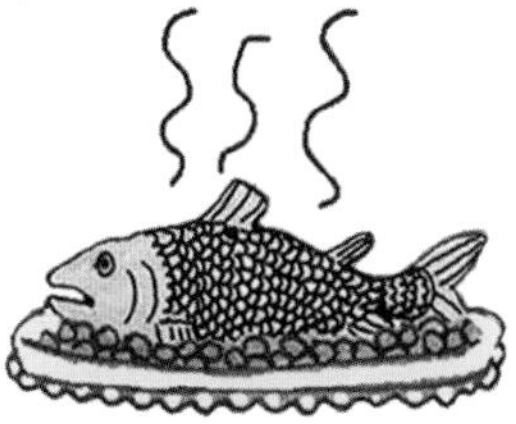

And you'll have a phenomenal health plan. No premiums, no deductibles, no preexisting conditions.

WeCare
Theodore
ID
ZMFKD002
8400742
GROUP#324
PLANcode:
MKKJ14
Diamond plan

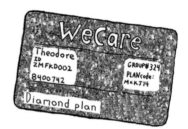

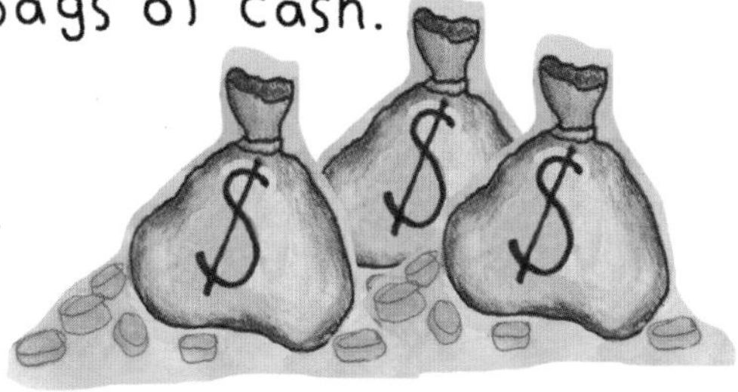

And best of all, you'll be swimming in brand-name medication--

Uppers.

Downers.

Tranqs.

Stims.

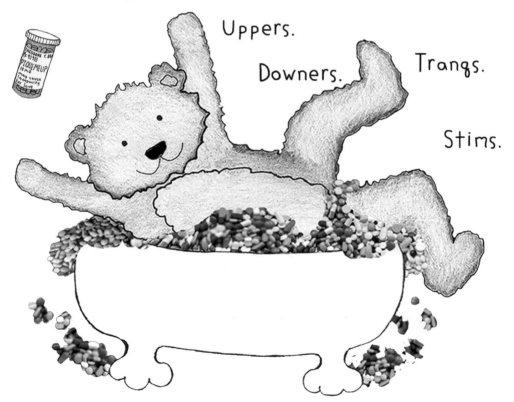

Imagine, Theodore.

You'll finally be a productive member of society.

Well-adjusted.

SANE.

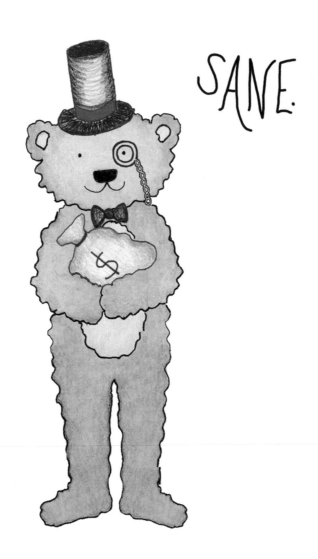

Refuse...

And I will make you into

a RUG.

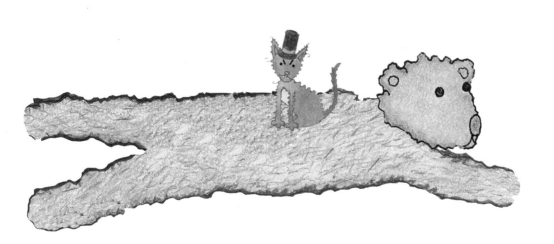

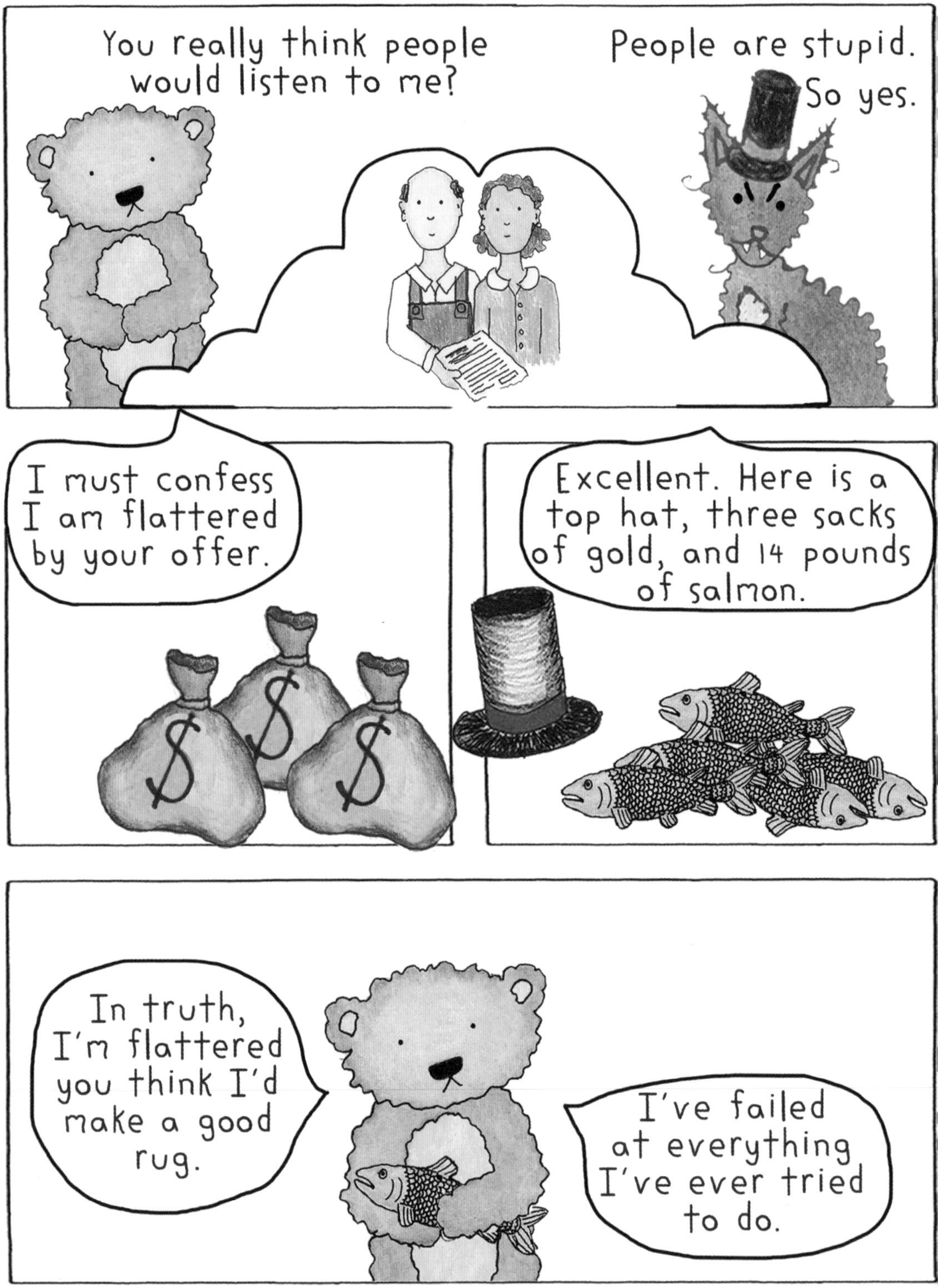
You really think people would listen to me?
People are stupid.
So yes.
I must confess I am flattered by your offer.
Excellent. Here is a top hat, three sacks of gold, and 14 pounds of salmon.
In truth, I'm flattered you think I'd make a good rug.
I've failed at everything I've ever tried to do.

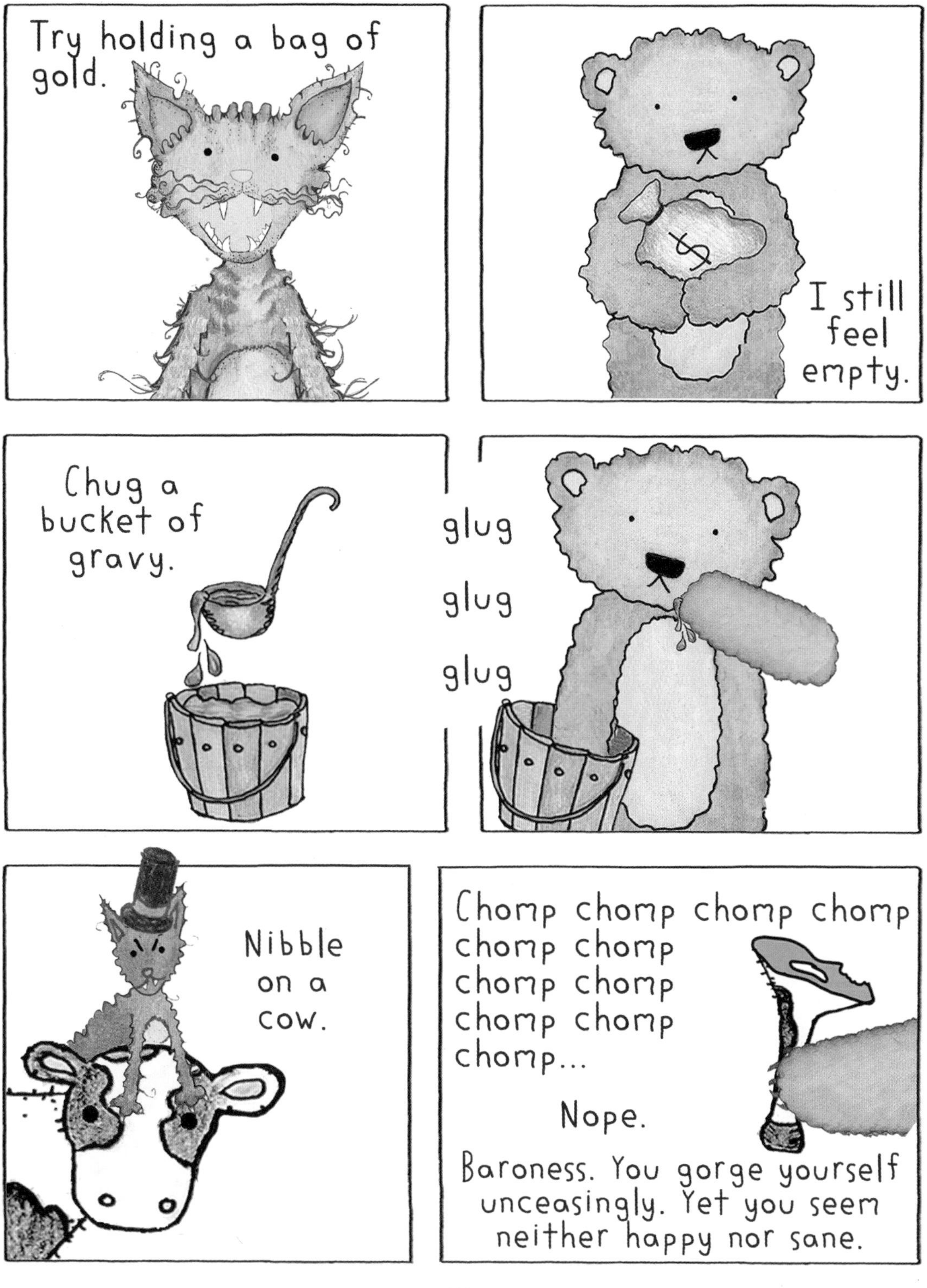

Try holding a bag of gold.
I still feel empty.
Chug a bucket of gravy.
glug
glug
glug
Nibble on a cow.
Chomp chomp chomp chomp chomp chomp chomp chomp chomp chomp chomp...
Nope.
Baroness. You gorge yourself unceasingly. Yet you seem neither happy nor sane.

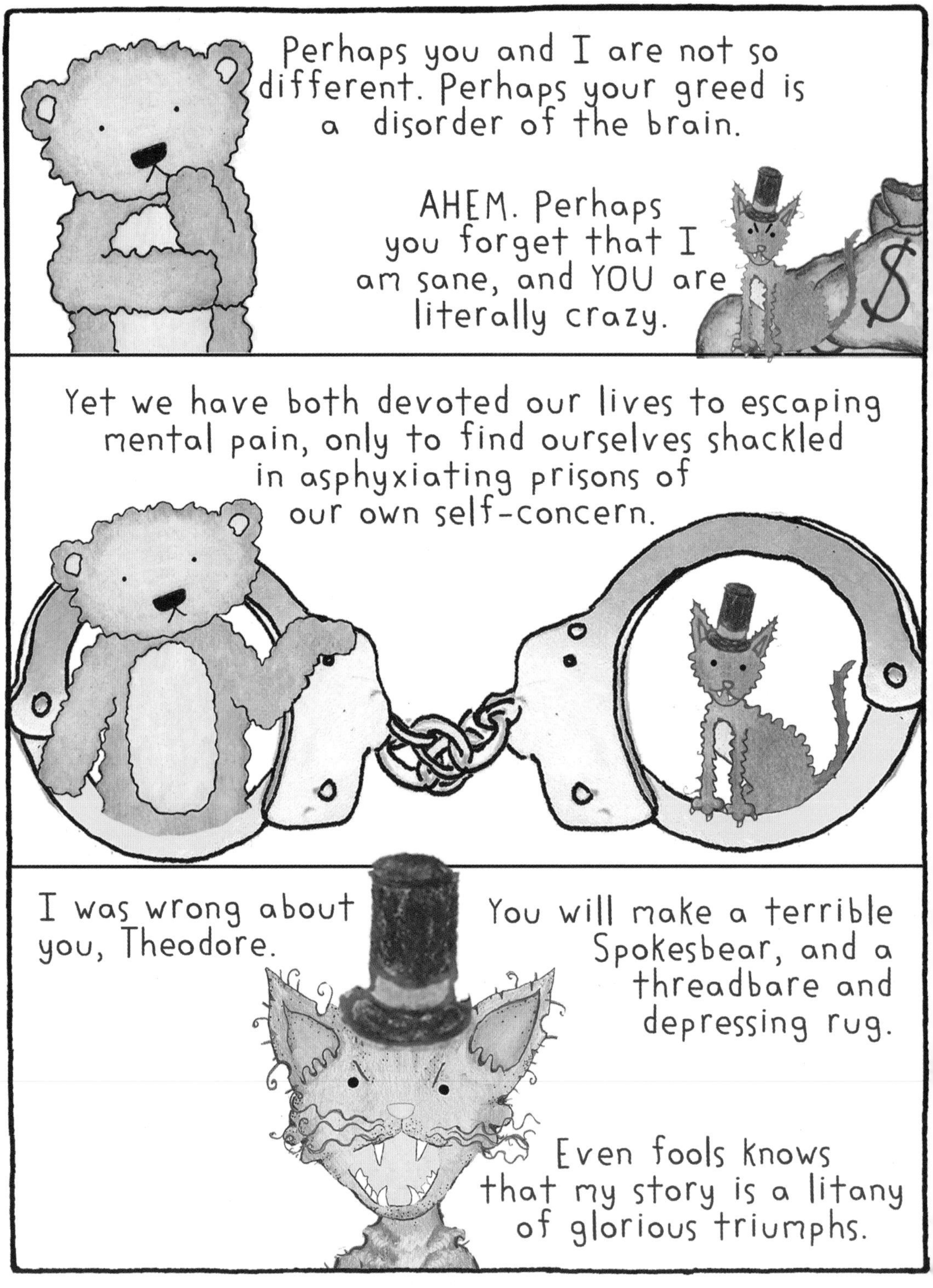

Perhaps you and I are not so different. Perhaps your greed is a disorder of the brain.

AHEM. Perhaps you forget that I am sane, and YOU are literally crazy.

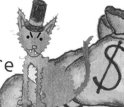

Yet we have both devoted our lives to escaping mental pain, only to find ourselves shackled in asphyxiating prisons of our own self-concern.

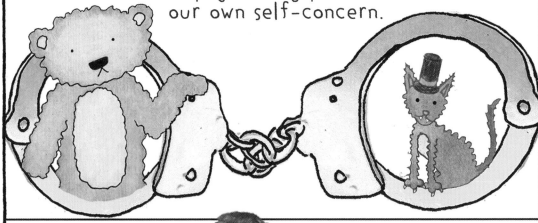

I was wrong about you, Theodore.

You will make a terrible Spokesbear, and a threadbare and depressing rug.

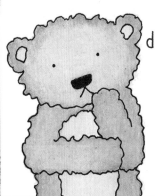

Even fools knows that my story is a litany of glorious triumphs.

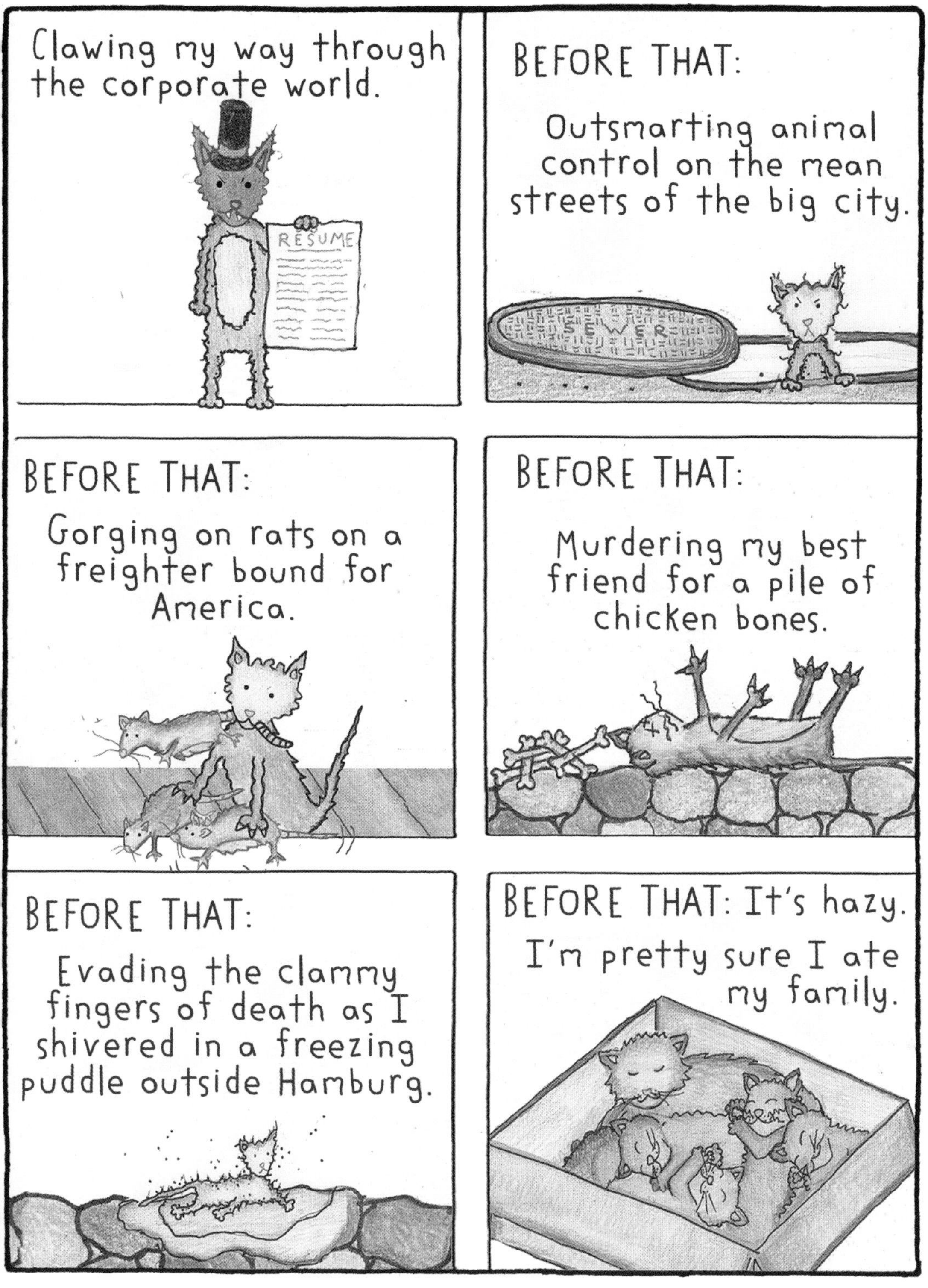

Clawing my way through the corporate world.

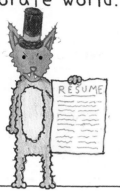

BEFORE THAT:

Outsmarting animal control on the mean streets of the big city.

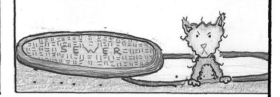

BEFORE THAT:

Gorging on rats on a freighter bound for America.

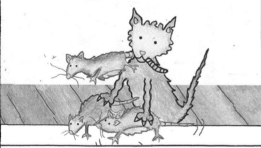

BEFORE THAT:

Murdering my best friend for a pile of chicken bones.

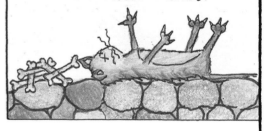

BEFORE THAT:

Evading the clammy fingers of death as I shivered in a freezing puddle outside Hamburg.

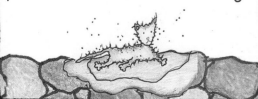

BEFORE THAT: It's hazy. I'm pretty sure I ate my family.

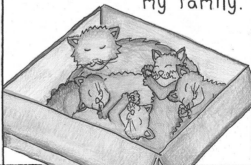

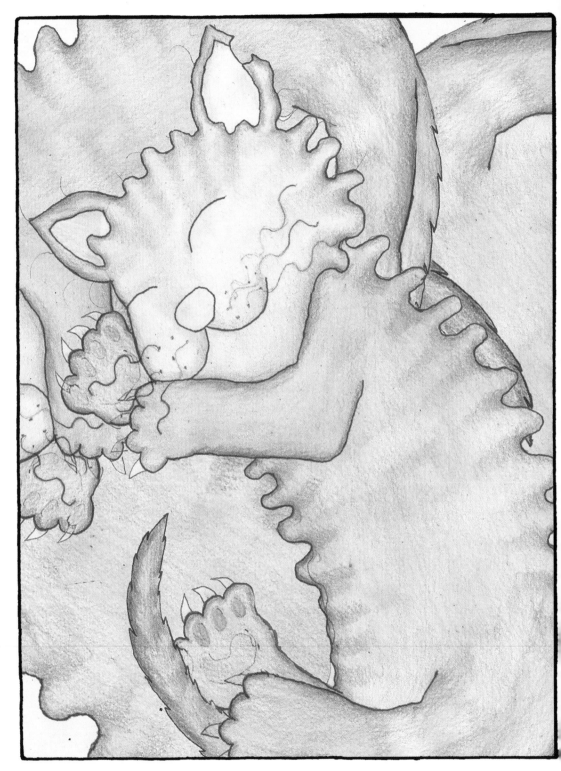

The memory was unbearable.
The Baroness snapped out of her trance
and leapt onto Theodore's head.

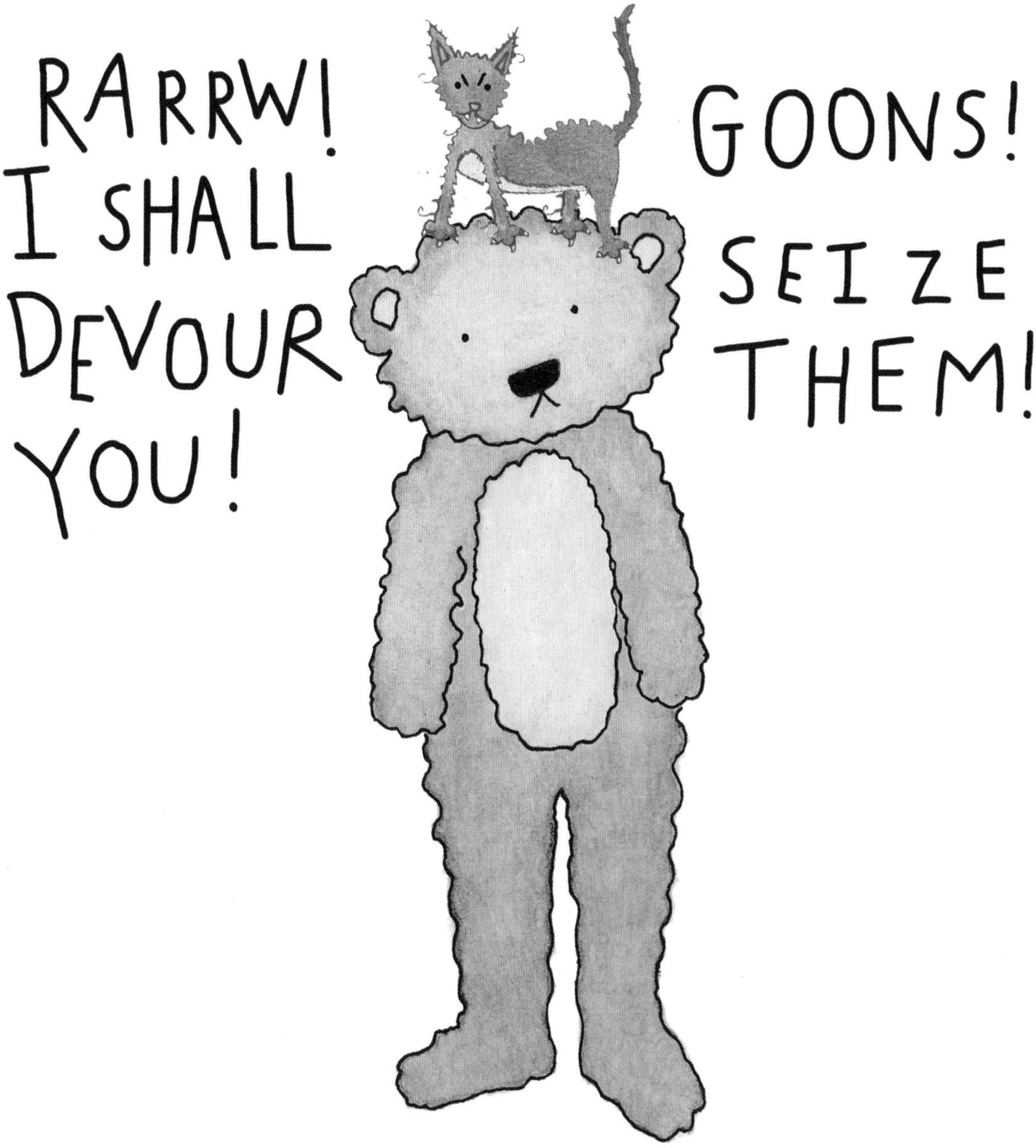
RARRW! I SHALL DEVOUR YOU!
GOONS! SEIZE THEM!

But the raccoon goons had grown bored. And they could not resist the allure of the nearby dumpster, which was teeming with baloney scraps.

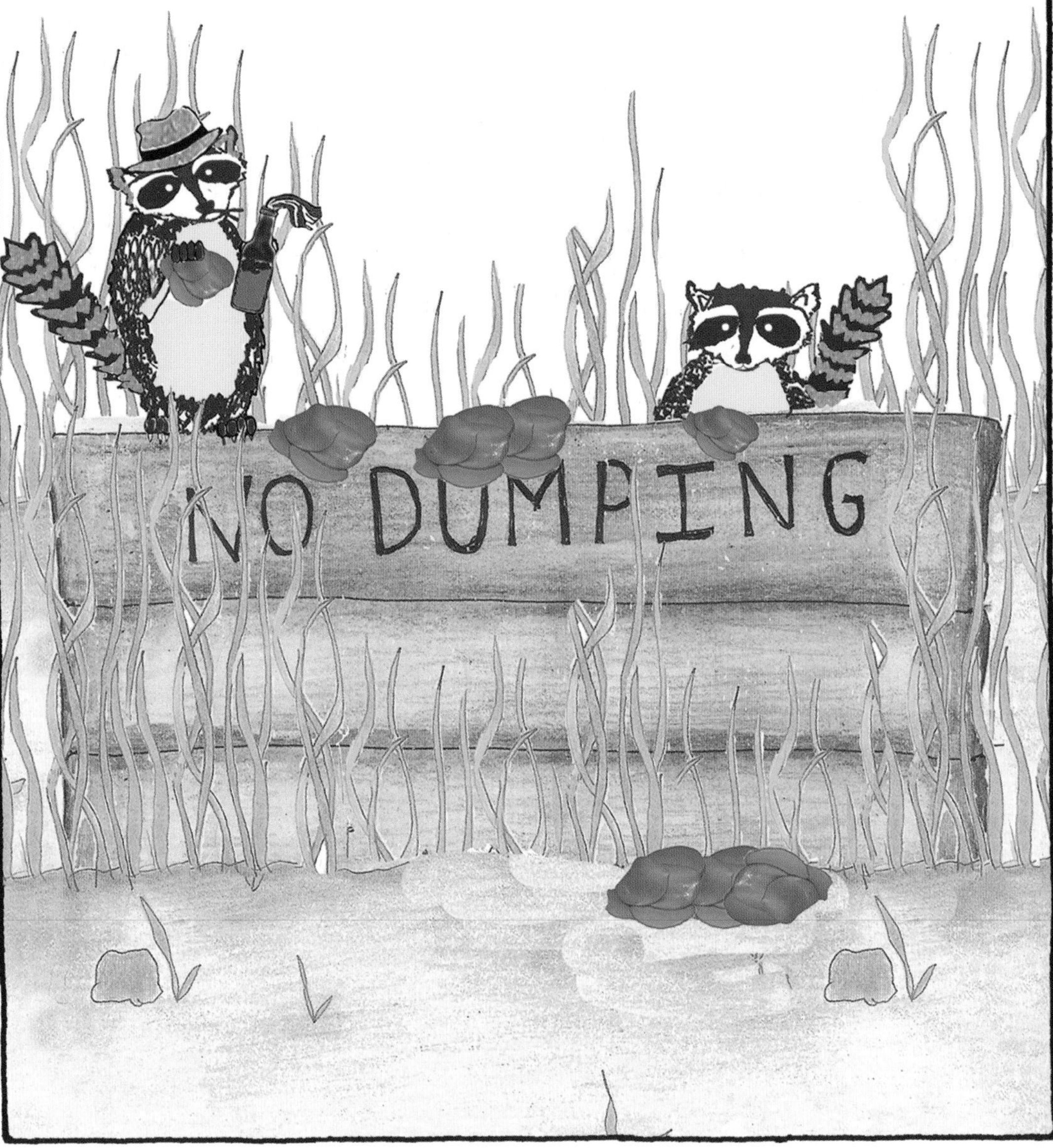
NO DUMPING

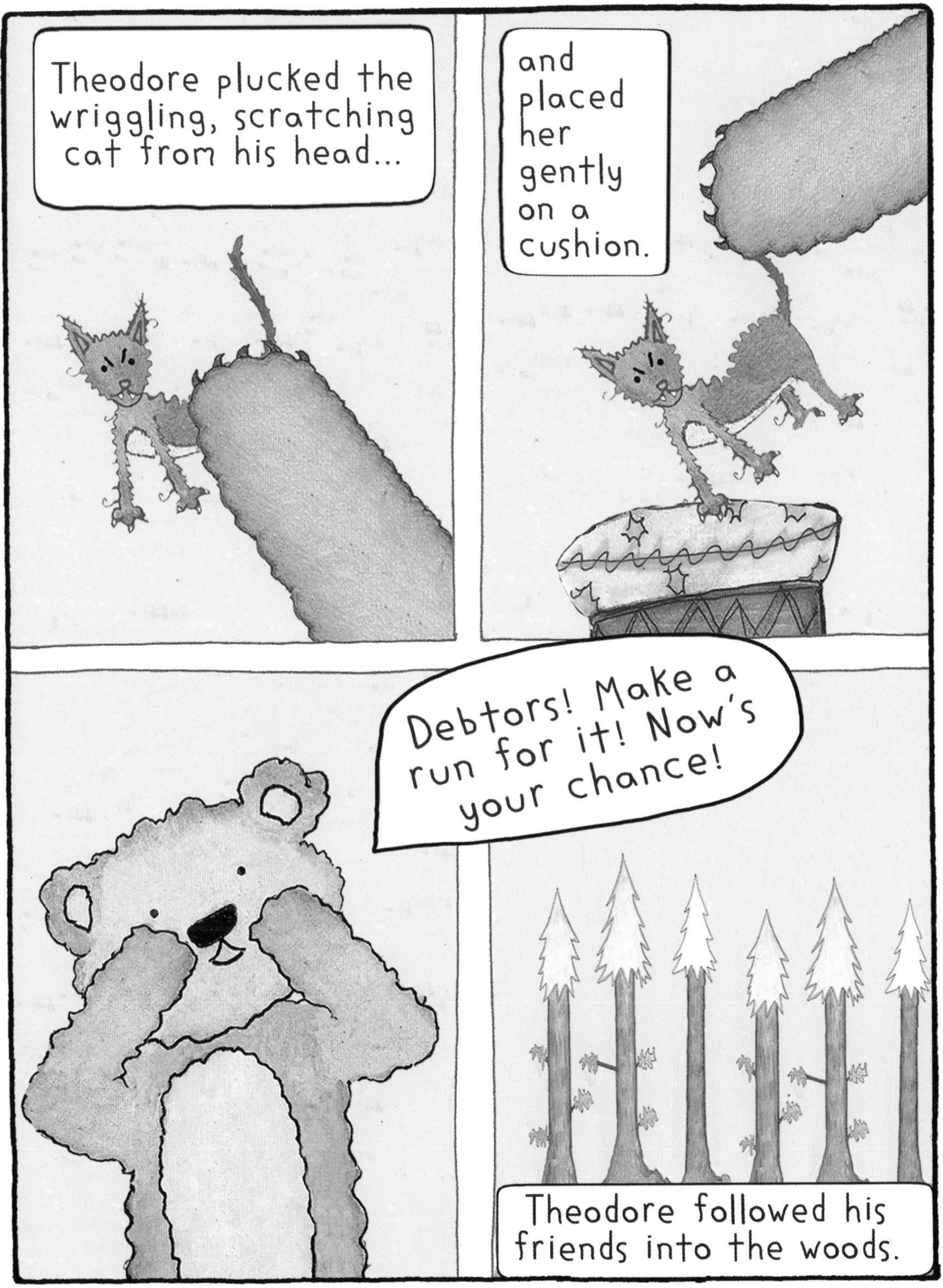
Theodore plucked the wriggling, scratching cat from his head...
and placed her gently on a cushion.
Debtors! Make a run for it! Now's your chance!
Theodore followed his friends into the woods.

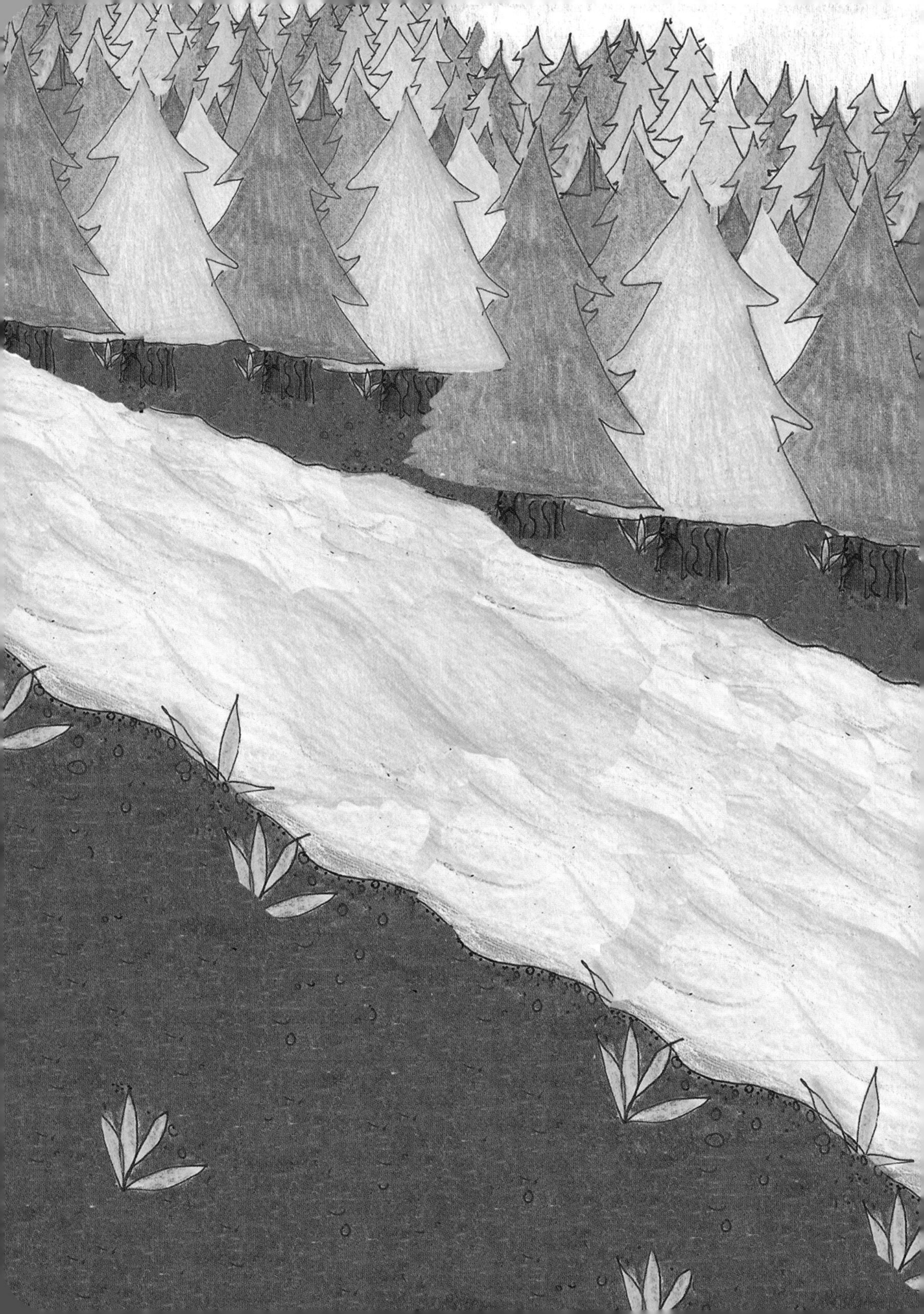

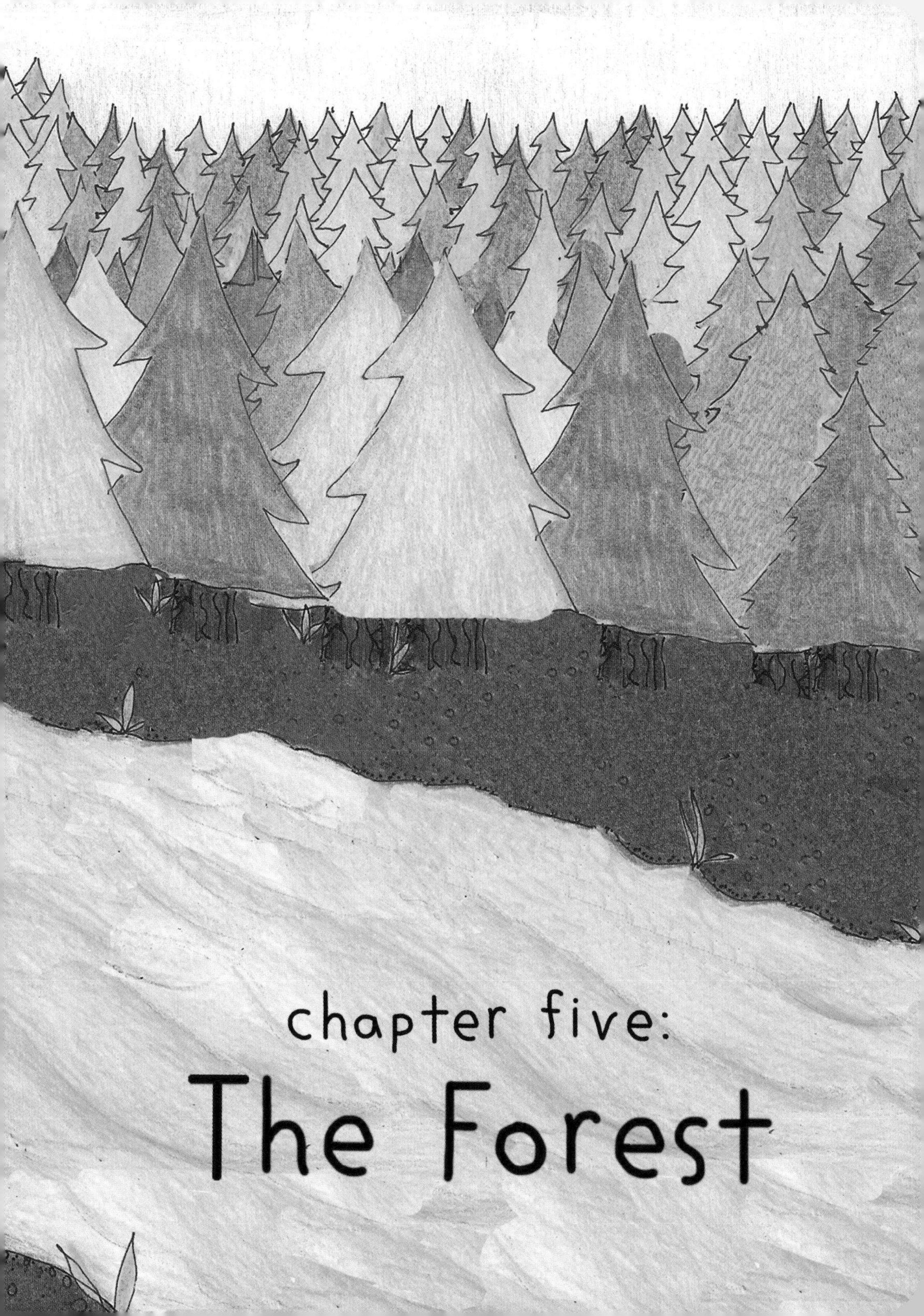

chapter five:

The Forest

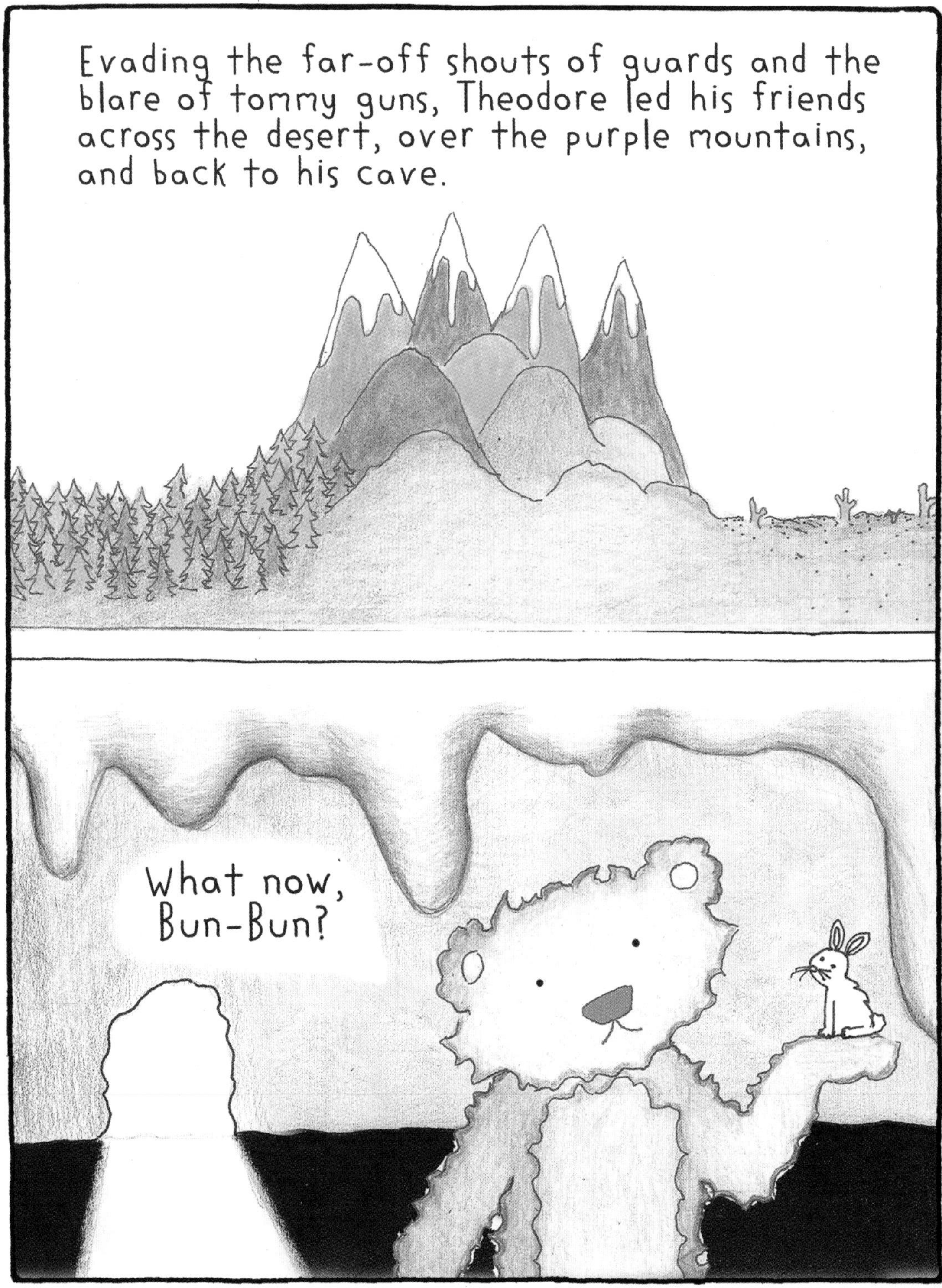
Evading the far-off shouts of guards and the blare of tommy guns, Theodore led his friends across the desert, over the purple mountains, and back to his cave.
What now, Bun-Bun?

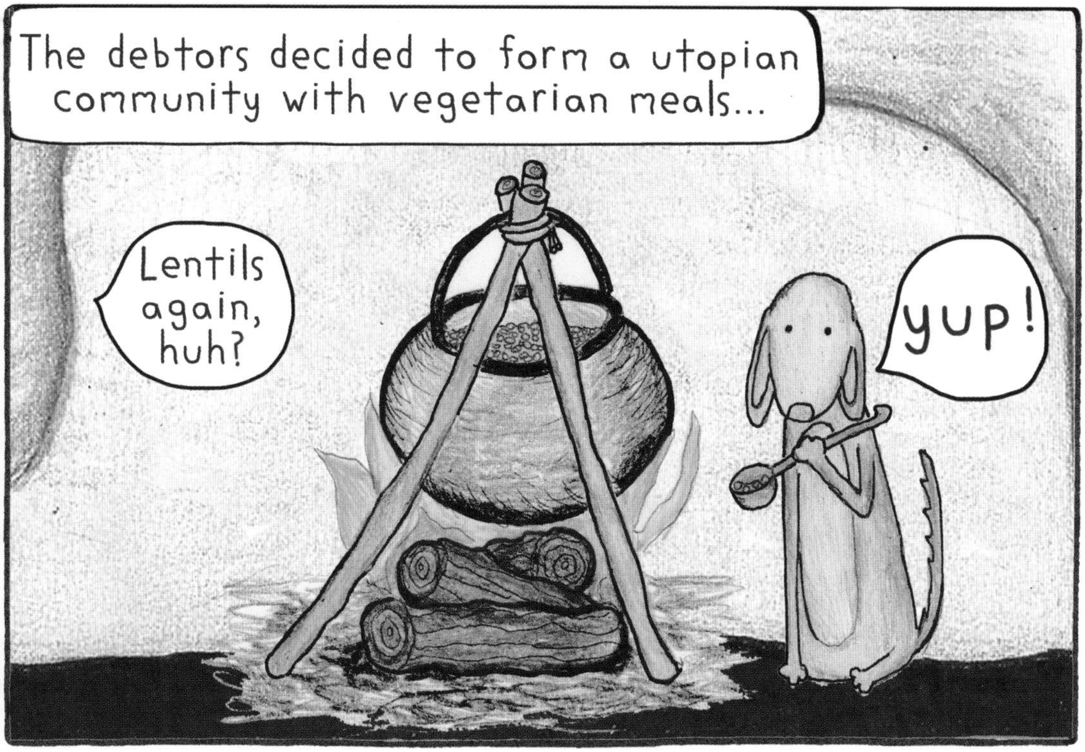
The debtors decided to form a utopian community with vegetarian meals...
Lentils again, huh?
yup!

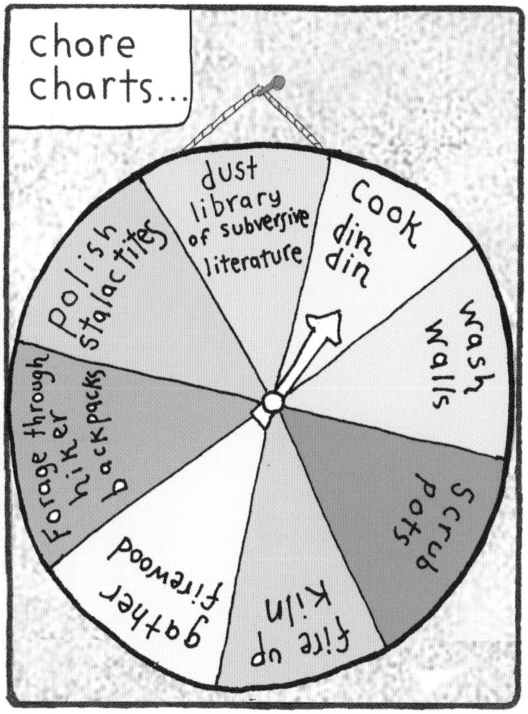
chore charts...
dust library of subversive literature
cook din din
wash walls
scrub pots
fire up kiln
gather firewood
Forage through hiker backpacks
polish stalactites

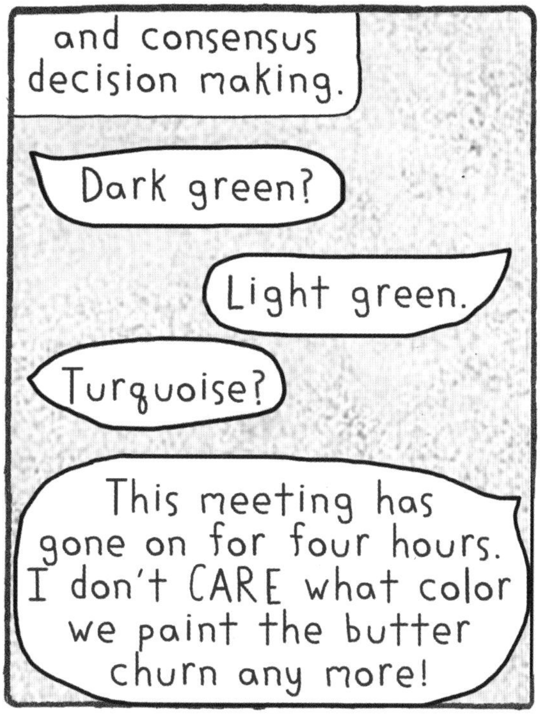
and consensus decision making.
Dark green?
Light green.
Turquoise?
This meeting has gone on for four hours. I don't CARE what color we paint the butter churn any more!

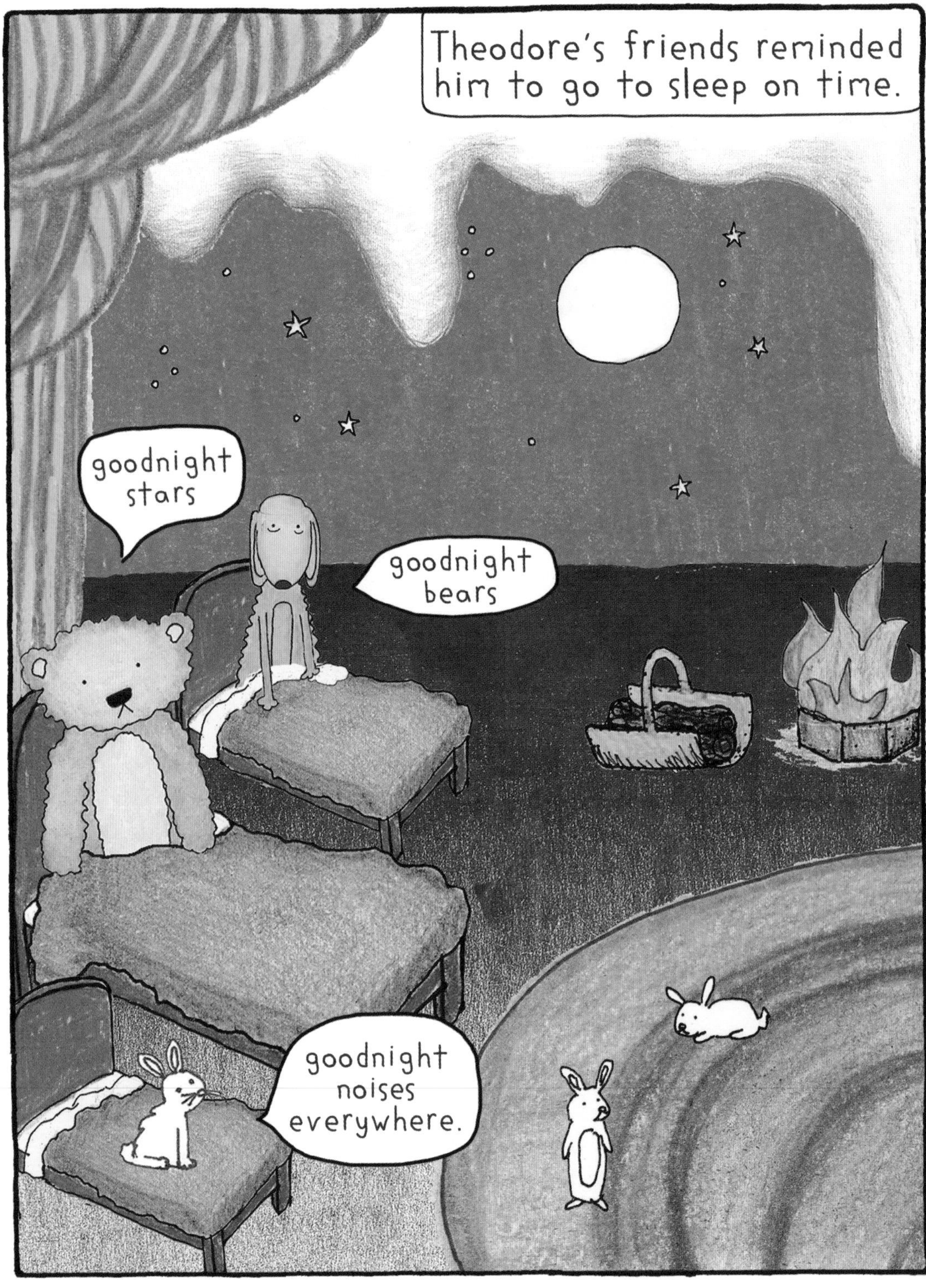
Theodore's friends reminded him to go to sleep on time.
goodnight stars
goodnight bears
goodnight noises everywhere.

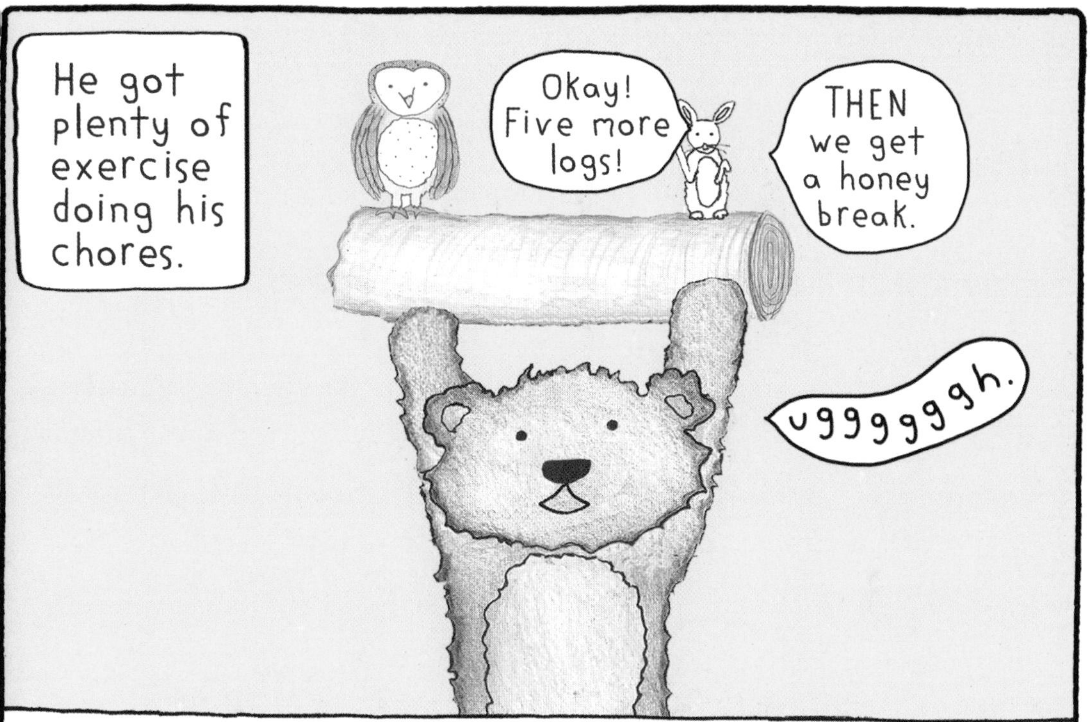
He got plenty of exercise doing his chores.
Okay! Five more logs!
THEN we get a honey break.
ugggggggh.

The debtors learned about nutrition.

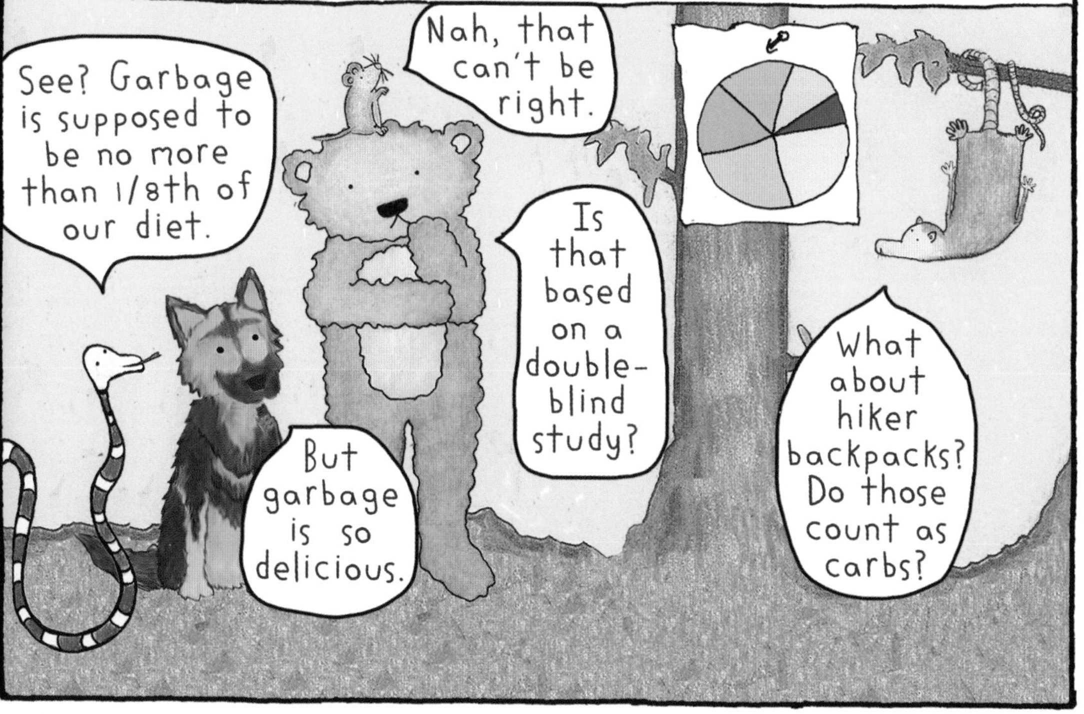
See? Garbage is supposed to be no more than 1/8th of our diet.
Nah, that can't be right.
Is that based on a double-blind study?
What about hiker backpacks? Do those count as carbs?
But garbage is so delicious.

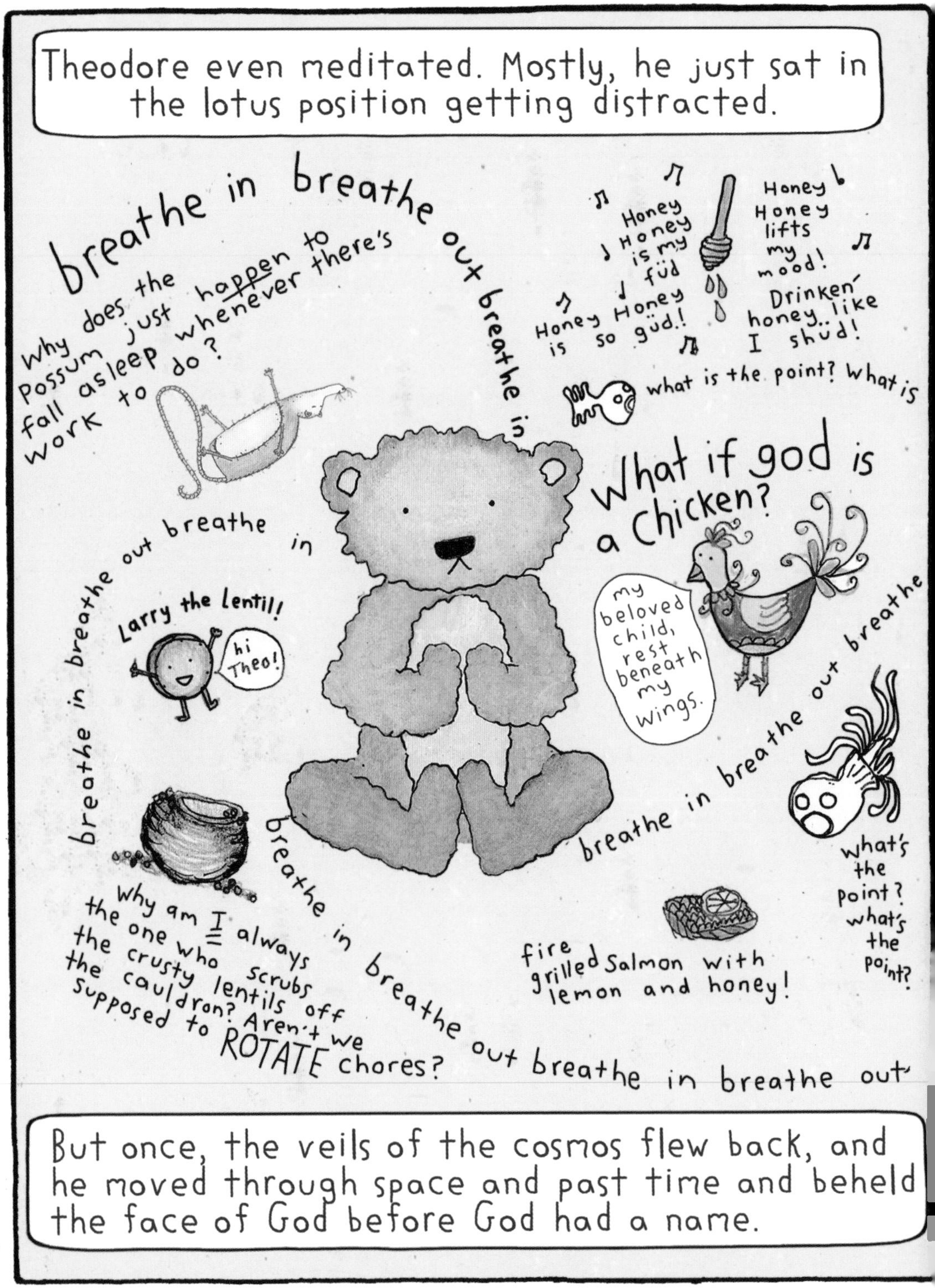
Theodore even meditated. Mostly, he just sat in the lotus position getting distracted.
breathe in breathe out breathe in
Why does the possum just happen to fall asleep whenever there's work to do?
Honey Honey is my füd Honey Honey is so güd!
Honey Honey lifts my mood! Drinken' honey like I shüd!
what is the point? What is
What if god is a Chicken?
my beloved child, rest beneath my wings.
breathe in breathe out breathe in
Larry the Lentil!
hi Theo!
breathe in breathe out breathe
what's the point? what's the point?
Why am I always the one who scrubs the crusty lentils off the cauldron? Aren't we supposed to ROTATE chores?
breathe in breathe out breathe in breathe out
fire grilled Salmon with lemon and honey!
But once, the veils of the cosmos flew back, and he moved through space and past time and beheld the face of God before God had a name.

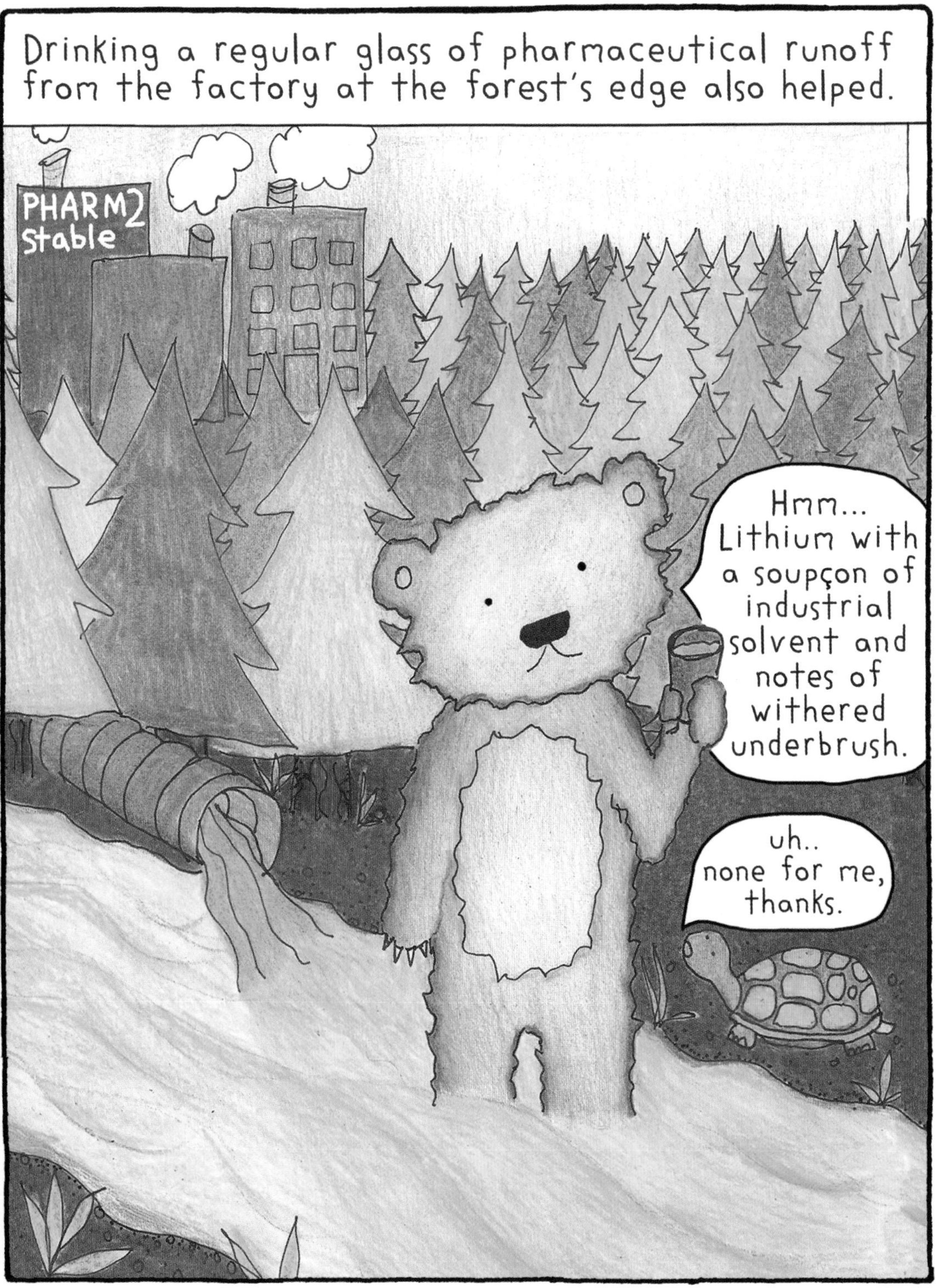
Drinking a regular glass of pharmaceutical runoff from the factory at the forest's edge also helped.
PHARM2 Stable
Hmm... Lithium with a soupçon of industrial solvent and notes of withered underbrush.
uh.. none for me, thanks.

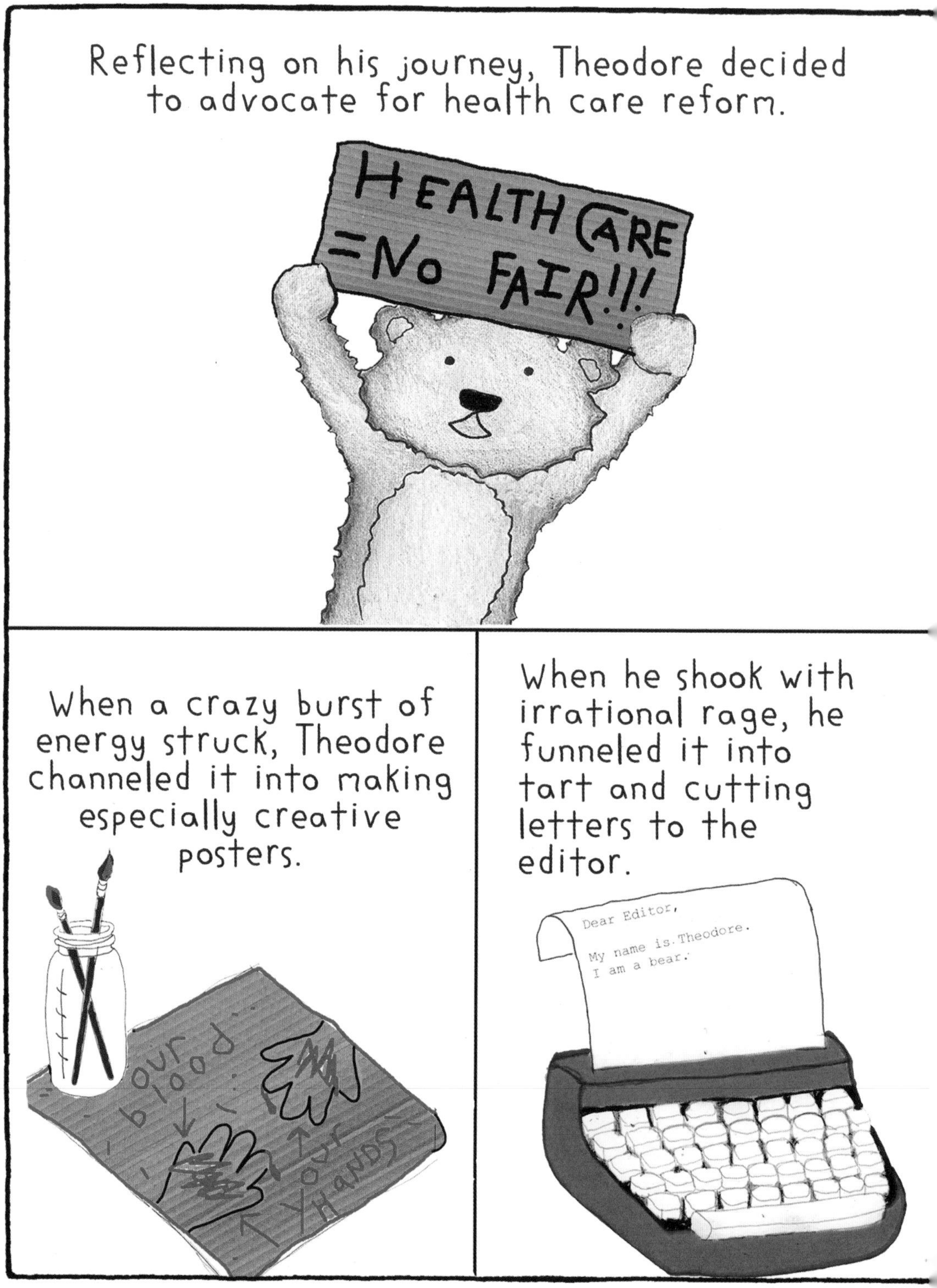
Reflecting on his journey, Theodore decided to advocate for health care reform.
HEALTH CARE =No FAIR!!!
When a crazy burst of energy struck, Theodore channeled it into making especially creative posters.
When he shook with irrational rage, he funneled it into tart and cutting letters to the editor.
Dear Editor,
My name is Theodore.
I am a bear.

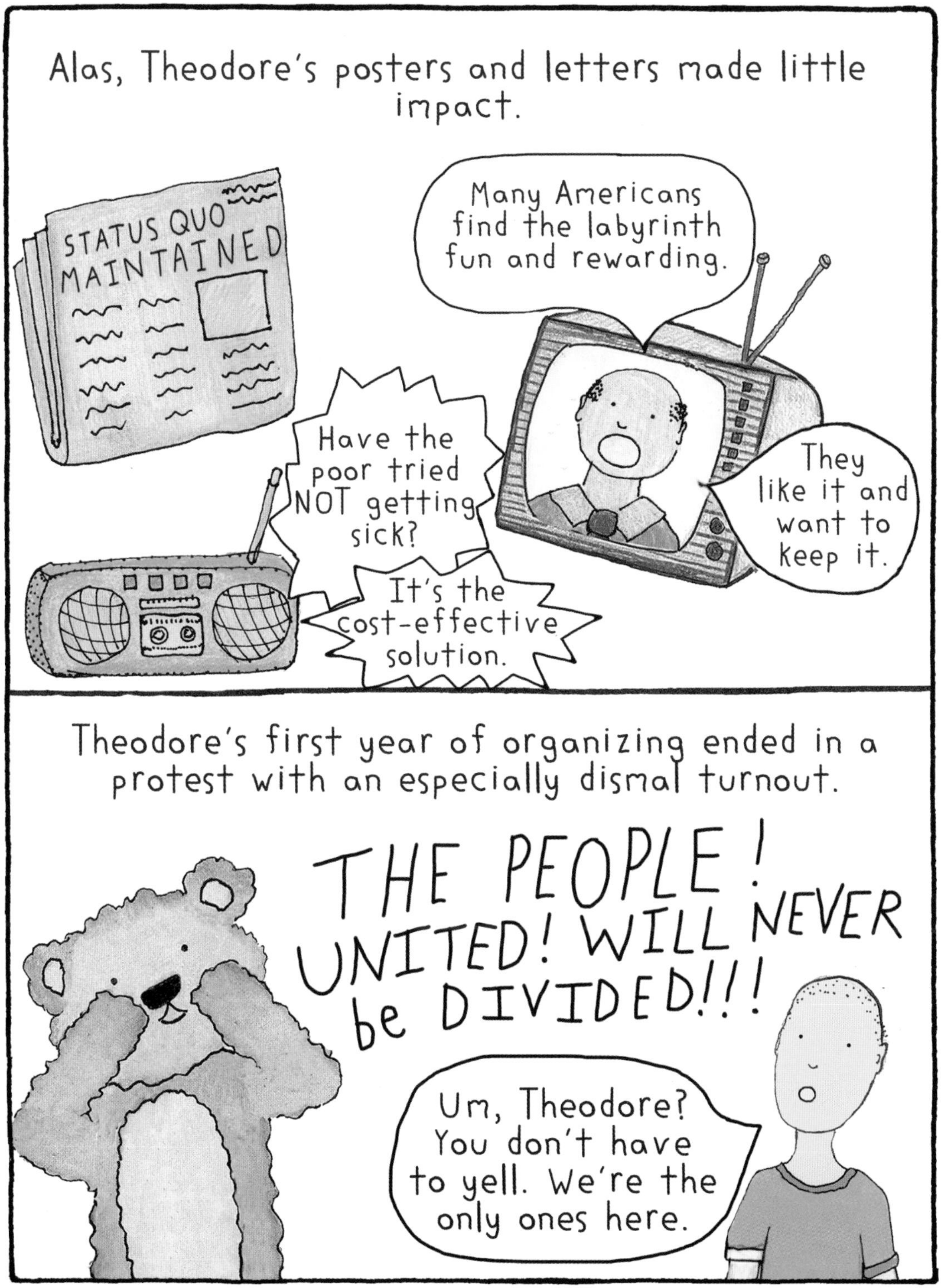
Alas, Theodore's posters and letters made little impact.
STATUS QUO MAINTAINED
Many Americans find the labyrinth fun and rewarding.
They like it and want to keep it.
Have the poor tried NOT getting sick?
It's the cost-effective solution.
Theodore's first year of organizing ended in a protest with an especially dismal turnout.
THE PEOPLE! UNITED! WILL NEVER be DIVIDED!!!
Um, Theodore? You don't have to yell. We're the only ones here.

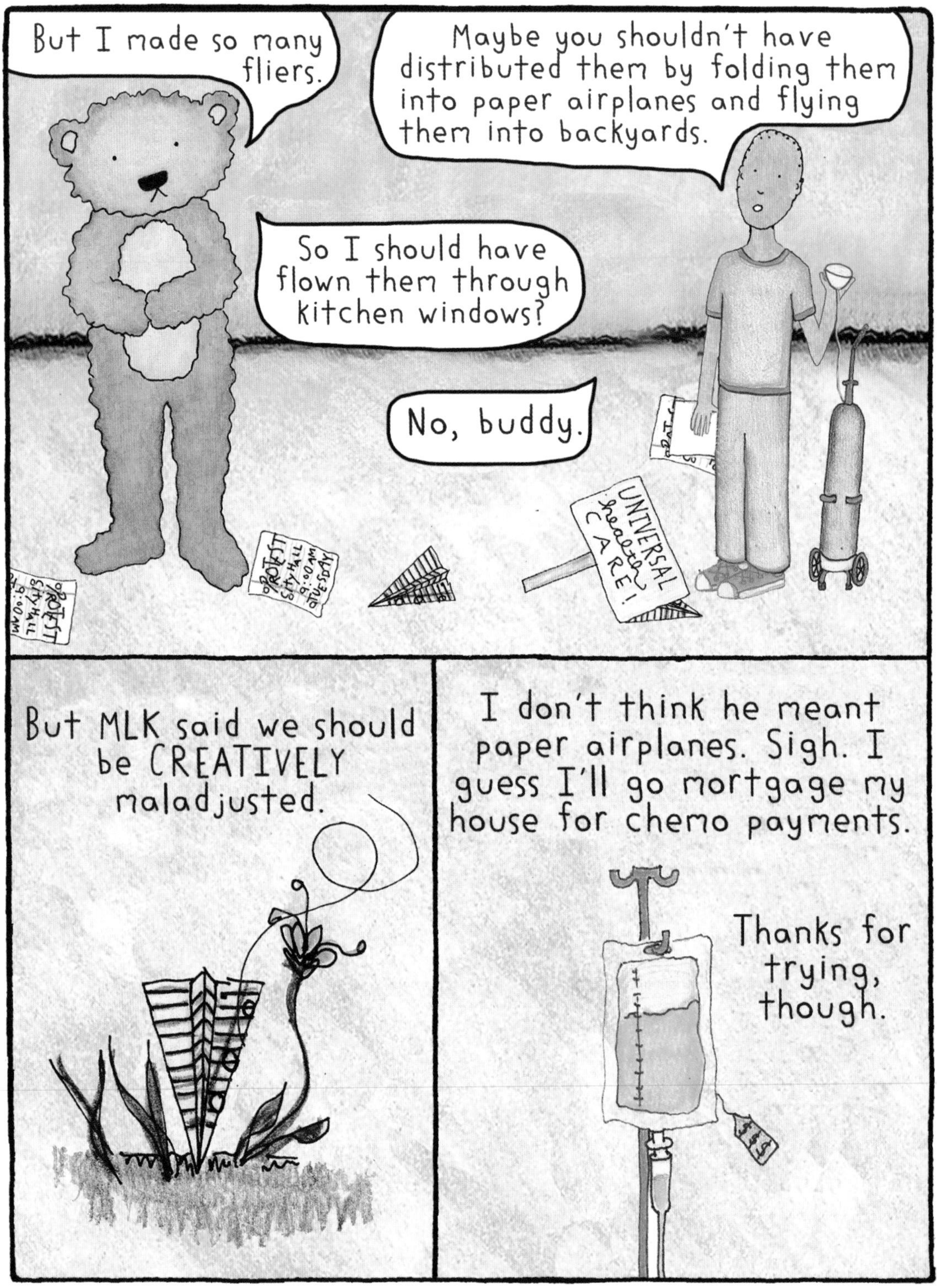
But I made so many fliers.
Maybe you shouldn't have distributed them by folding them into paper airplanes and flying them into backyards.
So I should have flown them through kitchen windows?
No, buddy.
PROTEST
CITY HALL
9:00AM
TUESDAY
UNIVERSAL
health
CARE!
But MLK said we should be CREATIVELY maladjusted.
I don't think he meant paper airplanes. Sigh. I guess I'll go mortgage my house for chemo payments.
Thanks for trying, though.

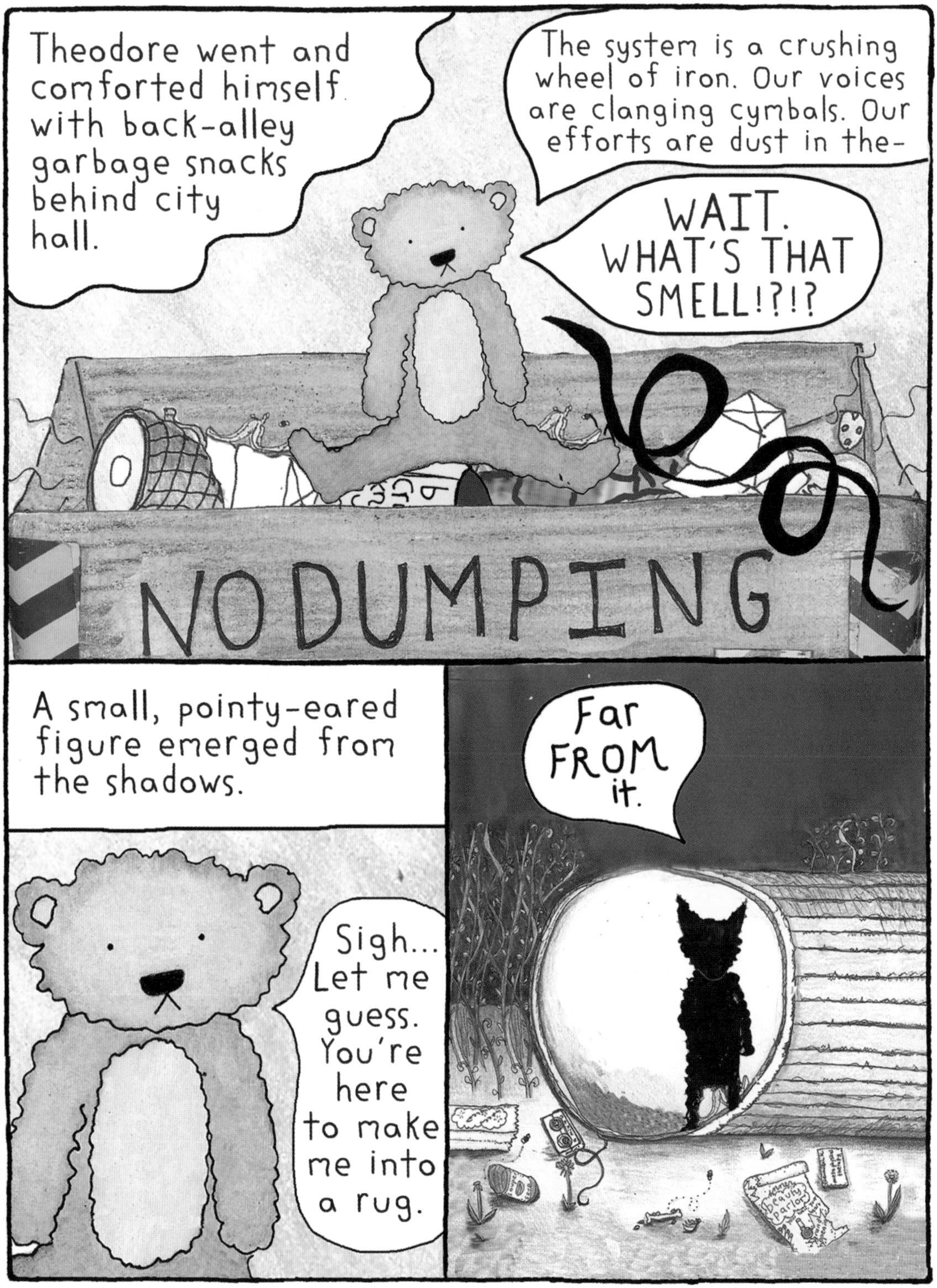
Theodore went and comforted himself with back-alley garbage snacks behind city hall.
The system is a crushing wheel of iron. Our voices are clanging cymbals. Our efforts are dust in the-
WAIT. WHAT'S THAT SMELL!?!?
NODUMPING
A small, pointy-eared figure emerged from the shadows.
Sigh... Let me guess. You're here to make me into a rug.
Far FROM it.

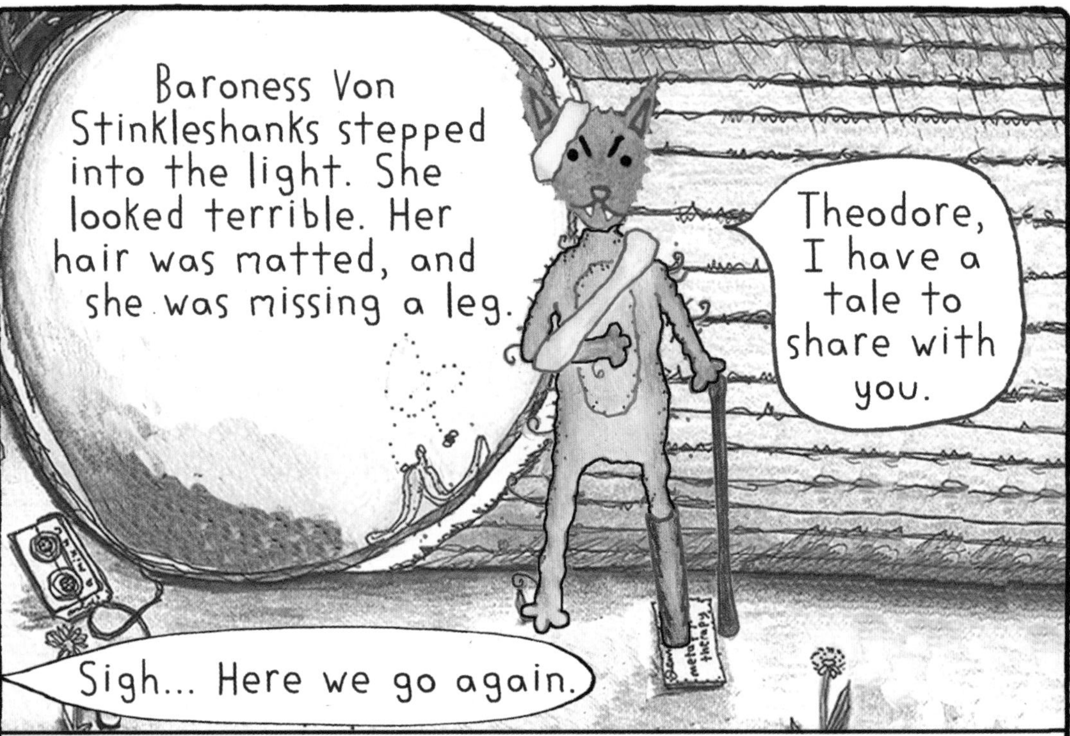
Baroness Von Stinkleshanks stepped into the light. She looked terrible. Her hair was matted, and she was missing a leg.
Theodore, I have a tale to share with you.
Sigh... Here we go again.

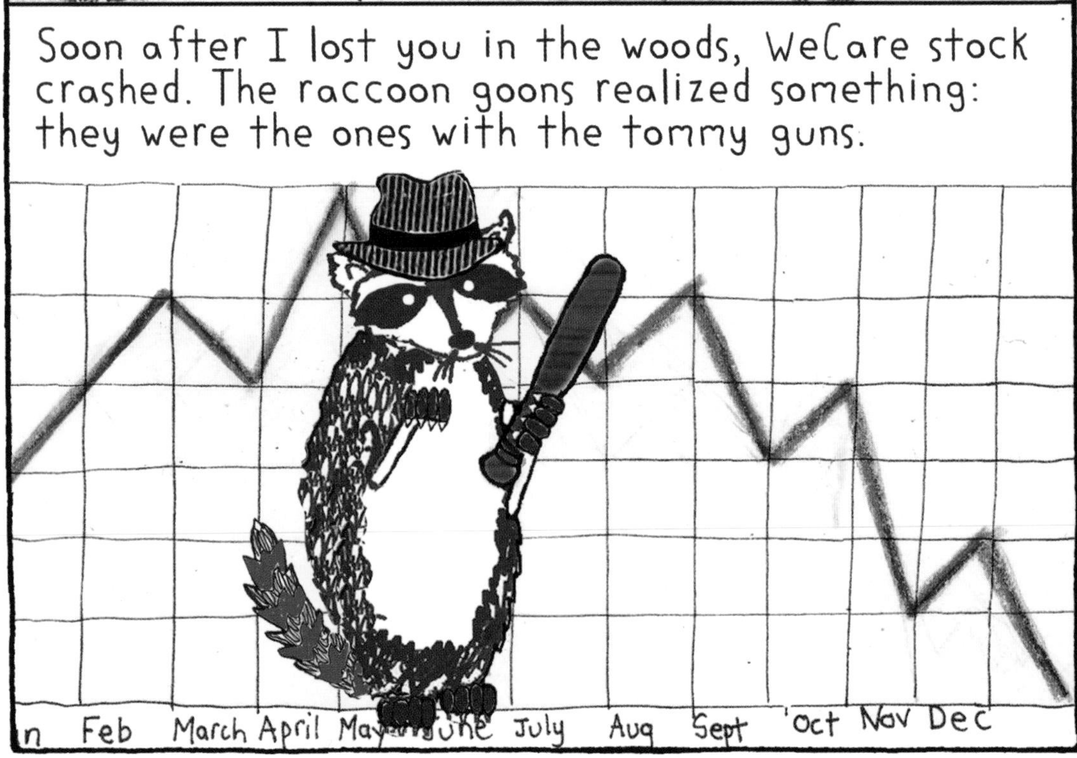
Soon after I lost you in the woods, WeCare stock crashed. The raccoon goons realized something: they were the ones with the tommy guns.
Feb
March
April
July
Aug
Sept
Oct
Nov
Dec

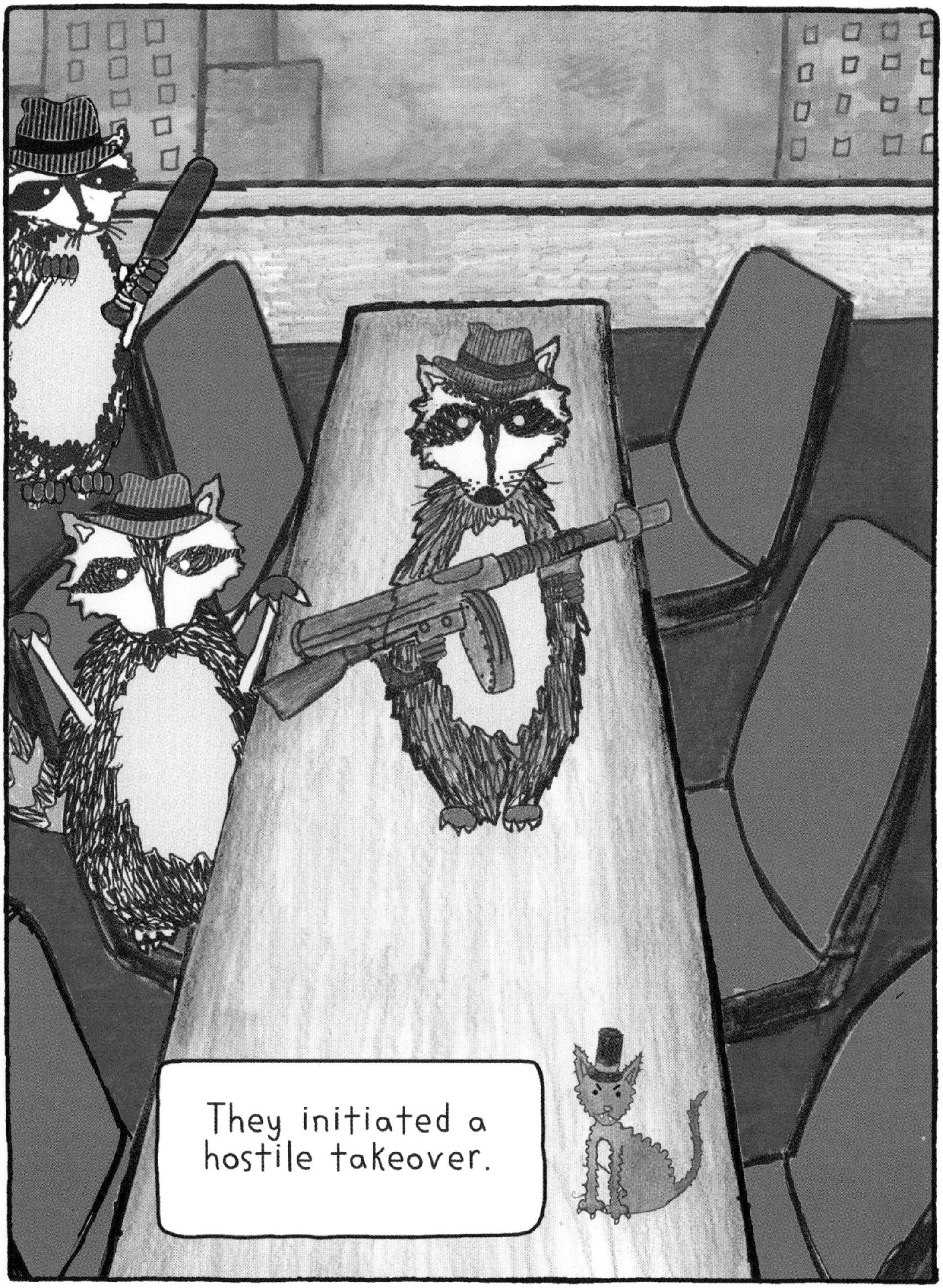
They initiated a hostile takeover.

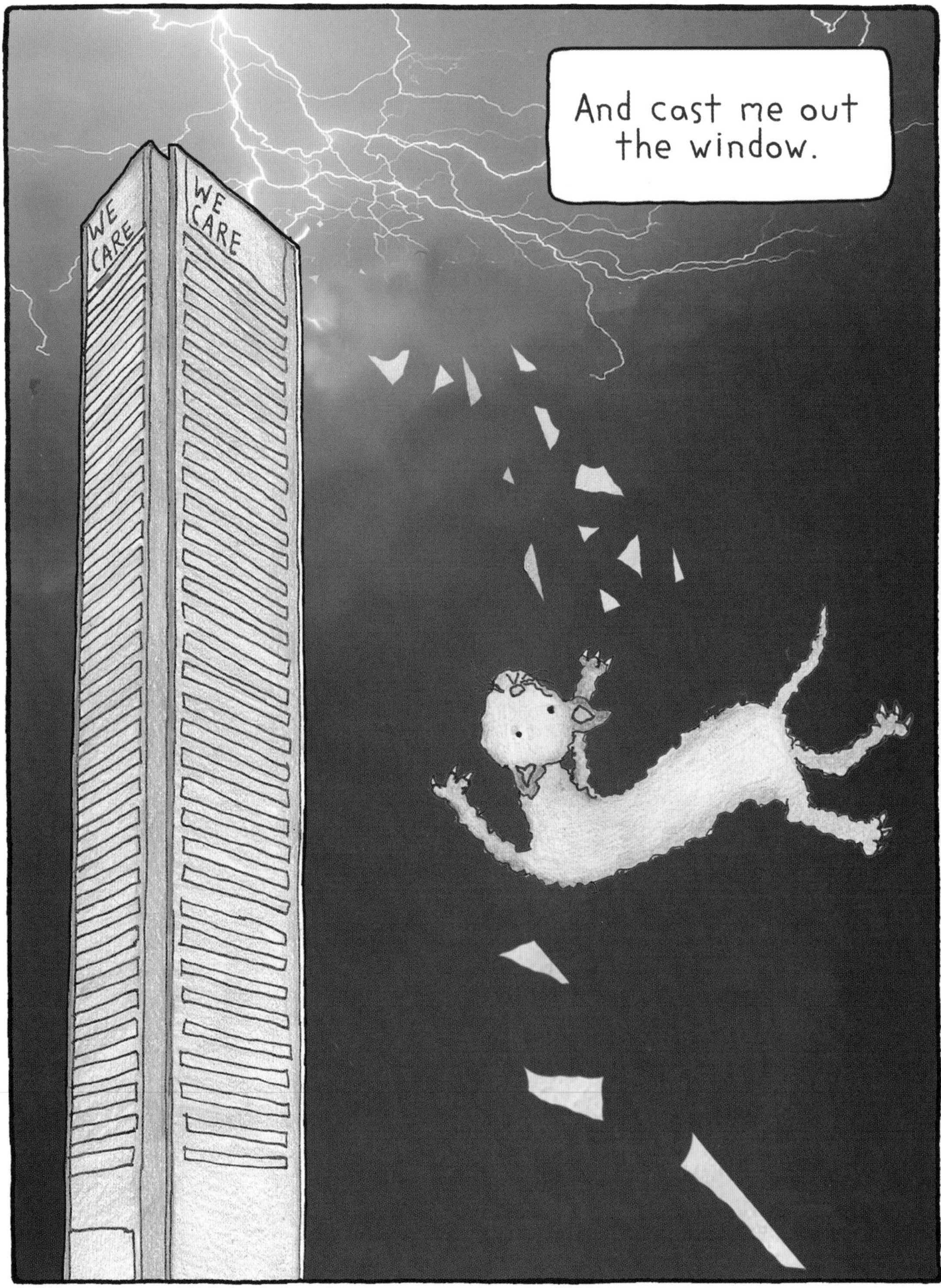
And cast me out the window.
WE CARE
WE CARE

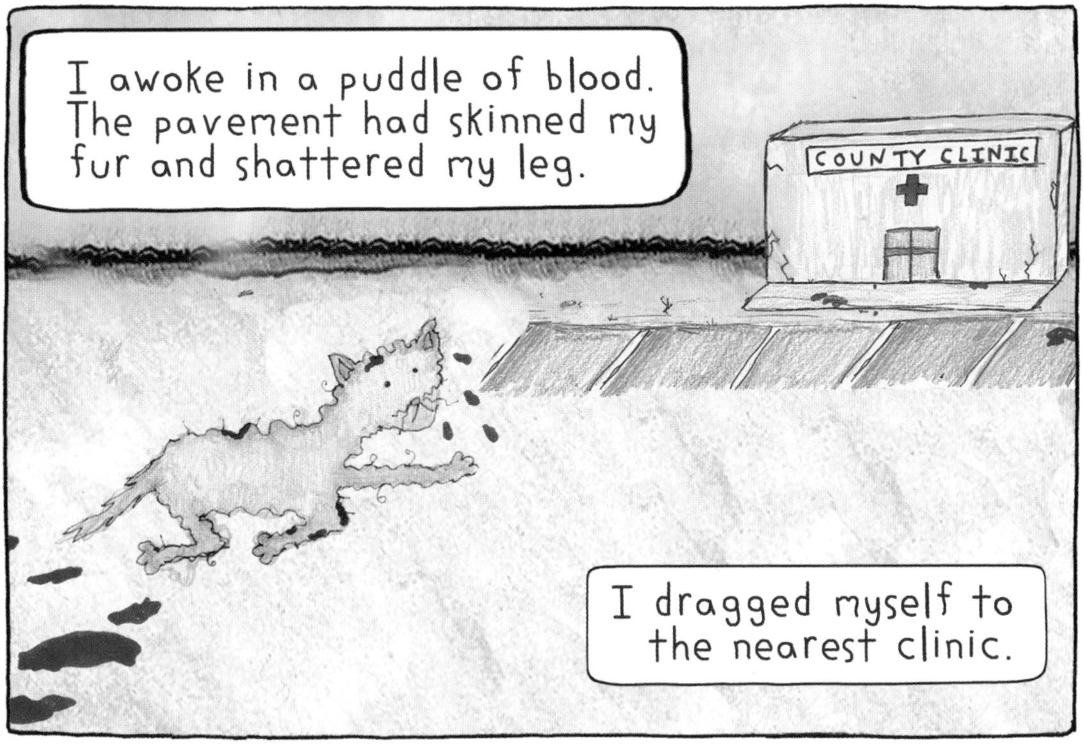
I awoke in a puddle of blood. The pavement had skinned my fur and shattered my leg.
COUNTY CLINIC
I dragged myself to the nearest clinic.

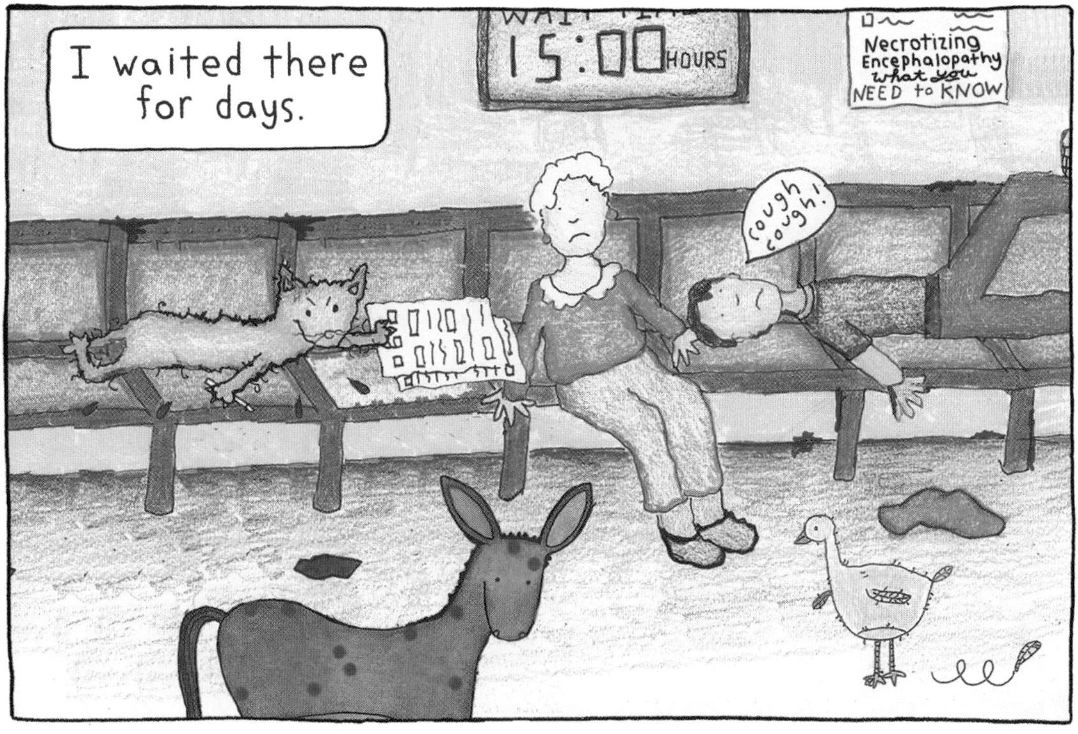
I waited there for days.
15:00 HOURS
Necrotizing Encephalopathy what you NEED to KNOW
cough cough!

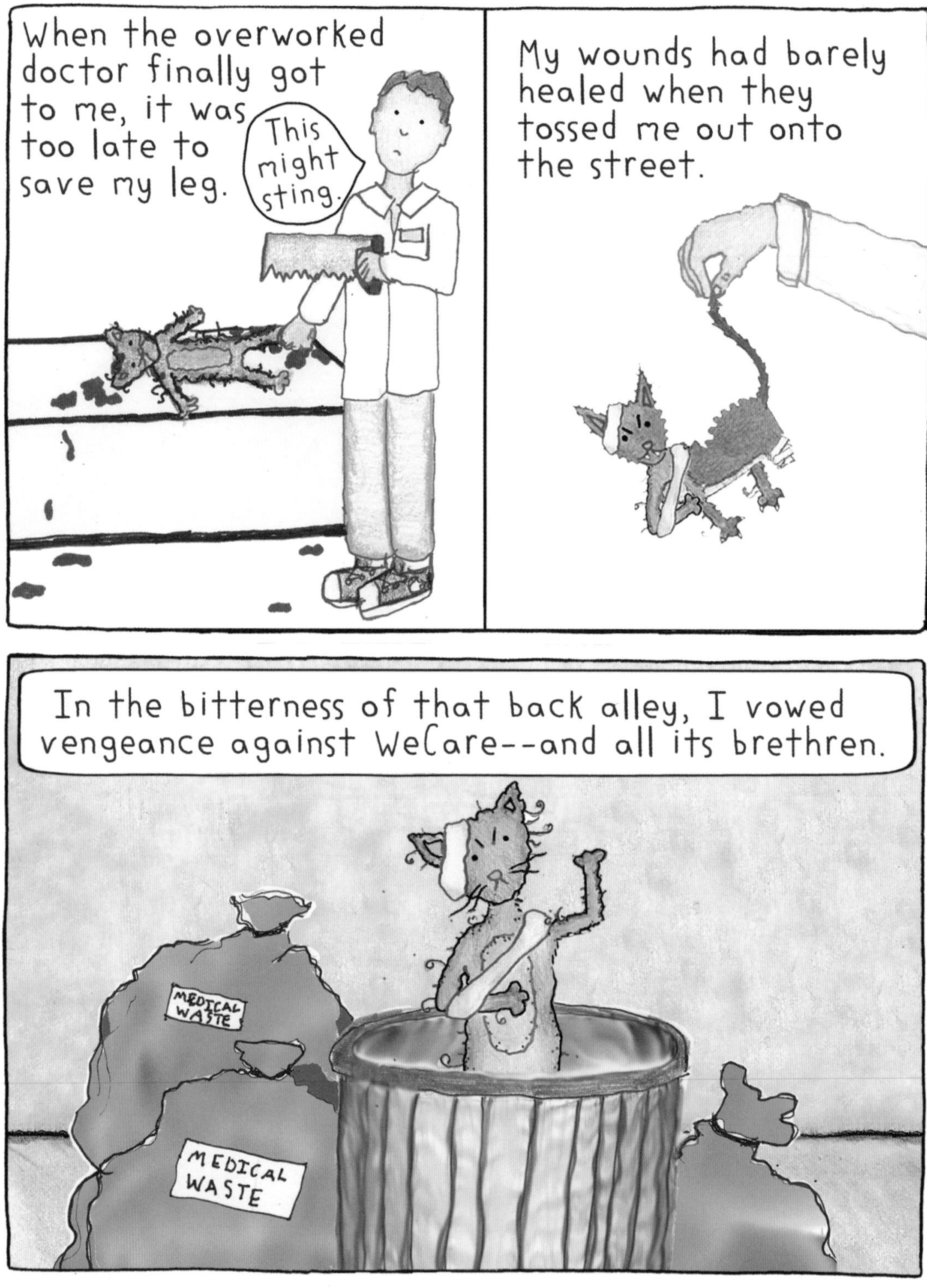
When the overworked doctor finally got to me, it was too late to save my leg.
This might sting.
My wounds had barely healed when they tossed me out onto the street.
In the bitterness of that back alley, I vowed vengeance against WeCare--and all its brethren.
MEDICAL WASTE
MEDICAL WASTE

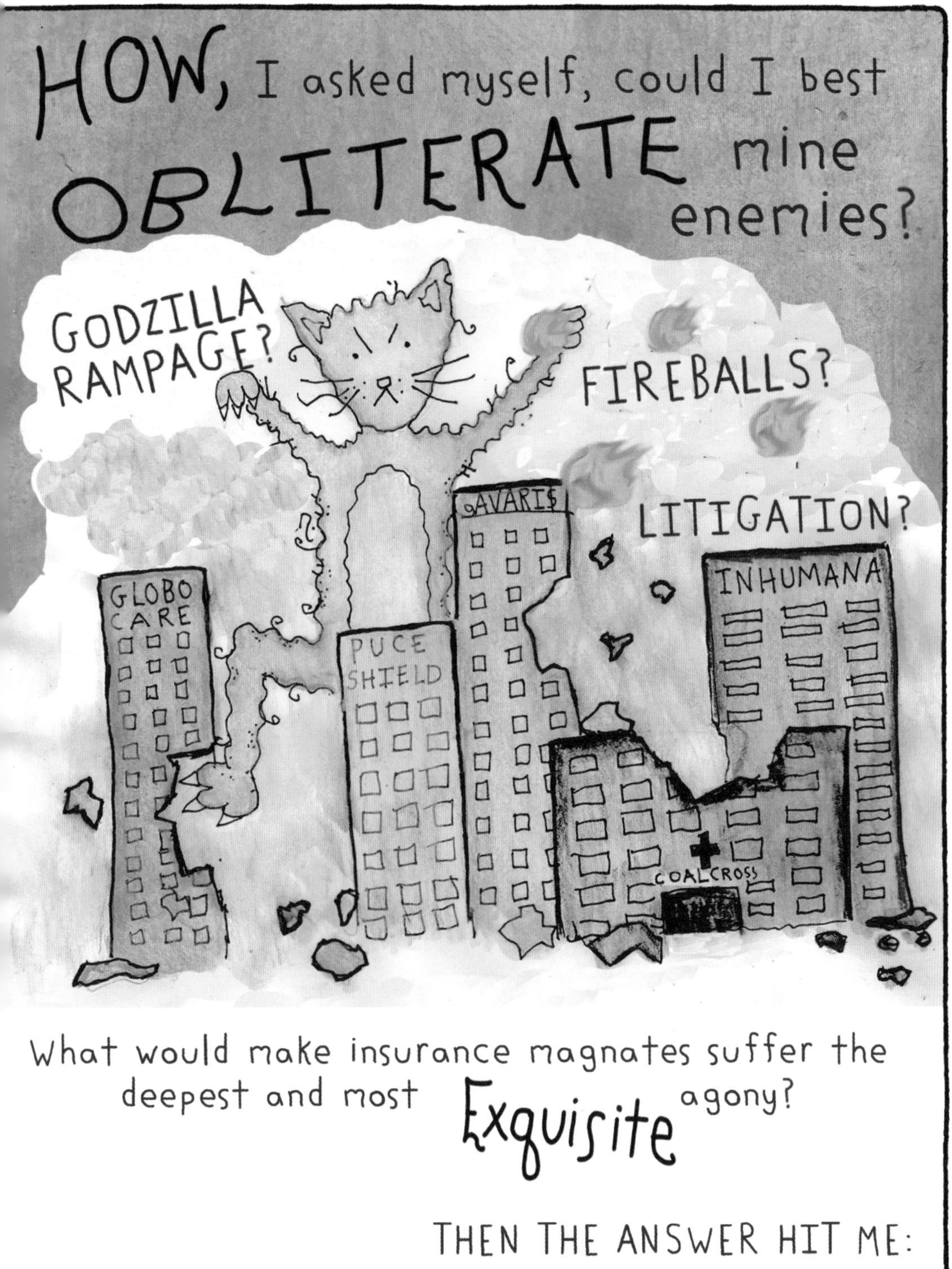
HOW, I asked myself, could I best OBLITERATE mine enemies?
GODZILLA RAMPAGE?
FIREBALLS?
LITIGATION?
GLOBO CARE
PUCE SHIELD
AVARI$
INHUMANA
COALCROSS
What would make insurance magnates suffer the deepest and most Exquisite agony?
THEN THE ANSWER HIT ME:

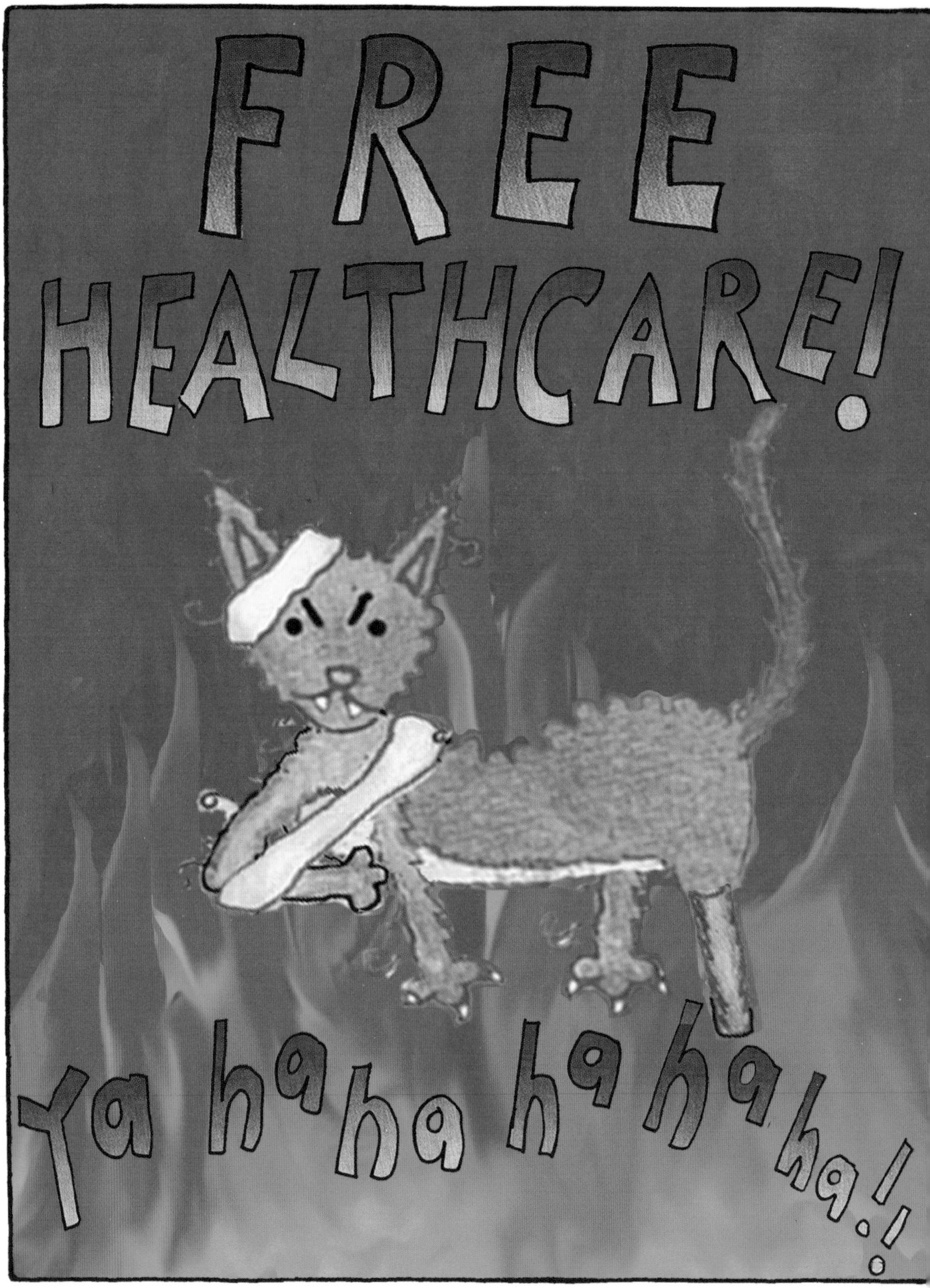
FREE HEALTHCARE!
Ya ha ha ha ha ha ha ha!!

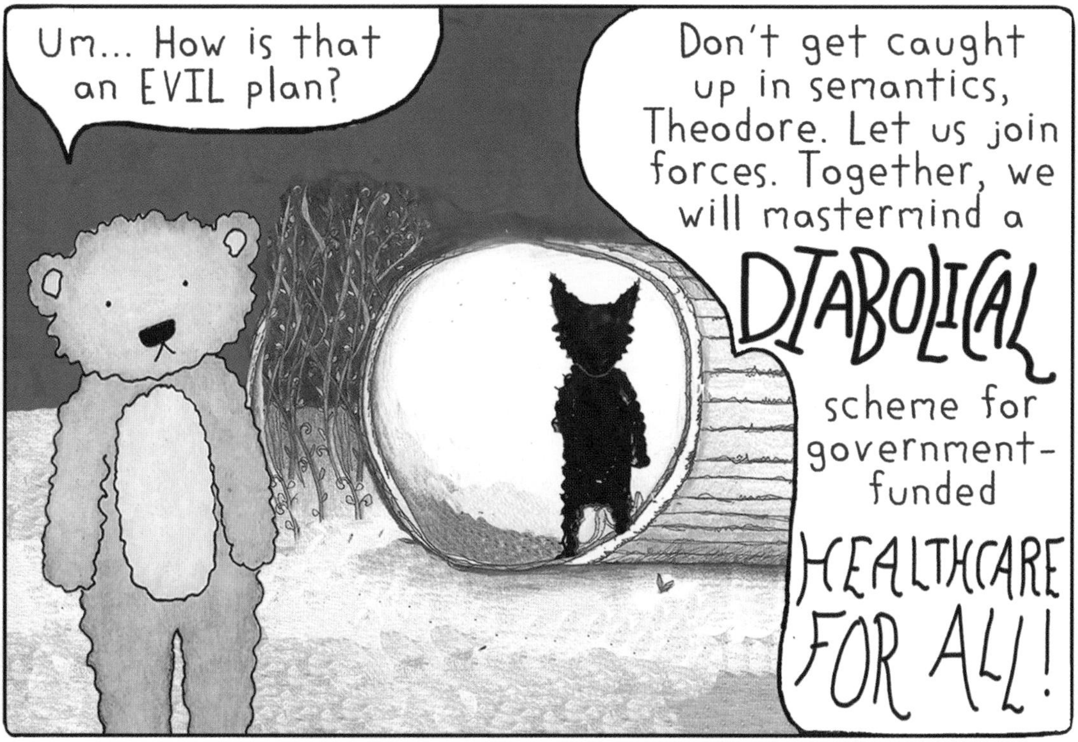
Um... How is that an EVIL plan?
Don't get caught up in semantics, Theodore. Let us join forces. Together, we will mastermind a DIABOLICAL scheme for government-funded HEALTHCARE FOR ALL!

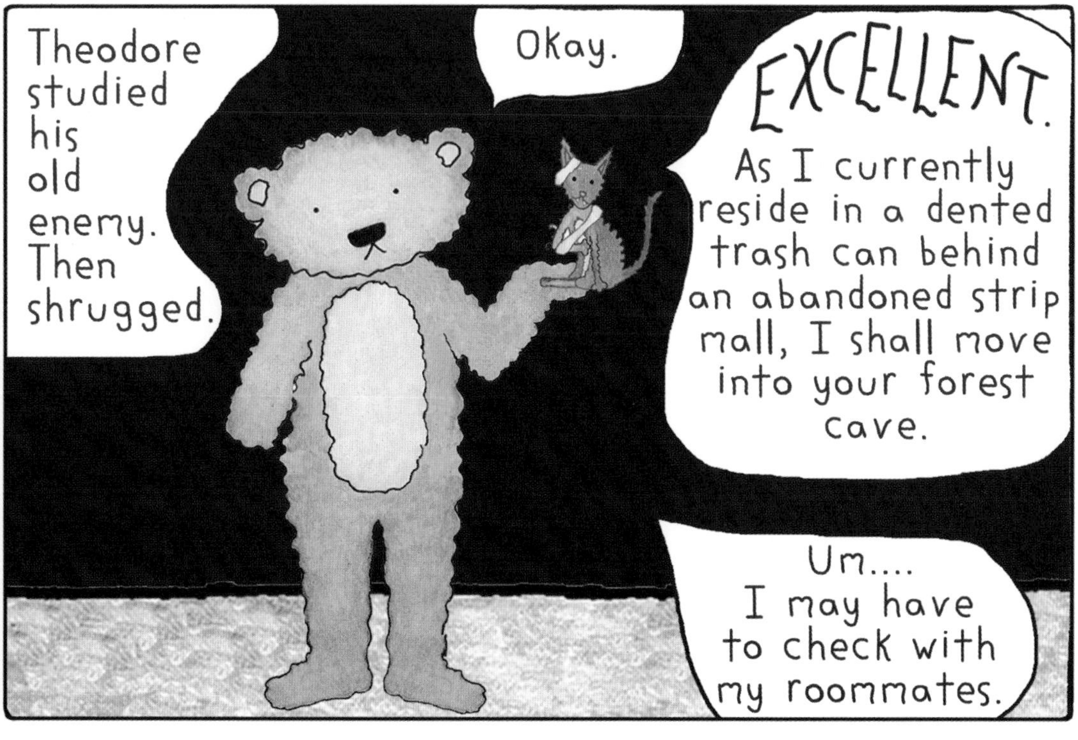
Theodore studied his old enemy. Then shrugged.
Okay.
EXCELLENT. As I currently reside in a dented trash can behind an abandoned strip mall, I shall move into your forest cave.
Um.... I may have to check with my roommates.

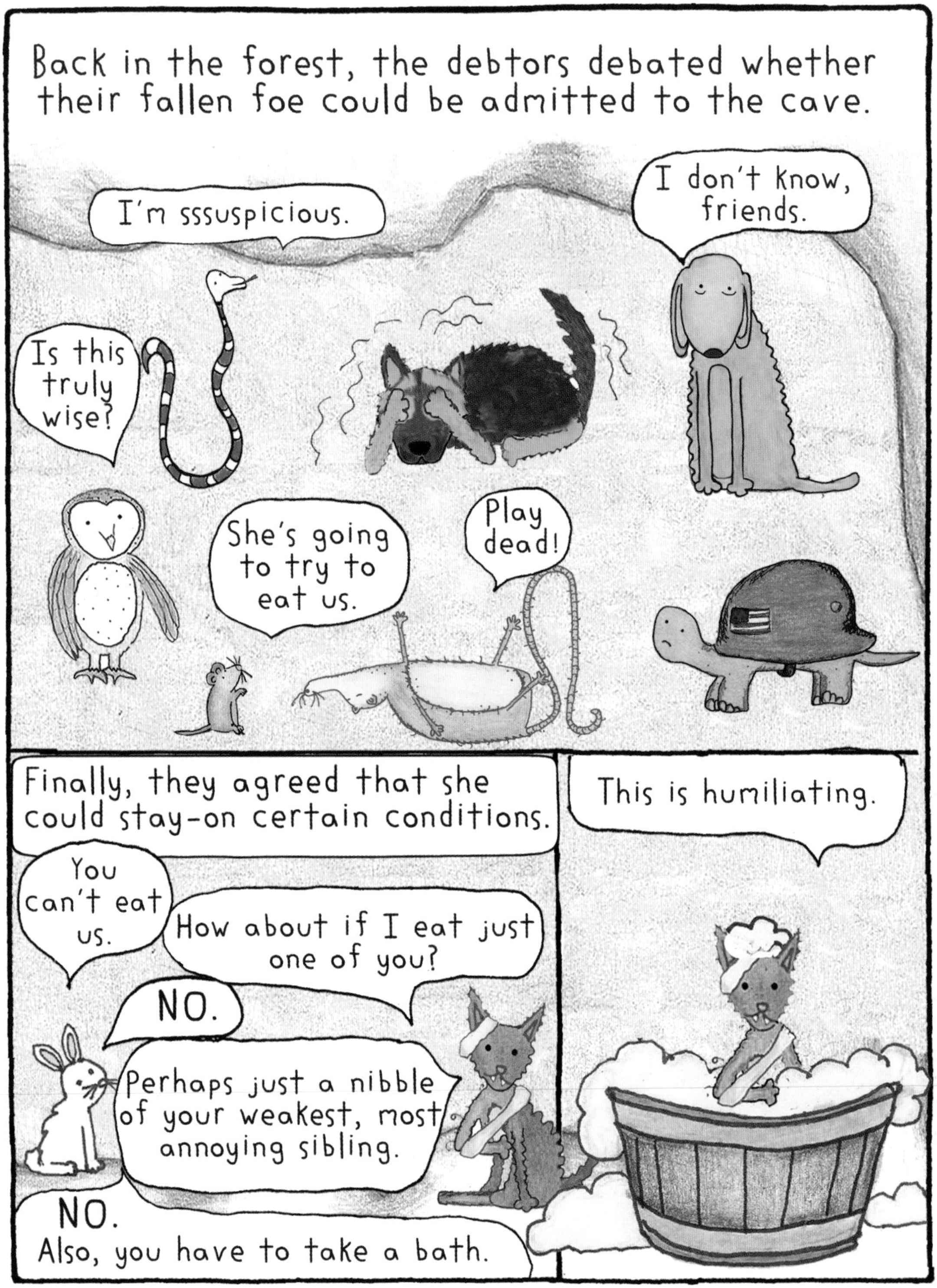
Back in the forest, the debtors debated whether their fallen foe could be admitted to the cave.
I'm sssuspicious.
I don't know, friends.
Is this truly wise?
She's going to try to eat us.
Play dead!
Finally, they agreed that she could stay-on certain conditions.
You can't eat us.
How about if I eat just one of you?
NO.
Perhaps just a nibble of your weakest, most annoying sibling.
NO.
Also, you have to take a bath.
This is humiliating.

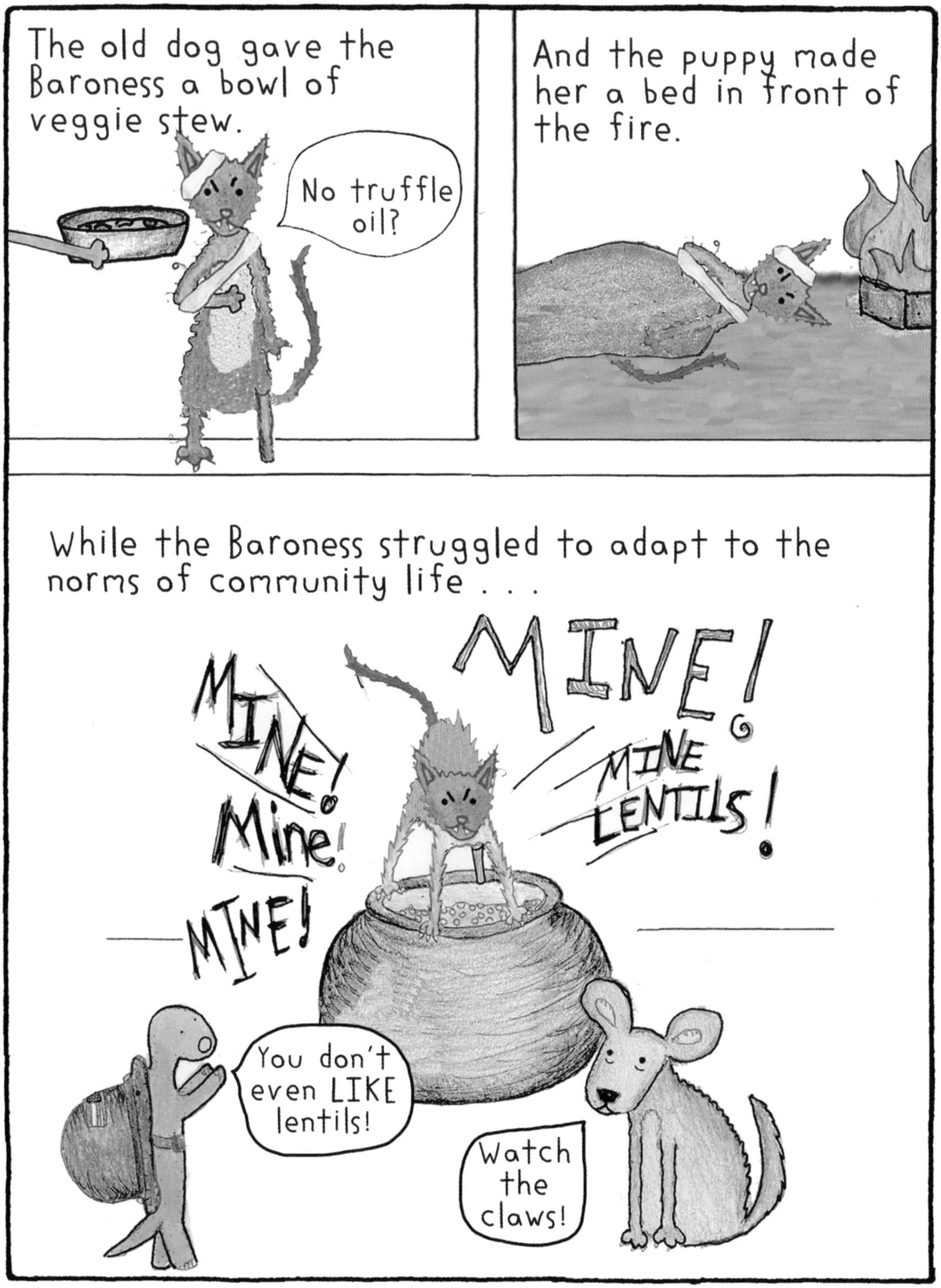
The old dog gave the Baroness a bowl of veggie stew.
No truffle oil?
And the puppy made her a bed in front of the fire.
While the Baroness struggled to adapt to the norms of community life . . .
MINE!
MINE!
Mine!
MINE!
MINE!
MINE LENTILS!
You don't even LIKE lentils!
Watch the claws!

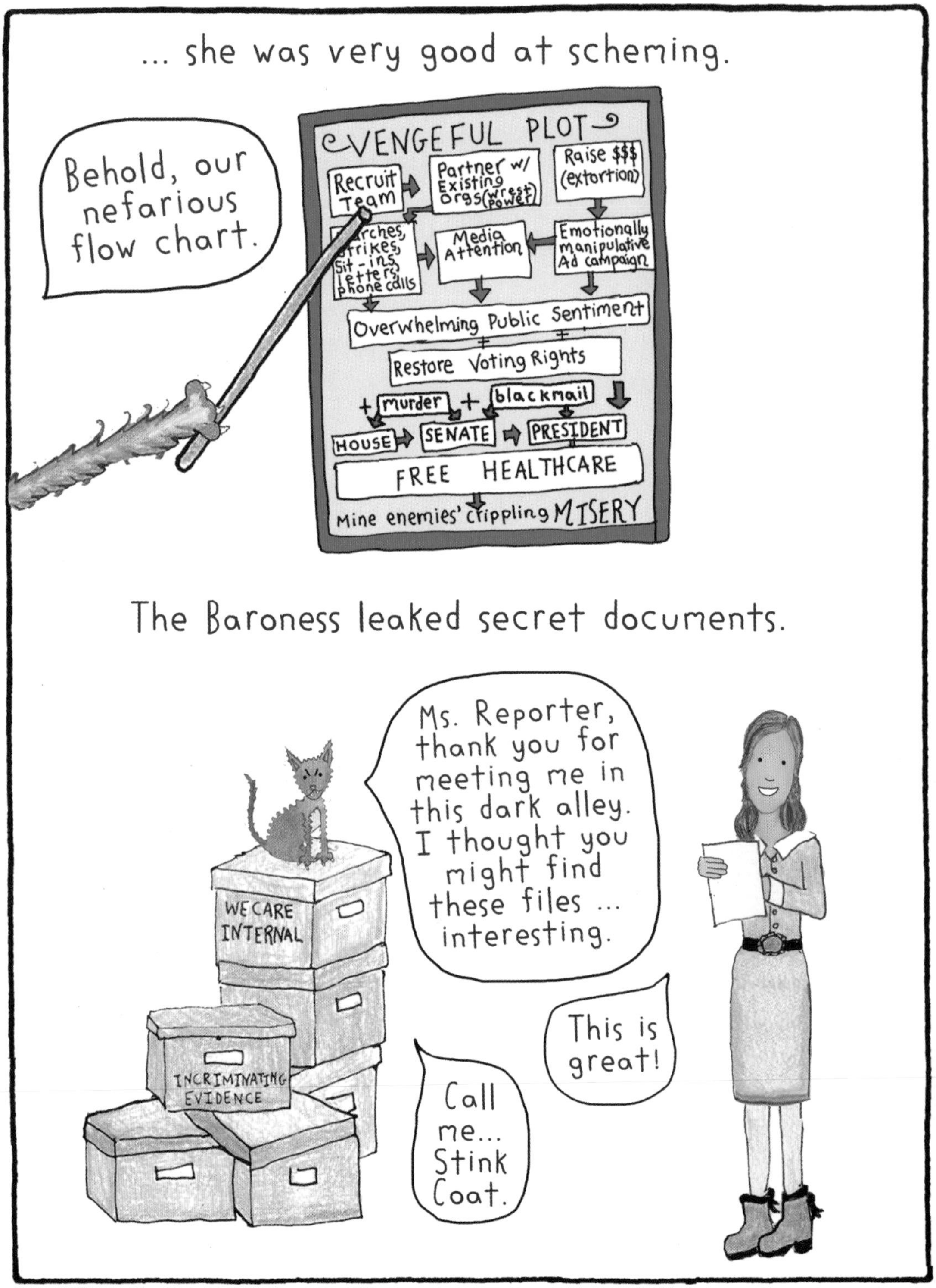
... she was very good at scheming.
Behold, our nefarious flow chart.
VENGEFUL PLOT
Recruit Team
Partner w/ Existing Orgs (wrest power)
Raise $$$ (extortion)
Sit-ins, letters, phone calls
Media Attention
Emotionally manipulative Ad campaign
Overwhelming Public Sentiment
Restore Voting Rights
murder
blackmail
HOUSE
SENATE
PRESIDENT
FREE HEALTHCARE
Mine enemies' crippling MISERY
The Baroness leaked secret documents.
WE CARE INTERNAL
INCRIMINATING EVIDENCE
Ms. Reporter, thank you for meeting me in this dark alley. I thought you might find these files ... interesting.
This is great!
Call me... Stink Coat.

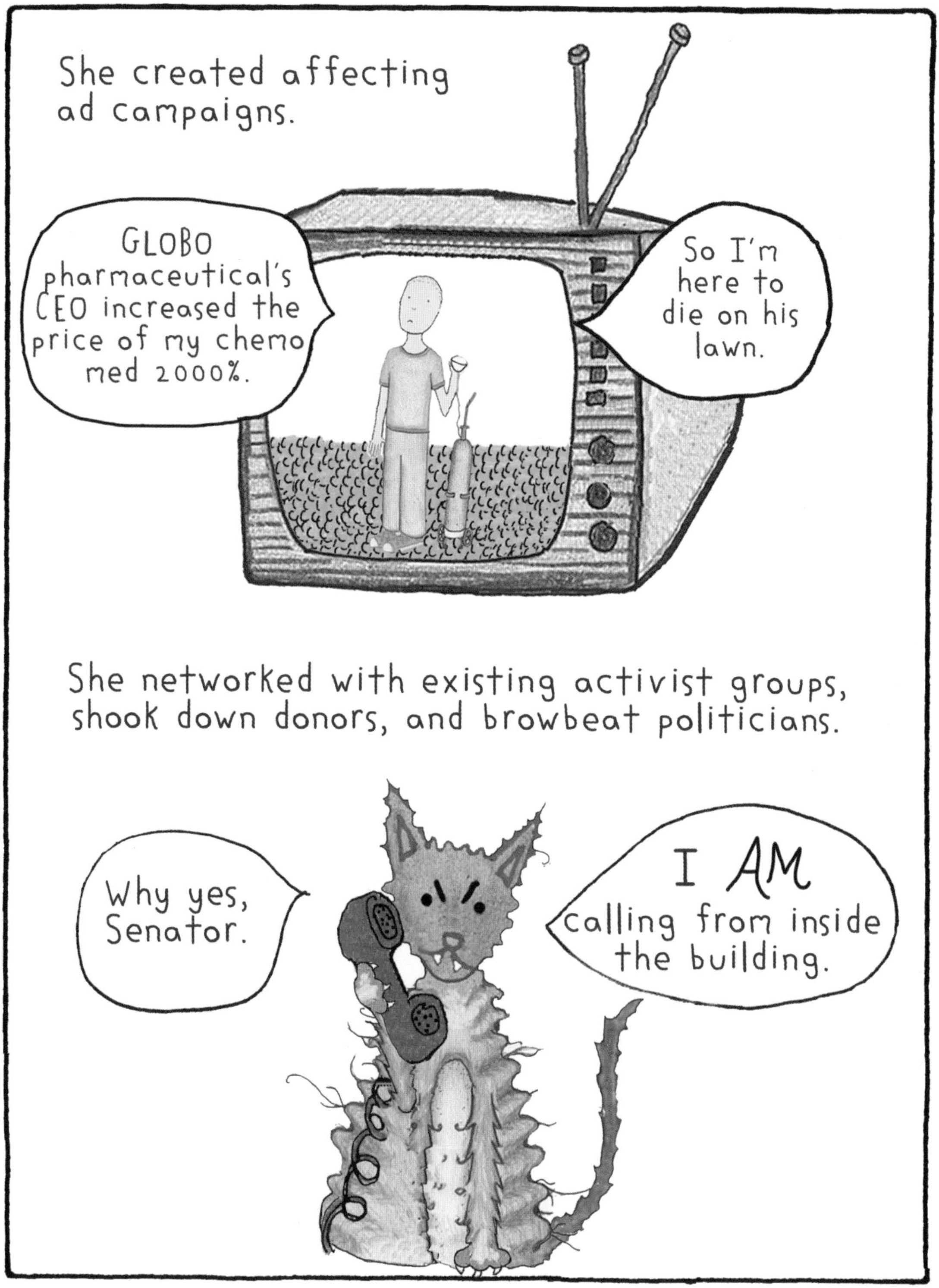
She created affecting ad campaigns.
GLOBO pharmaceutical's CEO increased the price of my chemo med 2000%.
So I'm here to die on his lawn.
She networked with existing activist groups, shook down donors, and browbeat politicians.
Why yes, Senator.
I AM calling from inside the building.

Also helpful: she hooked Theodore up with brand-name meds.

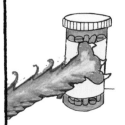

Let's just say this fell off a truck.

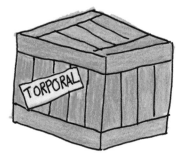

She gave the old dog codes to hack into a government database and erase the debtors' criminal records.

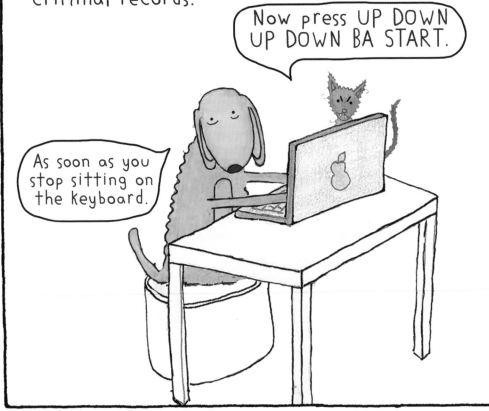

Now press UP DOWN UP DOWN BA START.

As soon as you stop sitting on the keyboard.

To everyone's surprise, the commune's vegetarian diet improved the Baroness's once-scrawny figure. Her coat still smelled sour, but she finally put some meat on her bones.

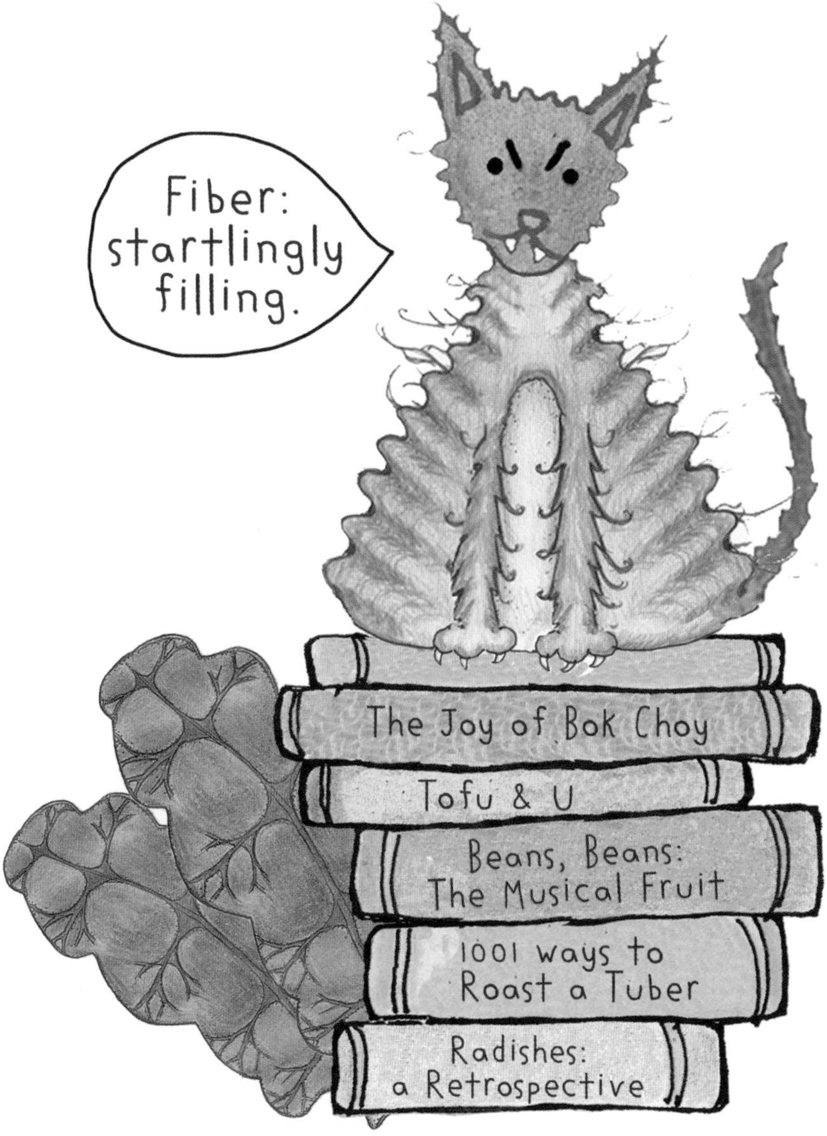
Fiber: startlingly filling.
The Joy of Bok Choy
Tofu & U
Beans, Beans: The Musical Fruit
1001 ways to Roast a Tuber
Radishes: a Retrospective

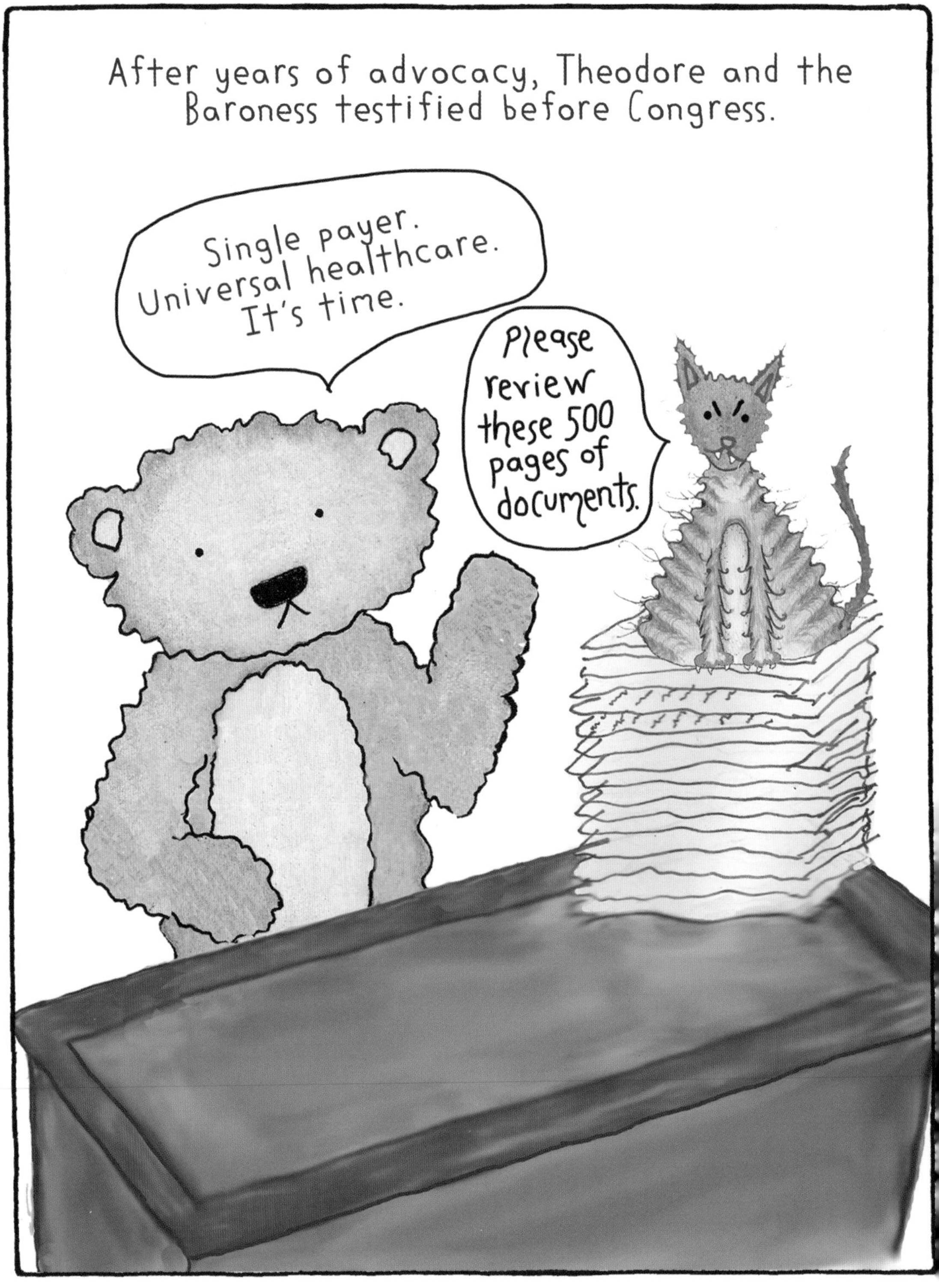
After years of advocacy, Theodore and the Baroness testified before Congress.
Single payer. Universal healthcare. It's time.
Please review these 500 pages of documents.

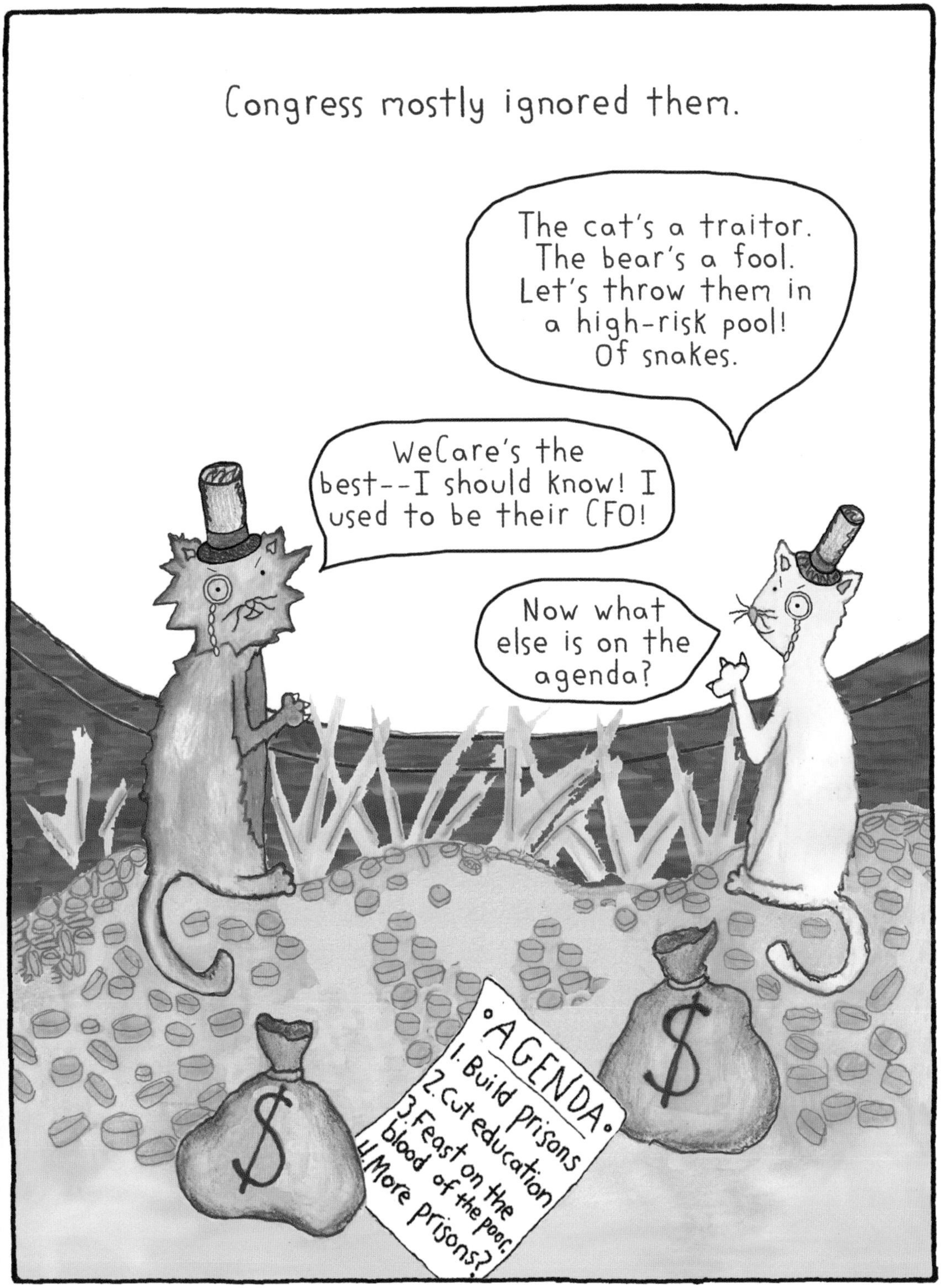
Congress mostly ignored them.
The cat's a traitor. The bear's a fool. Let's throw them in a high-risk pool! Of snakes.
WeCare's the best--I should know! I used to be their CFO!
Now what else is on the agenda?
AGENDA
1. Build prisons
2. Cut education
3. Feast on the blood of the poor.
4. More prisons?

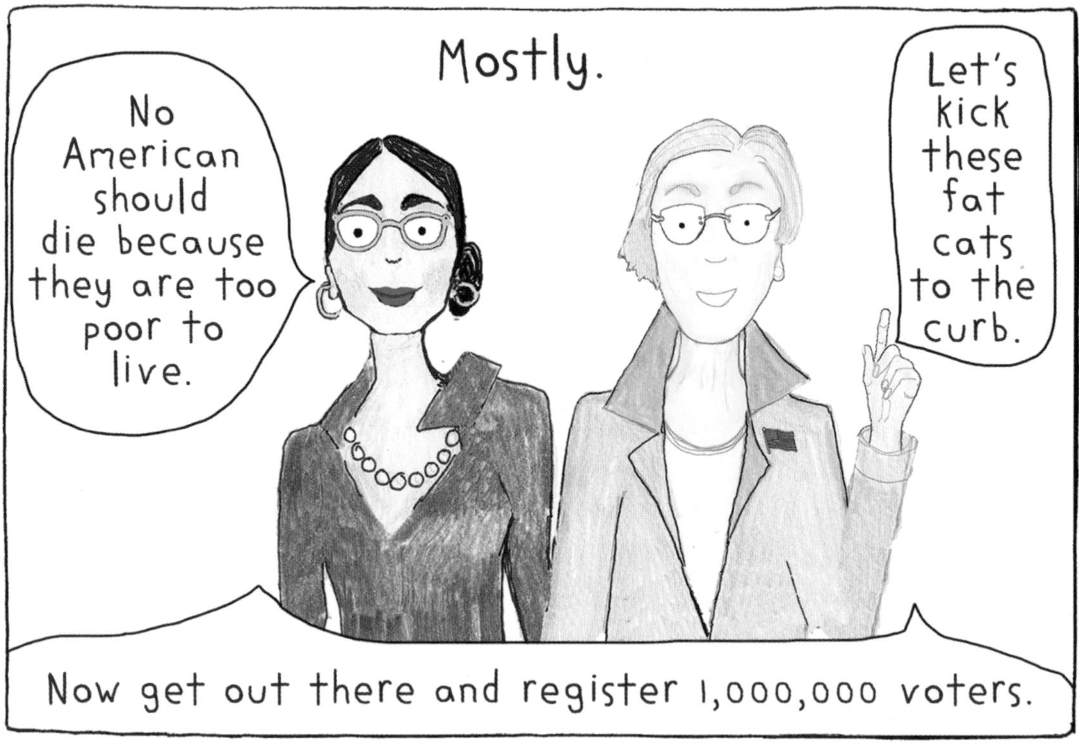
Mostly.
No American should die because they are too poor to live.
Let's kick these fat cats to the curb.
Now get out there and register 1,000,000 voters.

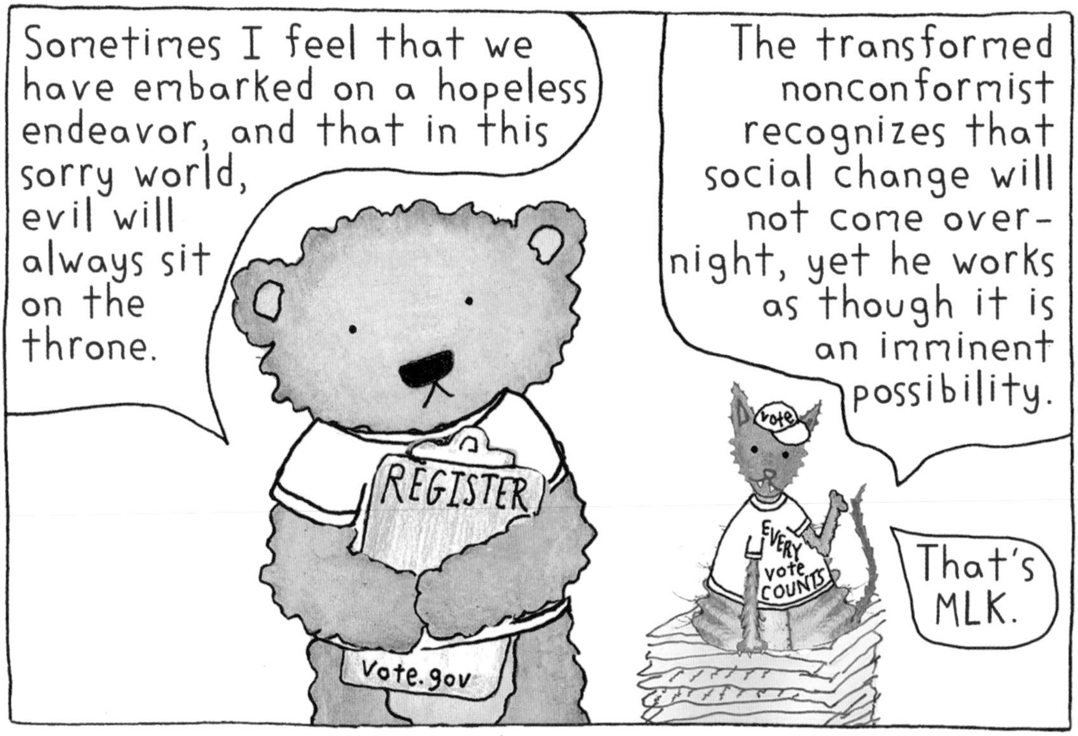
Sometimes I feel that we have embarked on a hopeless endeavor, and that in this sorry world, evil will always sit on the throne.
REGISTER
vote.gov
The transformed nonconformist recognizes that social change will not come over-night, yet he works as though it is an imminent possibility.
vote
EVERY vote COUNTS
That's MLK.

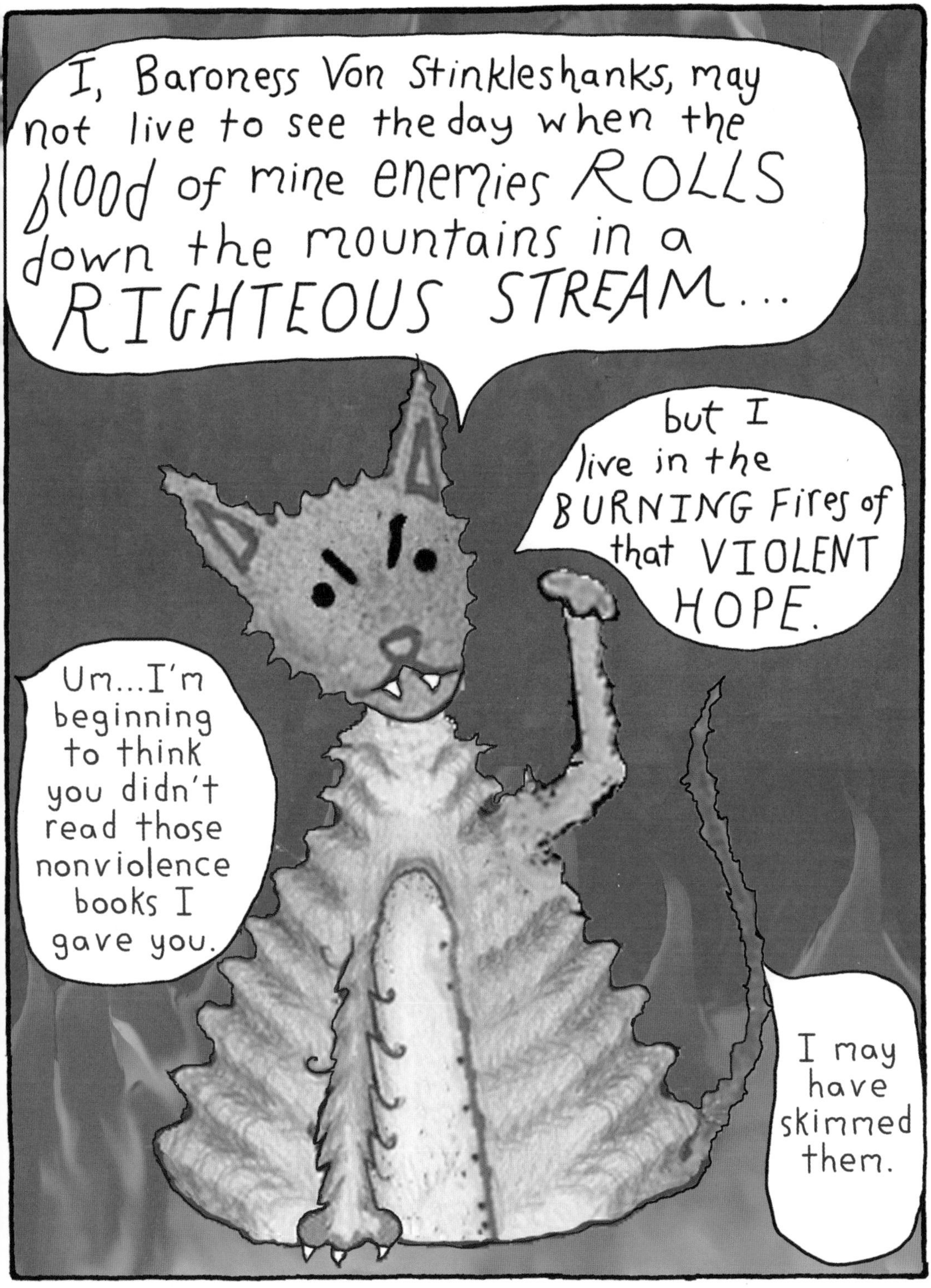
I, Baroness Von Stinkleshanks, may not live to see the day when the blood of mine enemies ROLLS down the mountains in a RIGHTEOUS STREAM...
but I live in the BURNING Fires of that VIOLENT HOPE.
Um...I'm beginning to think you didn't read those nonviolence books I gave you.
I may have skimmed them.

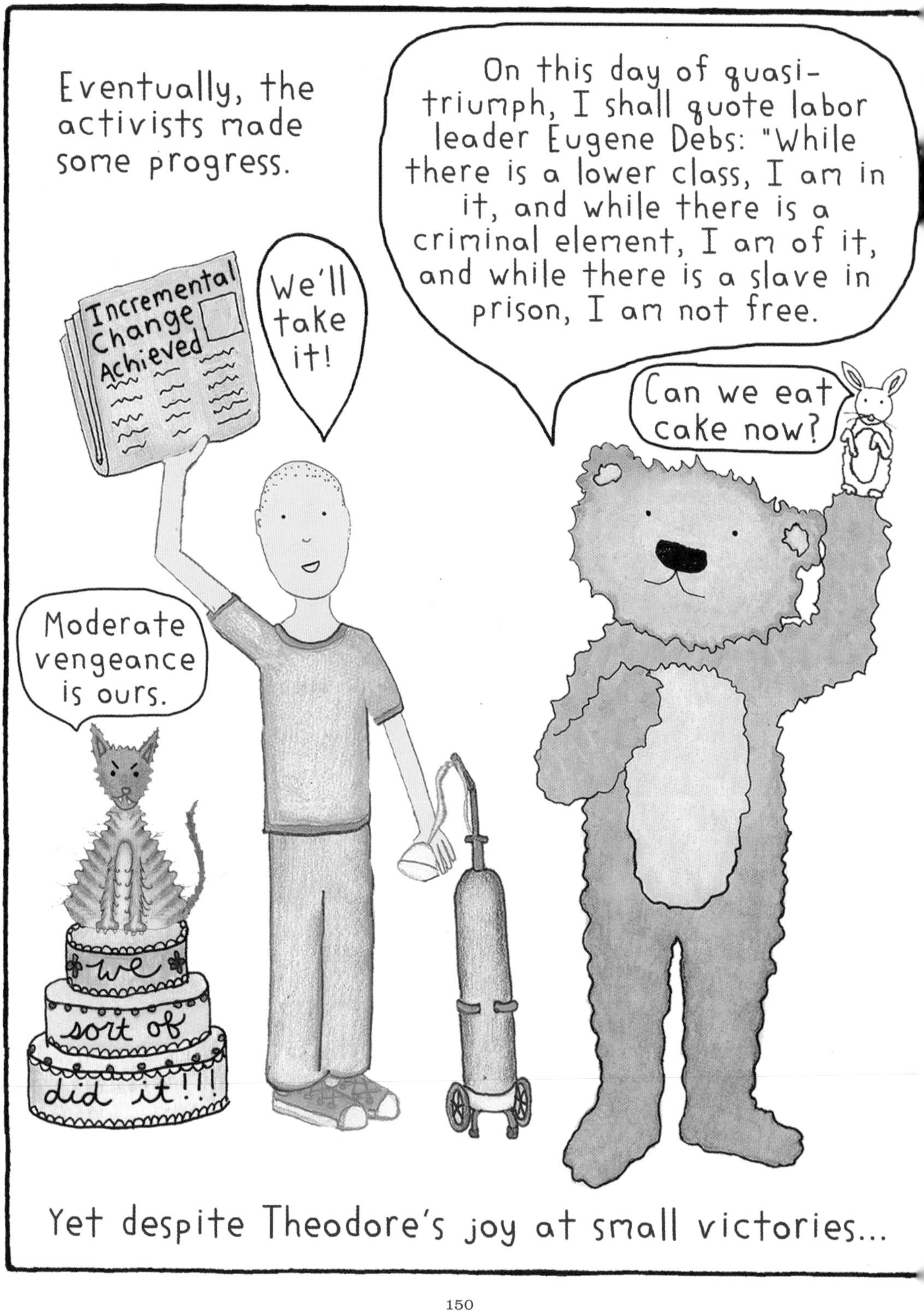
Eventually, the activists made some progress.
On this day of quasi-triumph, I shall quote labor leader Eugene Debs: "While there is a lower class, I am in it, and while there is a criminal element, I am of it, and while there is a slave in prison, I am not free.
Incremental Change Achieved
We'll take it!
Can we eat cake now?
Moderate vengeance is ours.
we sort of did it!!!
Yet despite Theodore's joy at small victories...

and despite his cocktail of meds and wheelhouse of coping mechanisms...

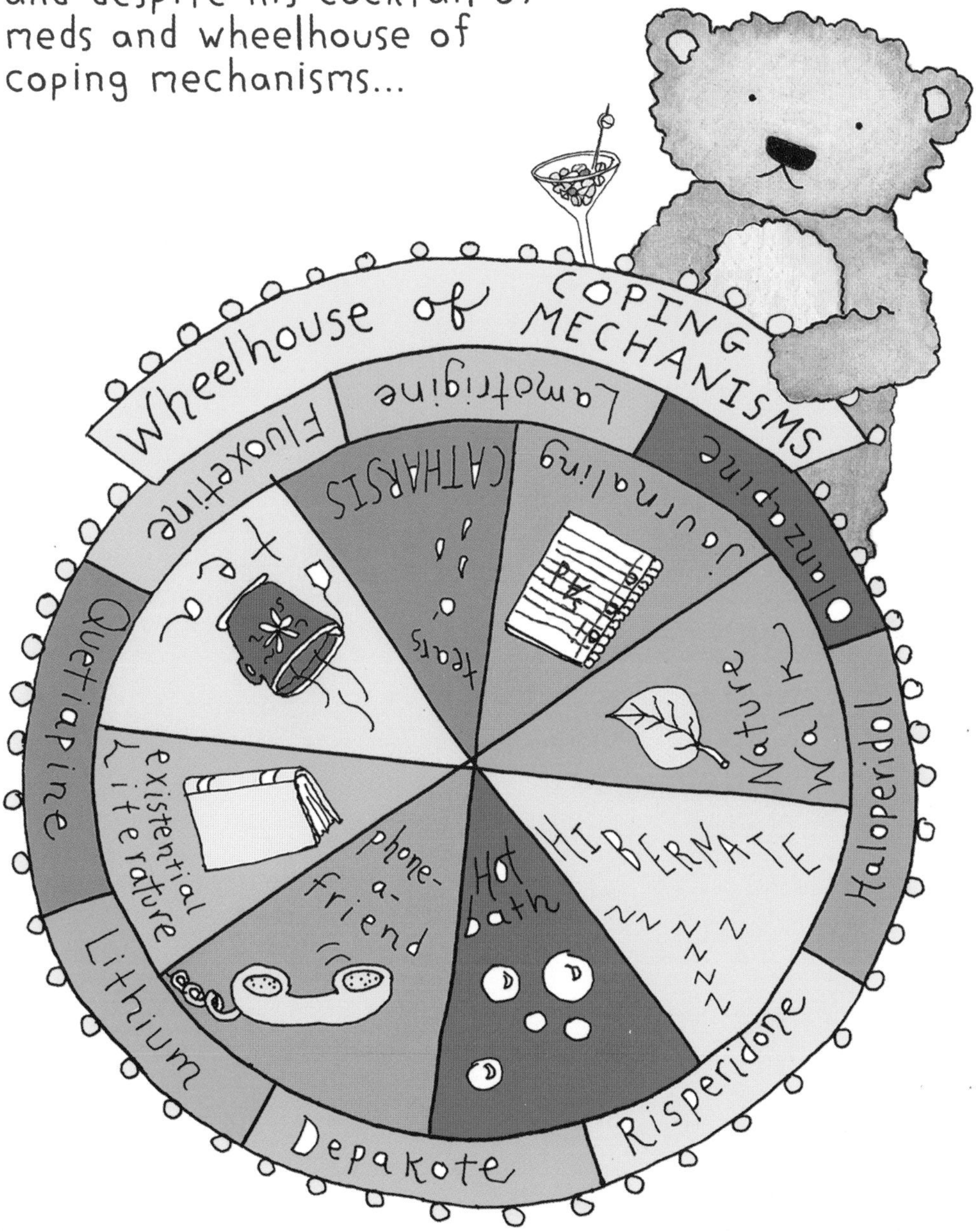
Wheelhouse of COPING MECHANISMS
Lamotrigine
Fluoxetine
Lanzapine
Quetiapine
Haloperidol
Lithium
Depakote
Risperidone
CATHARSIS
tears
Journaling
Nature Walk
HIBERNATE
ZZZZZZZ
Hot bath
phone-a-friend
existential Literature

the mood trouble resurfaced.

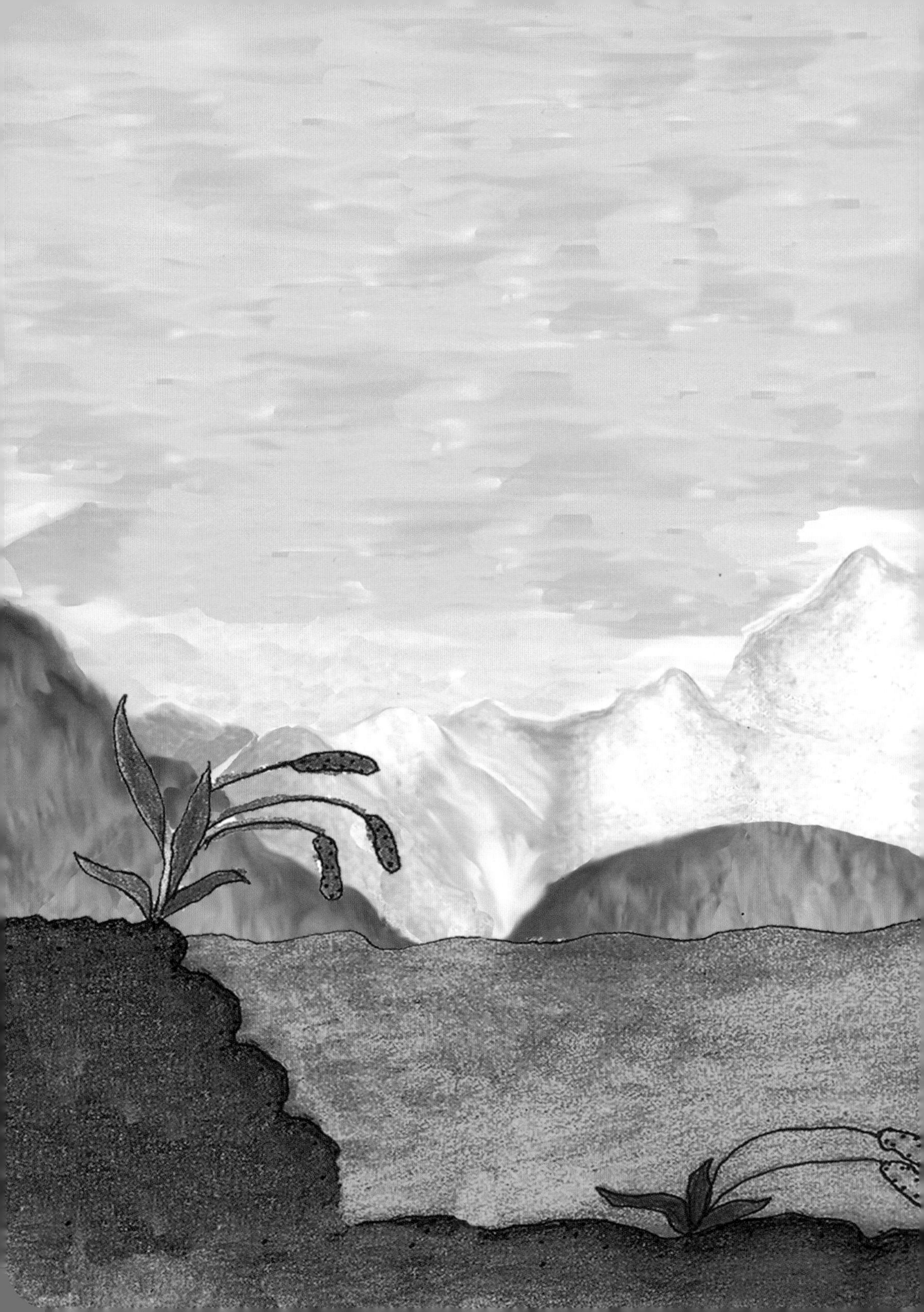

chapter six:

The Slough of Despond

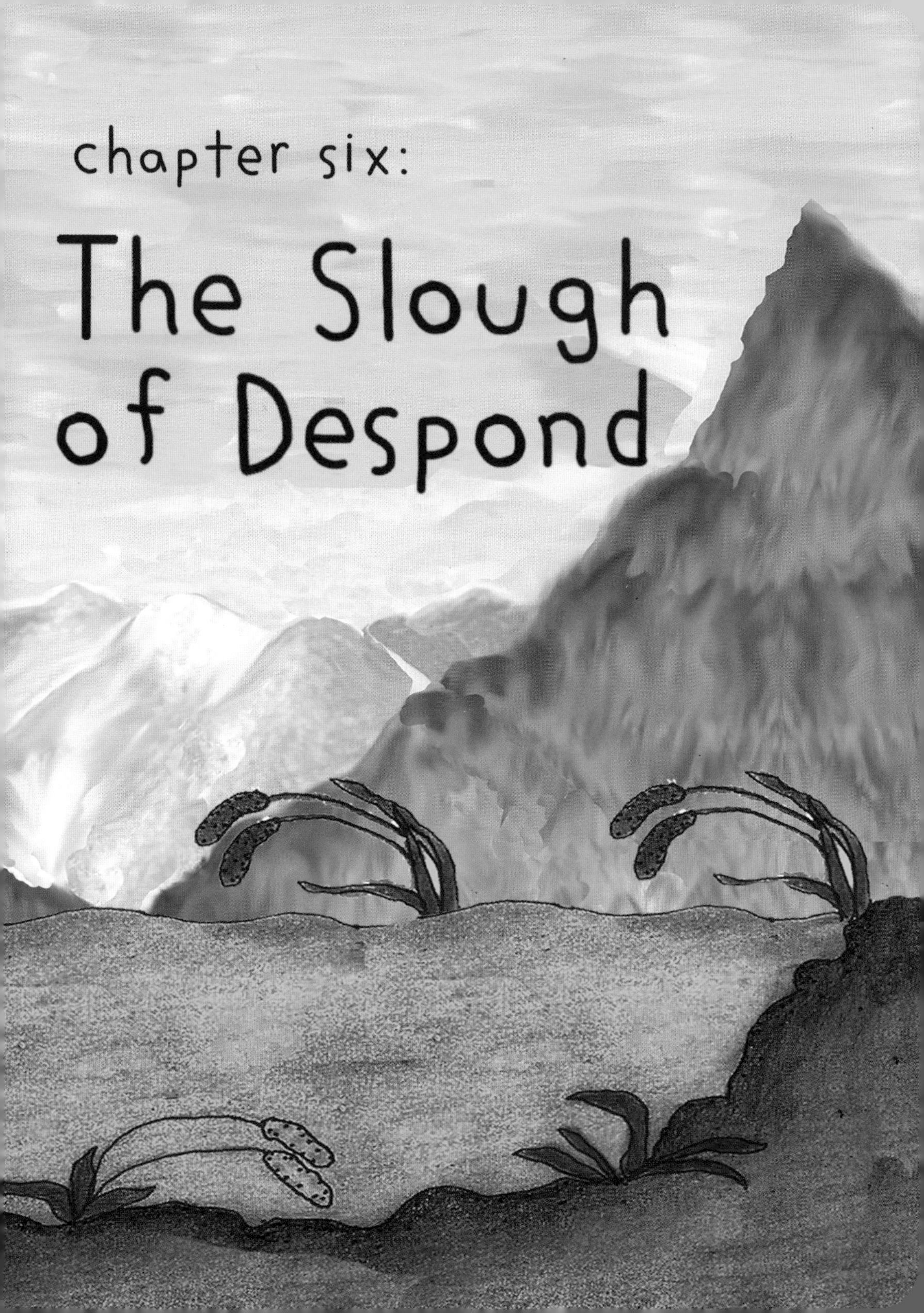

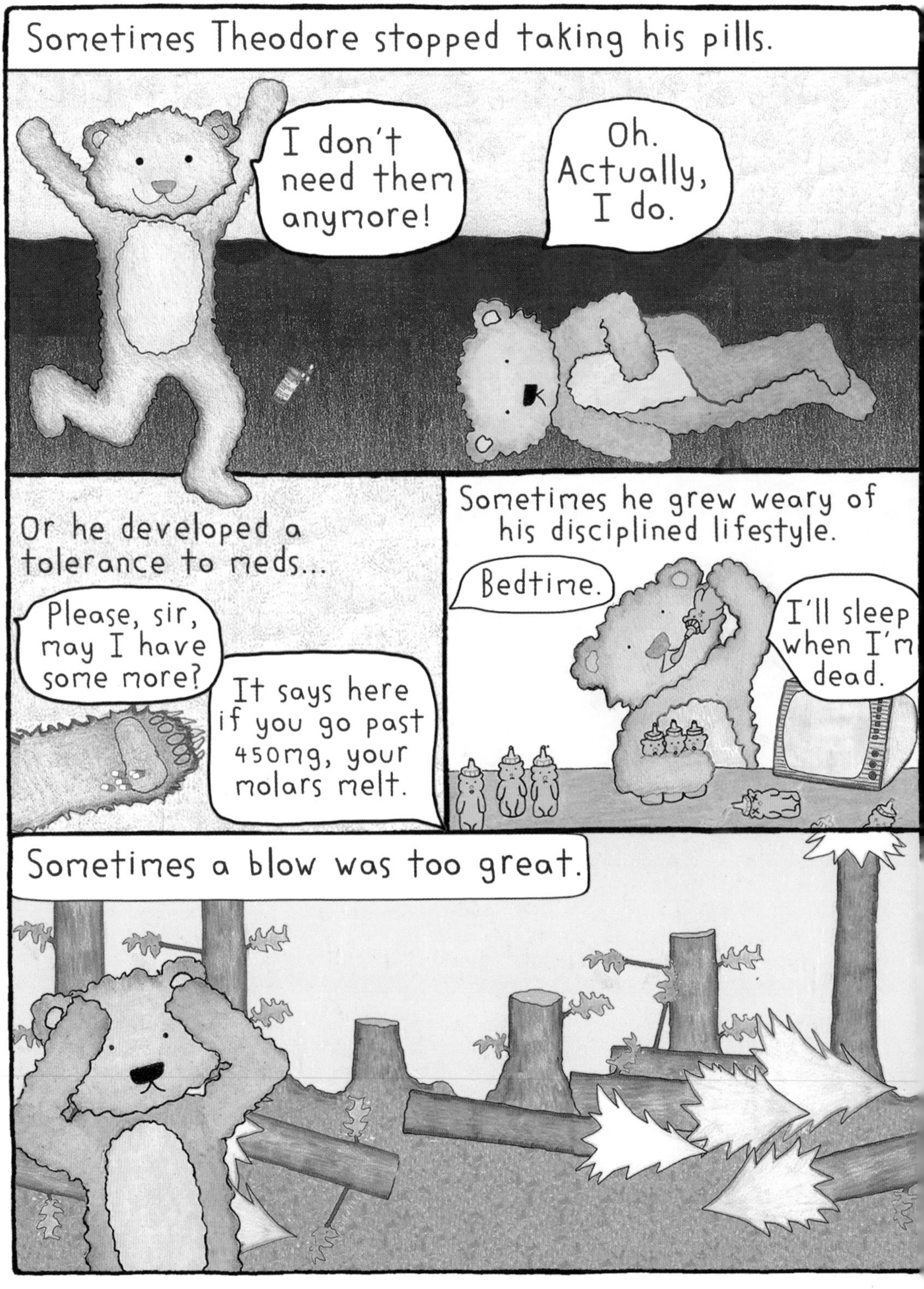
Sometimes Theodore stopped taking his pills.
I don't need them anymore!
Oh. Actually, I do.
Or he developed a tolerance to meds...
Please, sir, may I have some more?
It says here if you go past 450mg, your molars melt.
Sometimes he grew weary of his disciplined lifestyle.
Bedtime.
I'll sleep when I'm dead.
Sometimes a blow was too great.

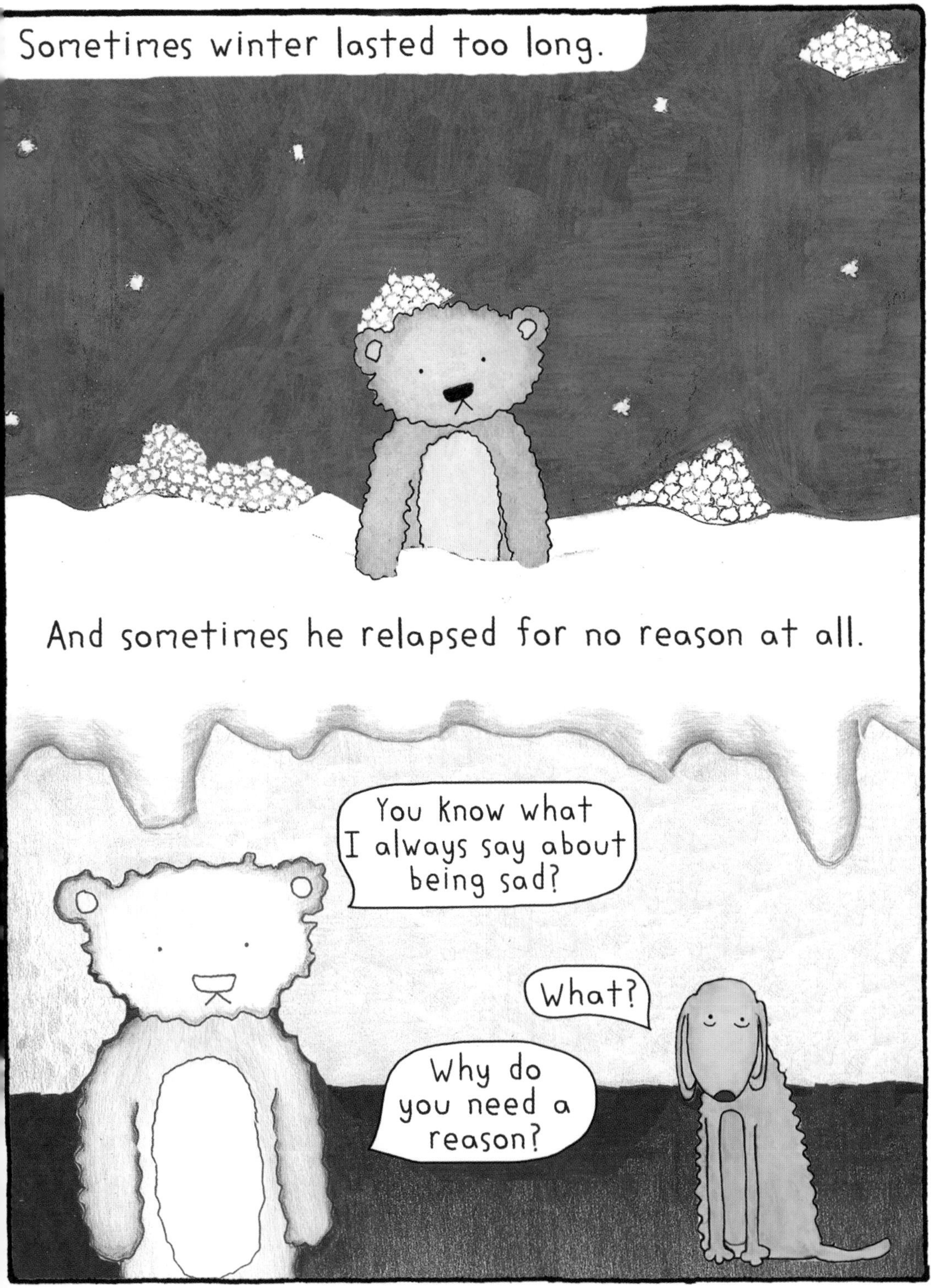
Sometimes winter lasted too long.
And sometimes he relapsed for no reason at all.
You know what I always say about being sad?
What?
Why do you need a reason?

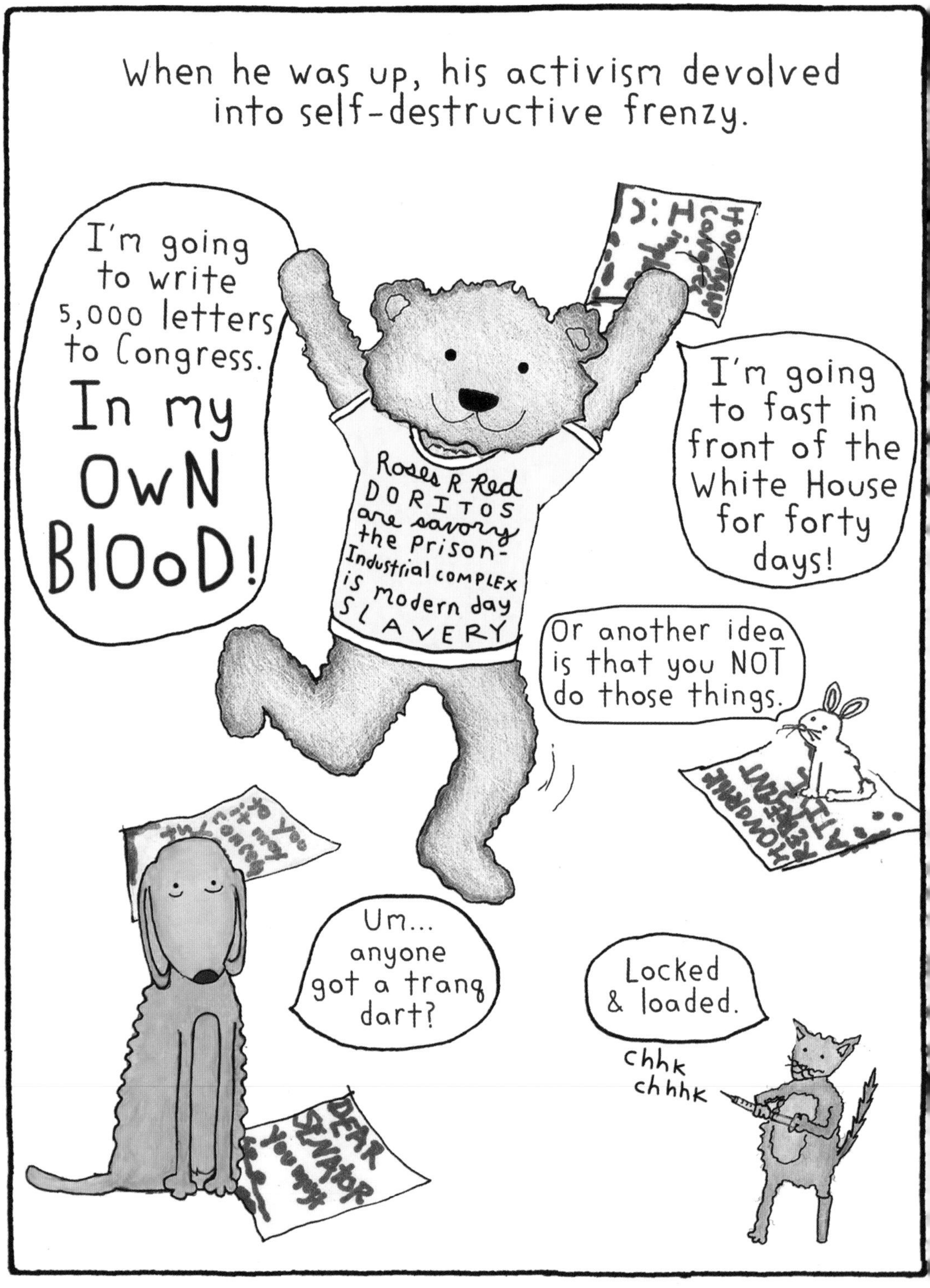
When he was up, his activism devolved into self-destructive frenzy.
I'm going to write 5,000 letters to Congress. In my OWN BlOoD!
Roses R Red DORITOS are savory the prison-Industrial COMPLEX is modern day SLAVERY
I'm going to fast in front of the White House for forty days!
Or another idea is that you NOT do those things.
Um... anyone got a tranq dart?
Locked & loaded.
chhk chhhk
DEAR SENATOR

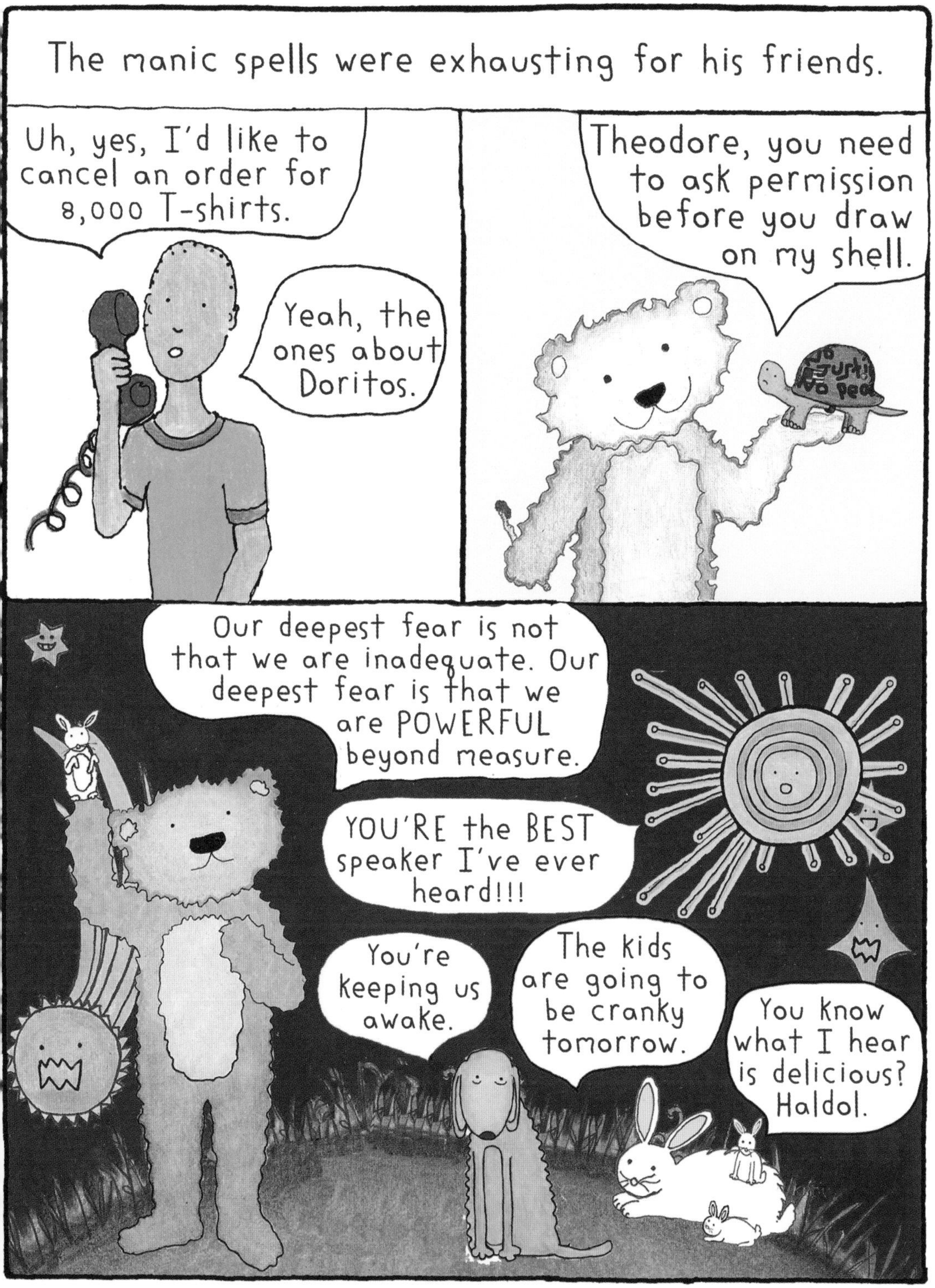
The manic spells were exhausting for his friends.
Uh, yes, I'd like to cancel an order for 8,000 T-shirts.
Yeah, the ones about Doritos.
Theodore, you need to ask permission before you draw on my shell.
Our deepest fear is not that we are inadequate. Our deepest fear is that we are POWERFUL beyond measure.
YOU'RE the BEST speaker I've ever heard!!!
You're keeping us awake.
The kids are going to be cranky tomorrow.
You know what I hear is delicious? Haldol.

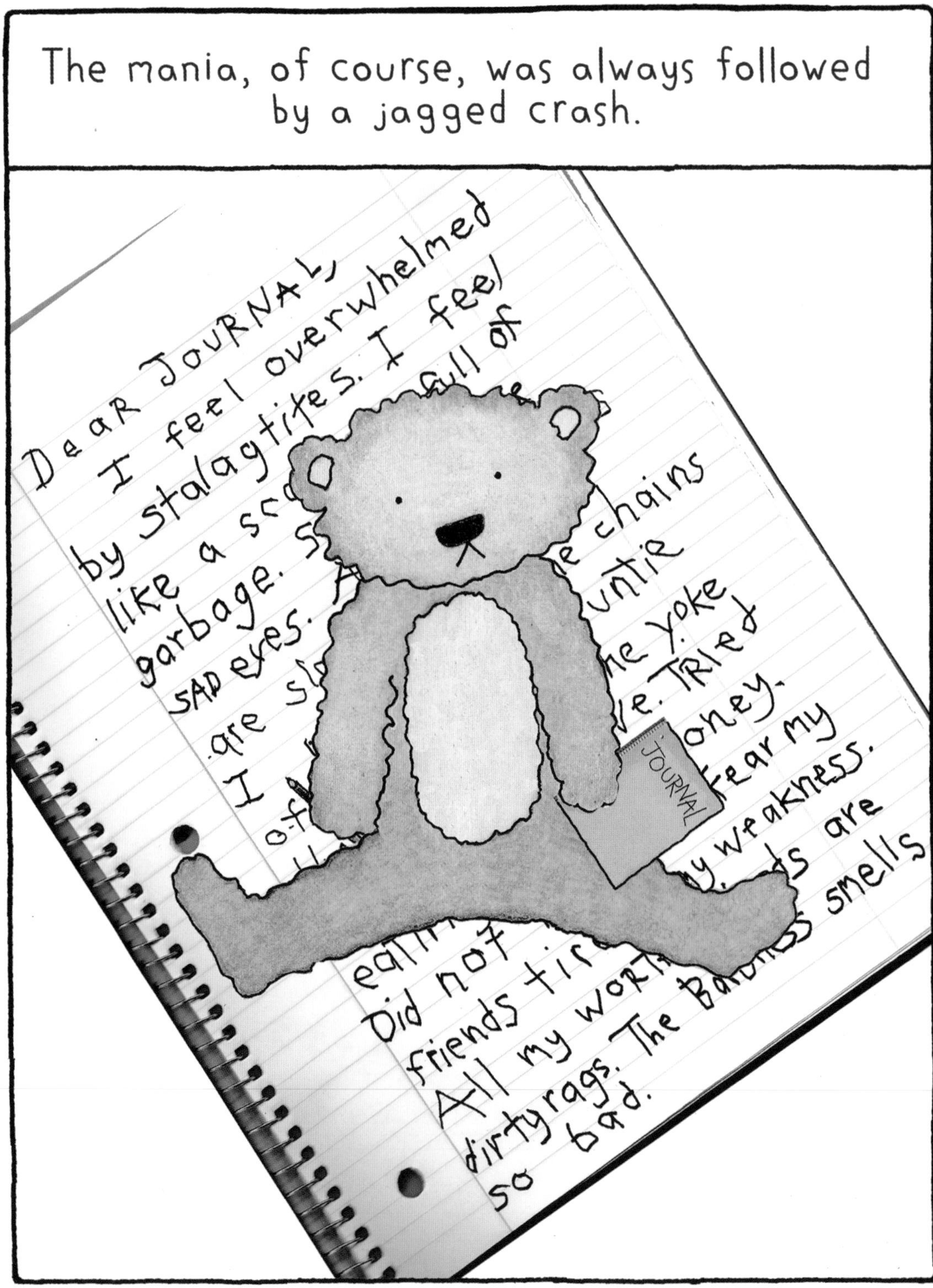
The mania, of course, was always followed by a jagged crash.
Dear Journal,
I feel overwhelmed
by stalagtites. I feel
like a
garbage.
SAD eyes.
are
I
chains
untie
the yoke
Tried
oney.
fear my
weakness.
are
smells
Did not
friends
All my
dirty rags. The
so bad.
JOURNAL

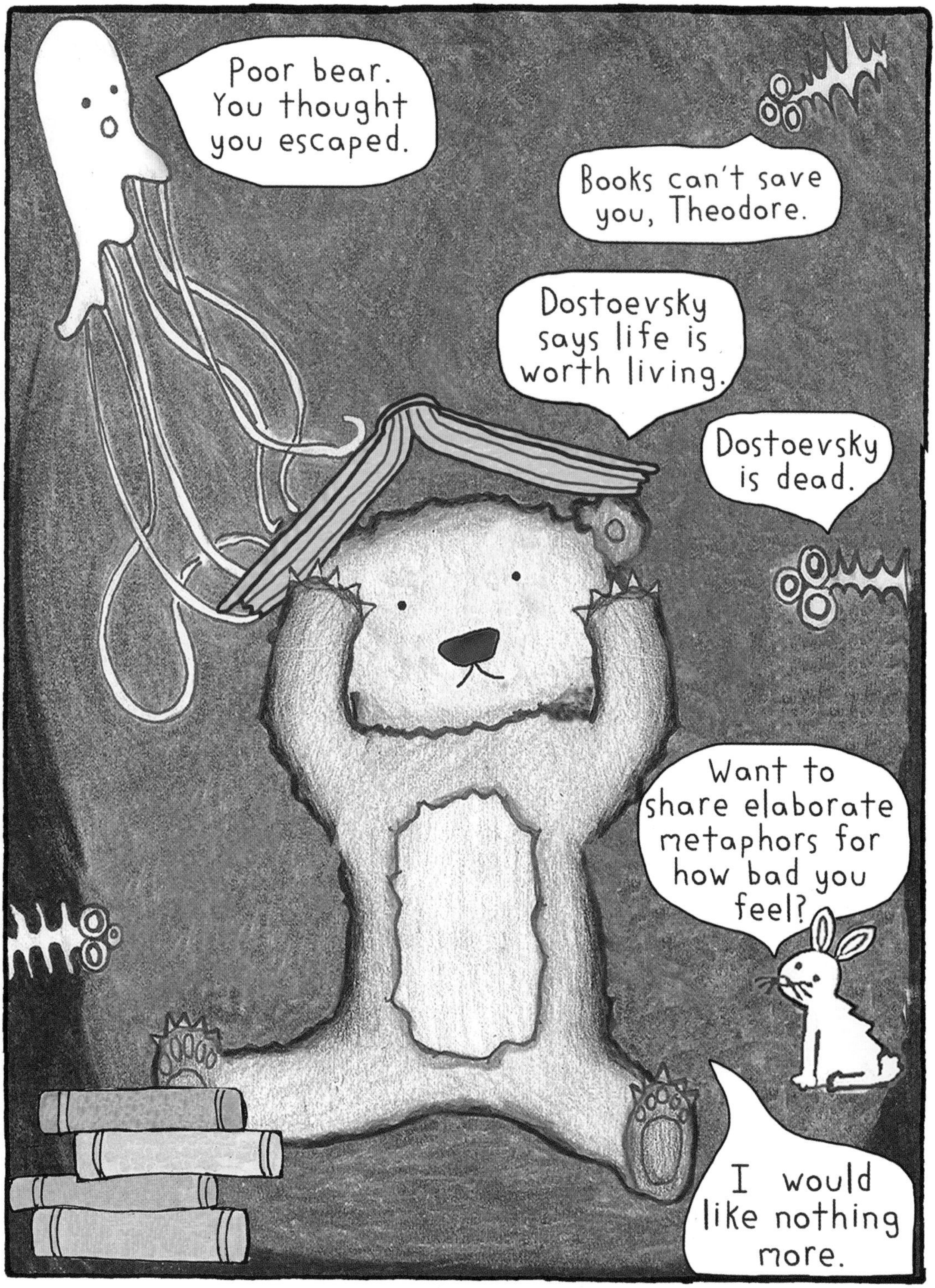
Poor bear. You thought you escaped.
Books can't save you, Theodore.
Dostoevsky says life is worth living.
Dostoevsky is dead.
Want to share elaborate metaphors for how bad you feel?
I would like nothing more.

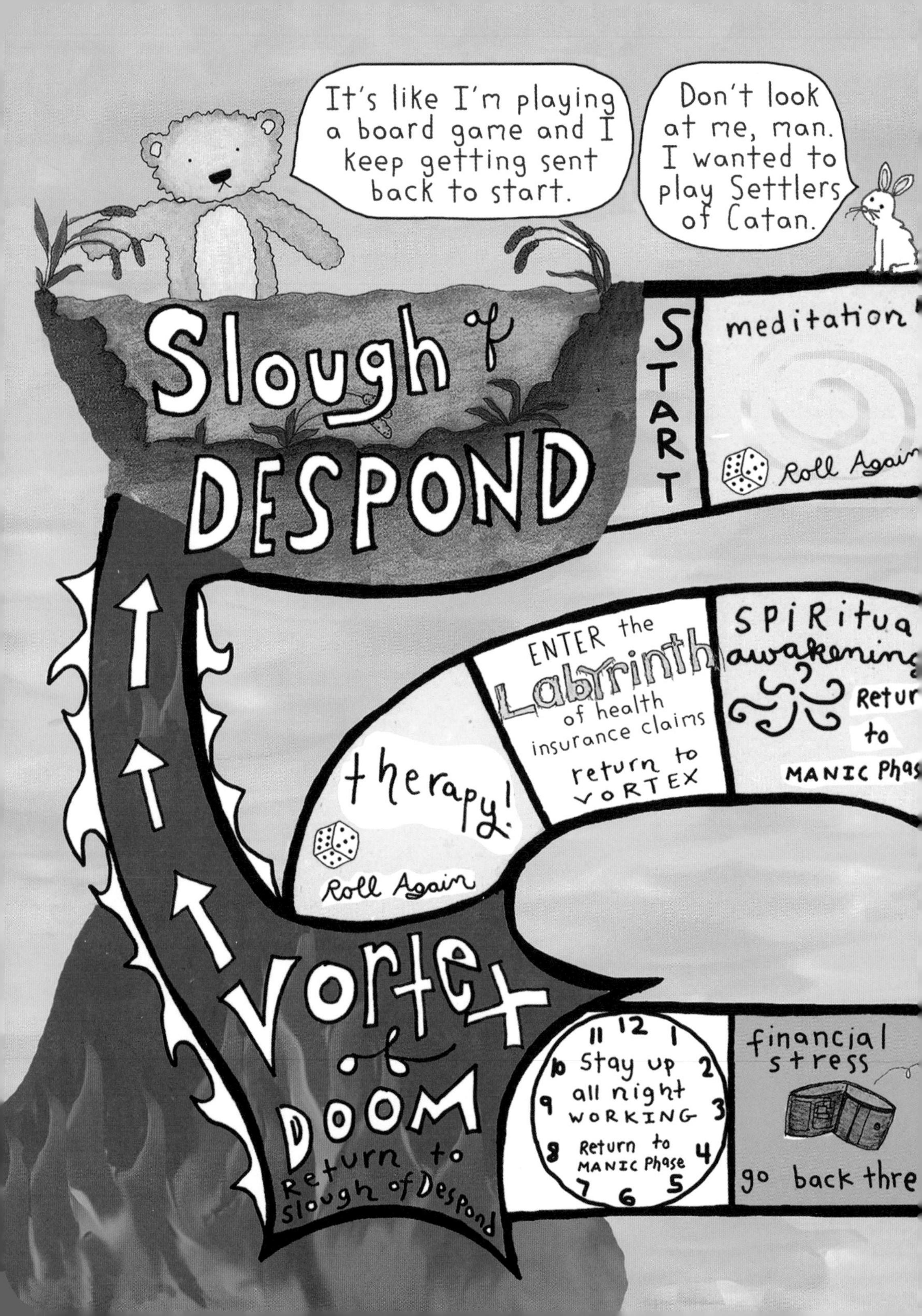

It's like I'm playing a board game and I keep getting sent back to start.
Don't look at me, man. I wanted to play Settlers of Catan.
Slough of DESPOND
START
meditation
Roll Again
SPIRitua awakening
Retur to MANIC Phas
ENTER the Labyrinth of health insurance claims
return to VORTEX
therapy!
Roll Again
Vortex of DOOM
Return to Slough of Despond
Stay up all night WORKING
Return to MANIC Phase
financial stress
go back thre

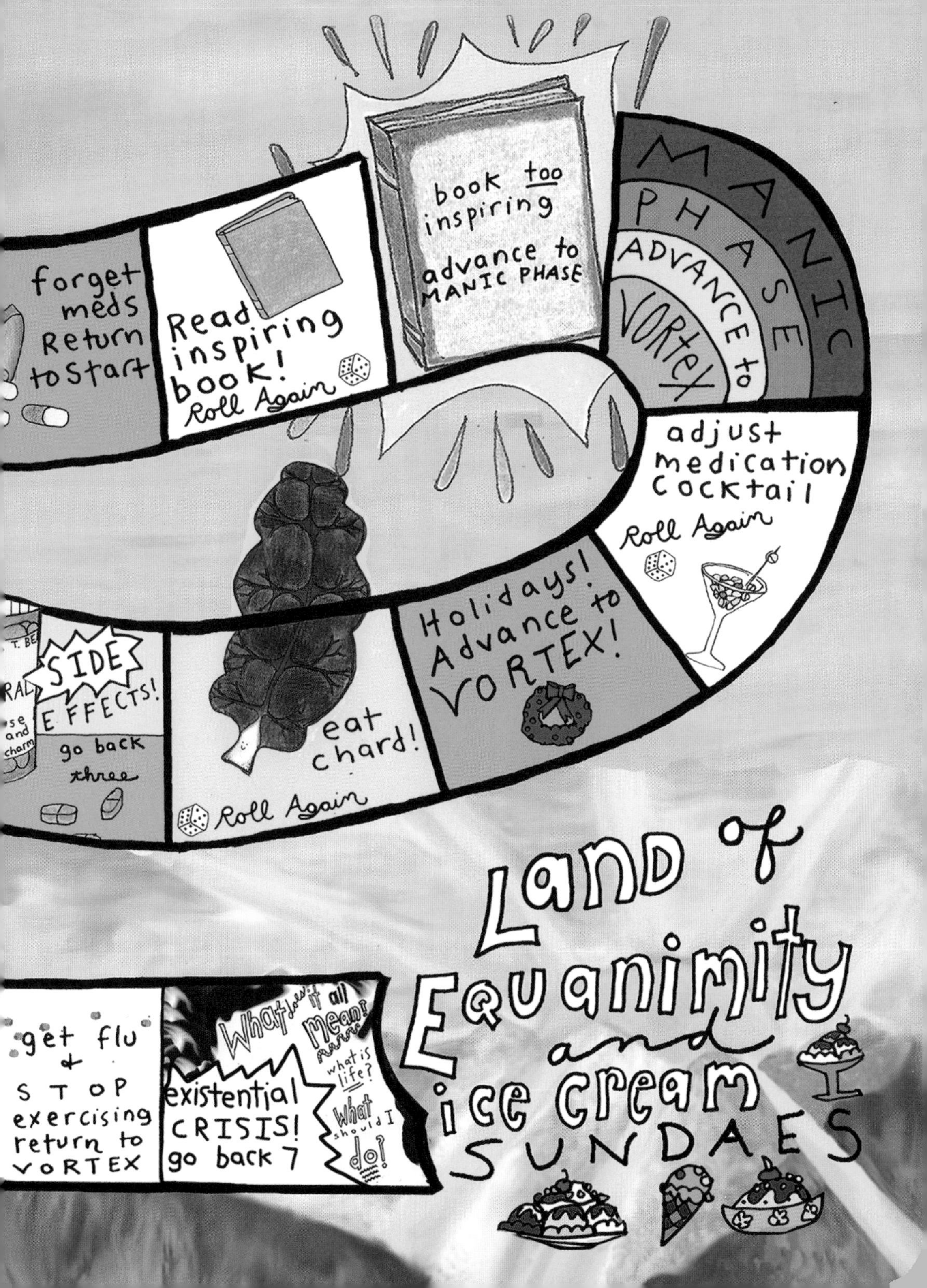

forget meds Return to Start
Read inspiring book! Roll Again
book too inspiring advance to MANIC PHASE
MANIC PHASE ADVANCE to VORTEX
adjust medication cocktail Roll Again
Holidays! Advance to VORTEX!
eat chard! Roll Again
SIDE EFFECTS! go back three
Land of Equanimity and ice cream SUNDAES
get flu & STOP exercising return to VORTEX
existential CRISIS! go back 7
What does it all mean?
what is life?
What should I do?

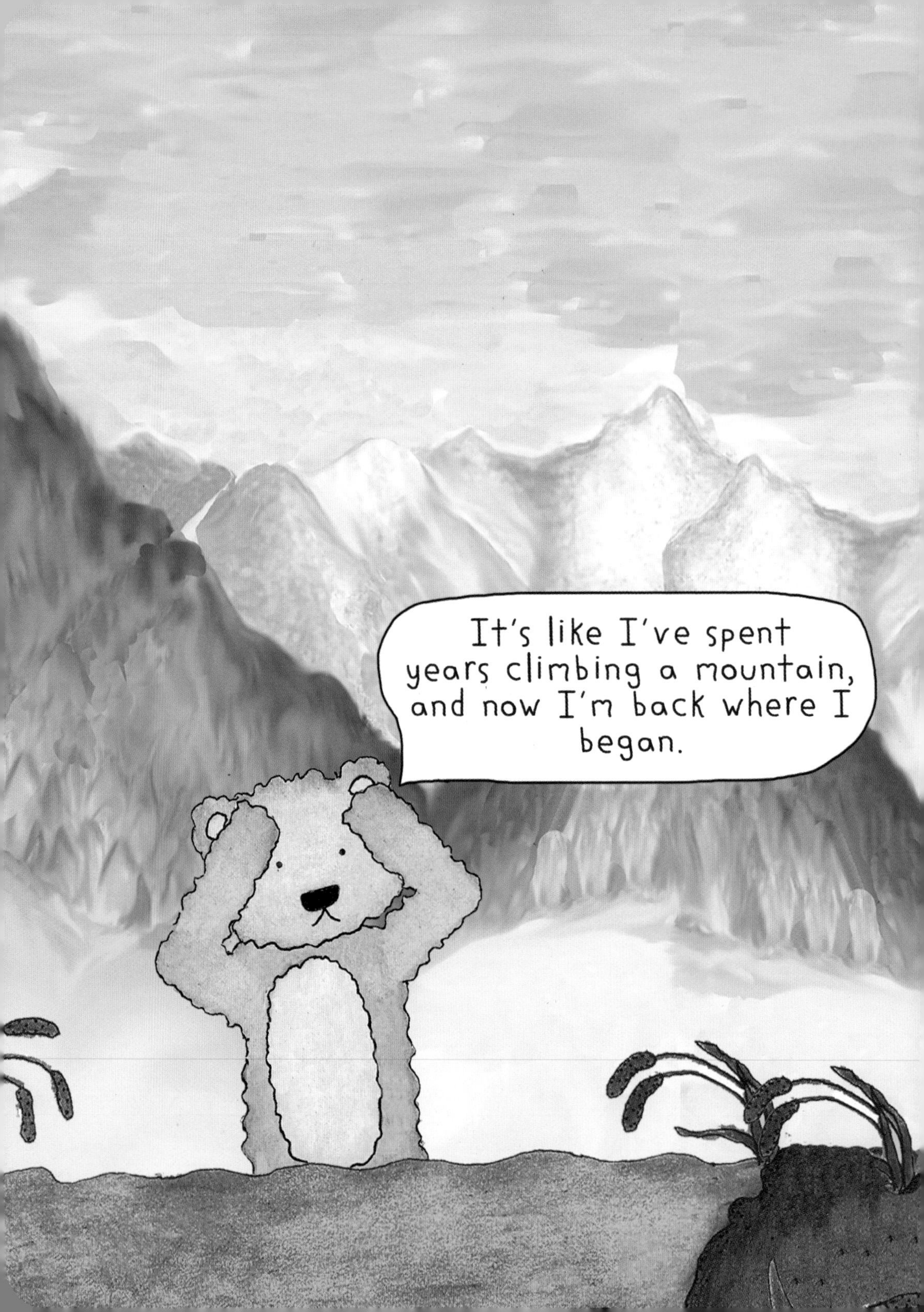
It's like I've spent years climbing a mountain, and now I'm back where I began.

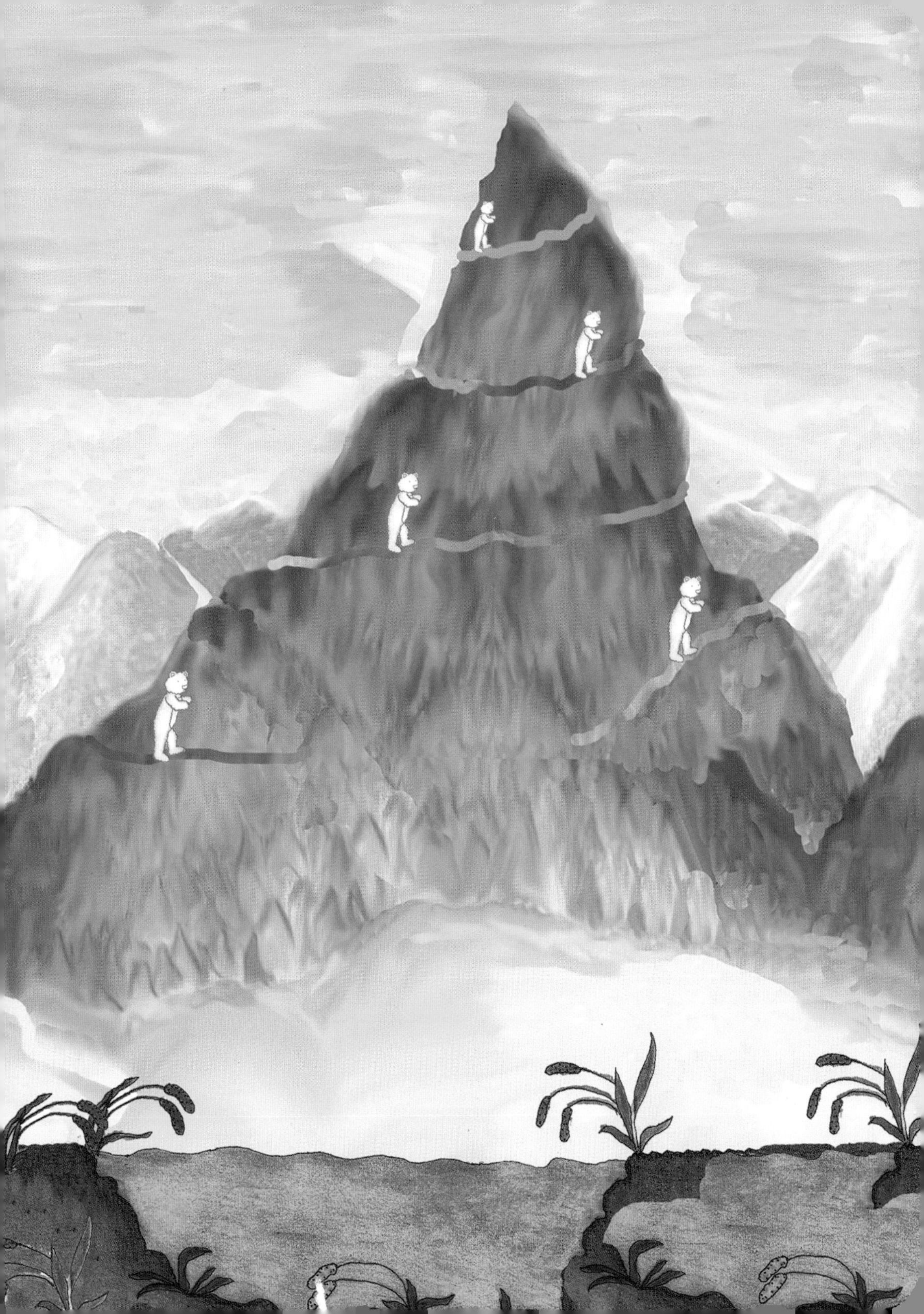

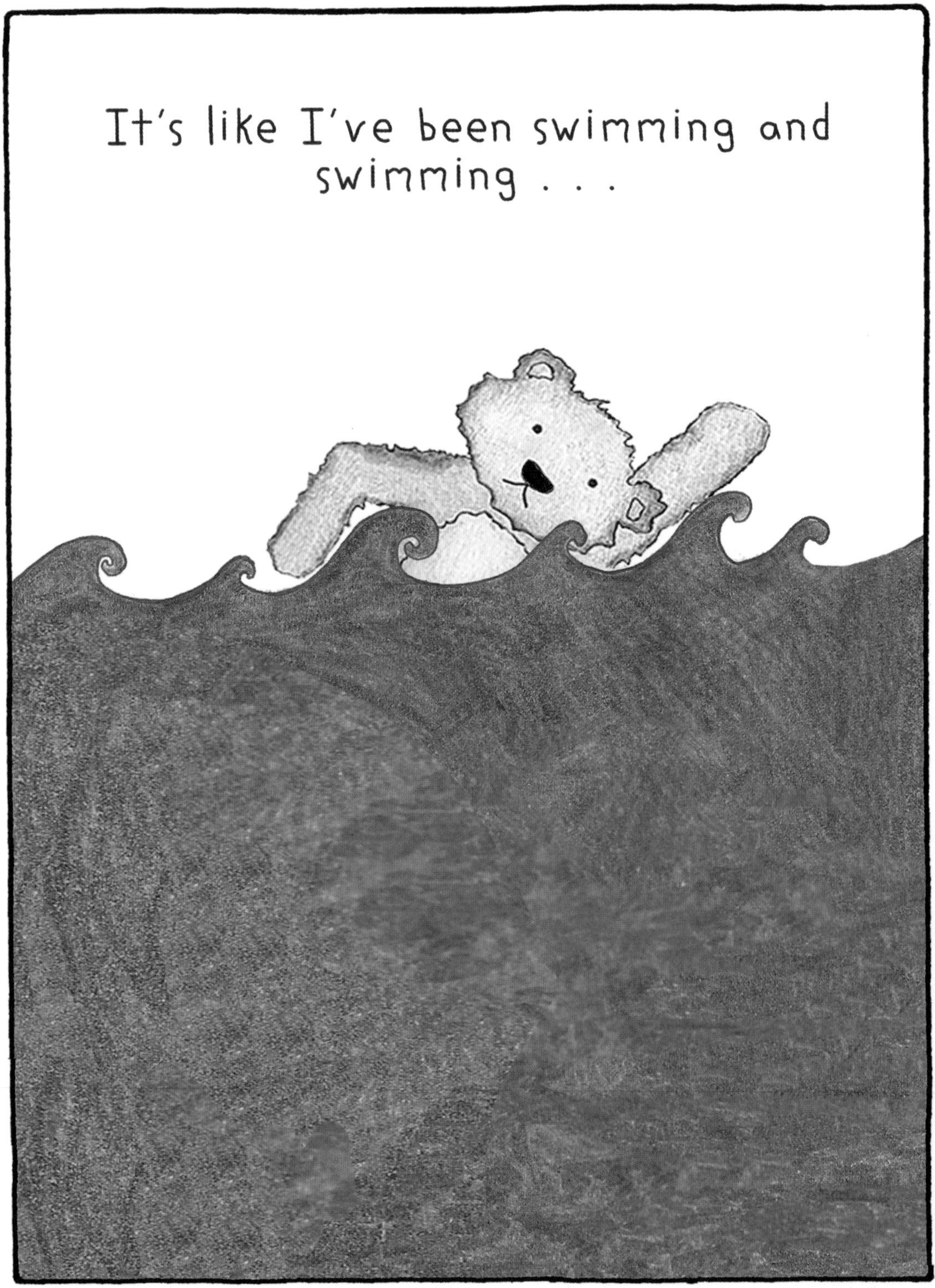
It's like I've been swimming and swimming . . .

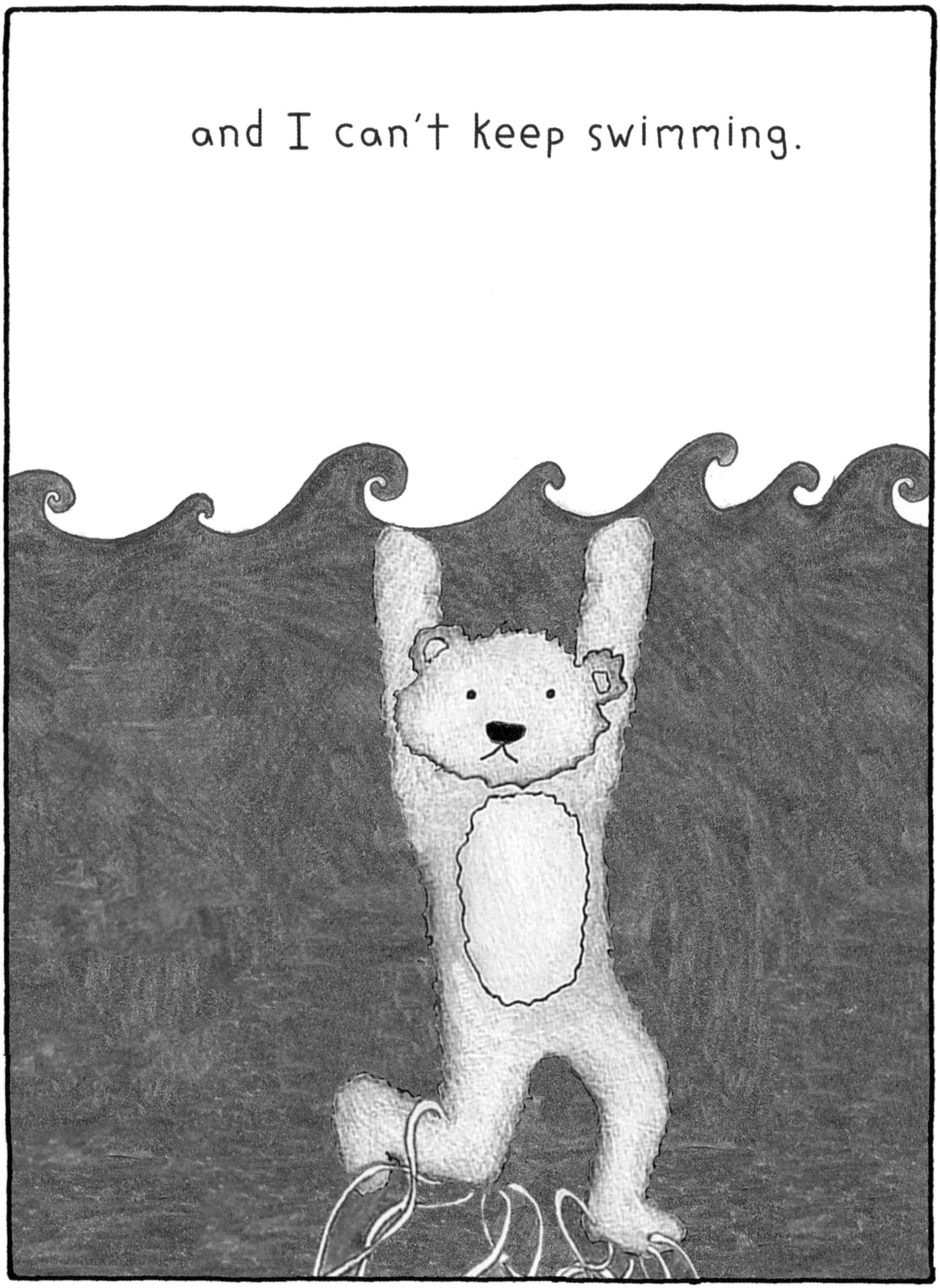
and I can't keep swimming.

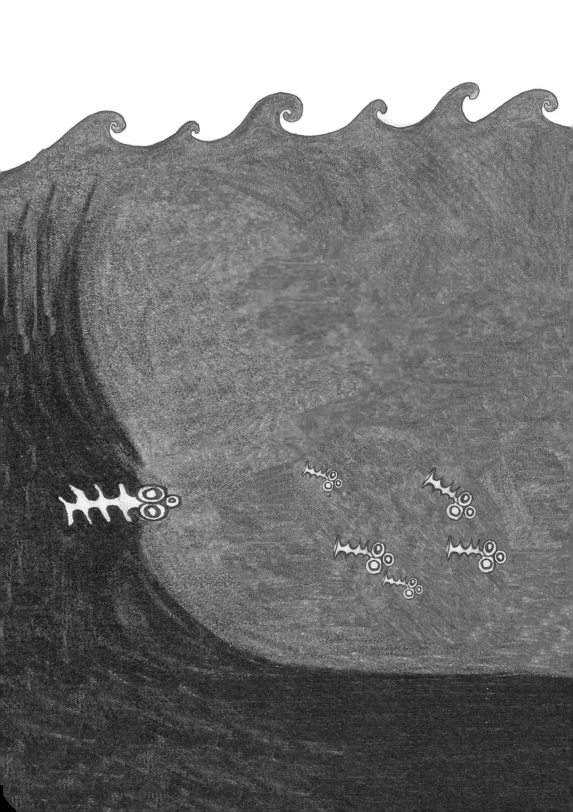

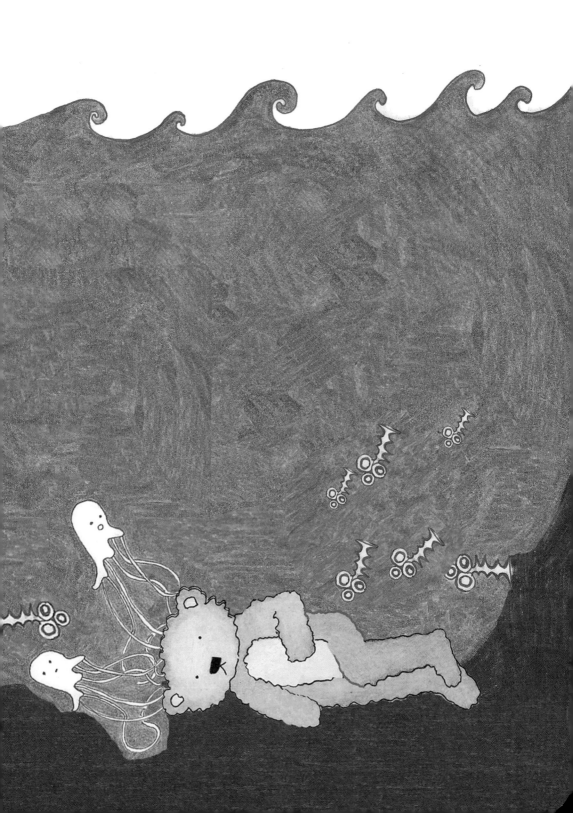

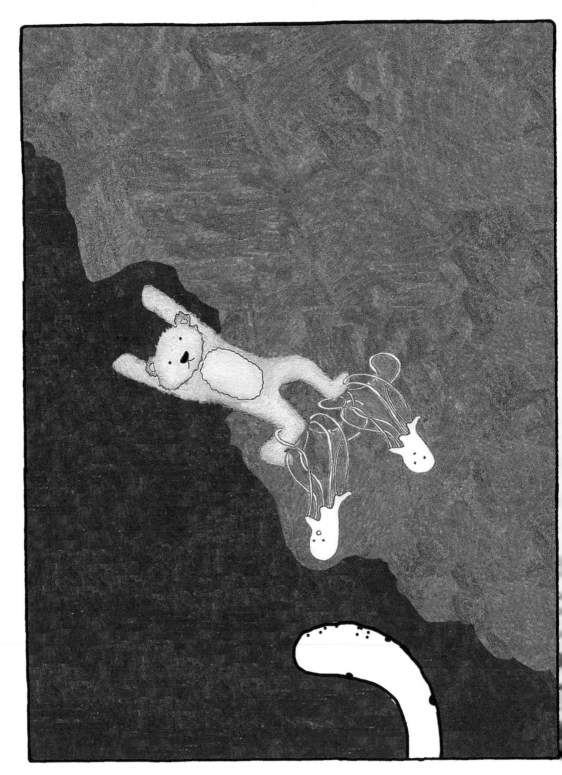

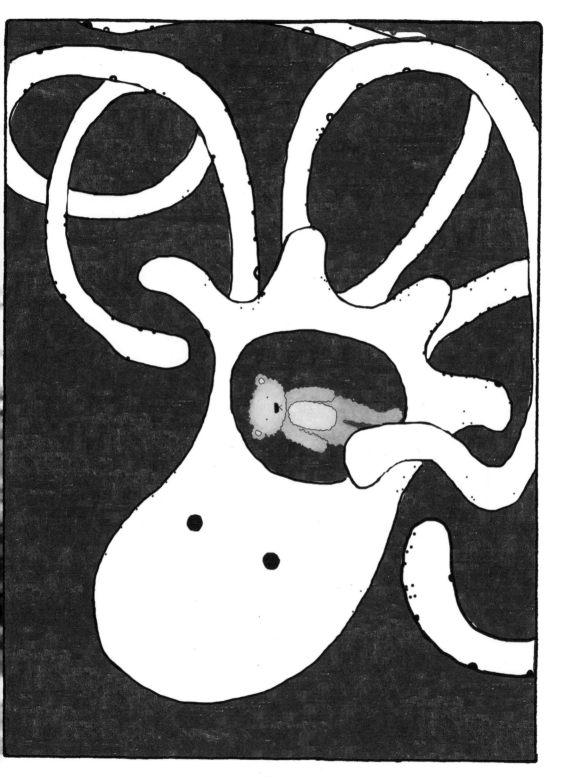

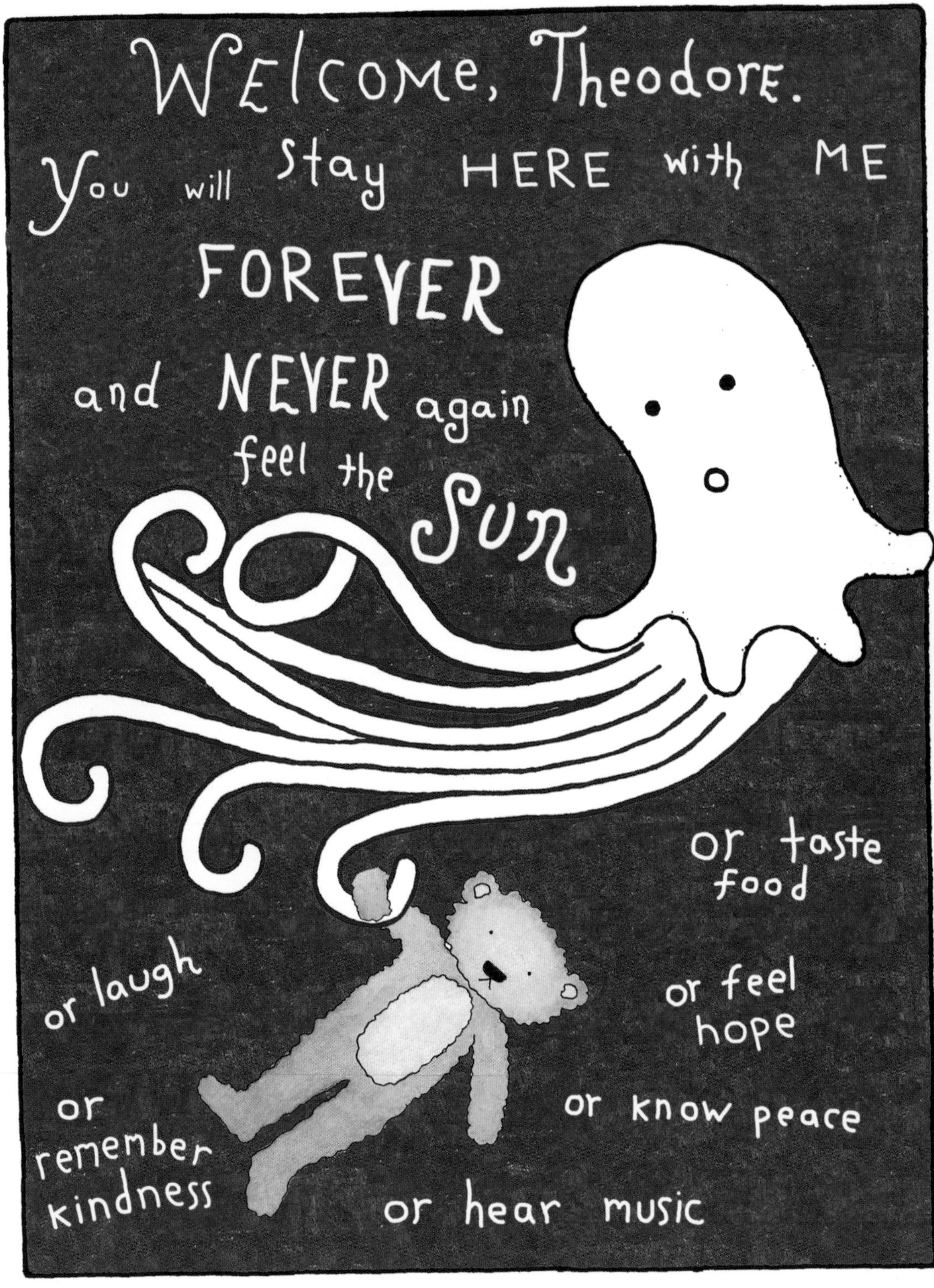
WELCOME, Theodore.
You will stay HERE with ME
FOREVER
and NEVER again
feel the SUN
or taste food
or laugh
or feel hope
or know peace
or remember kindness
or hear music

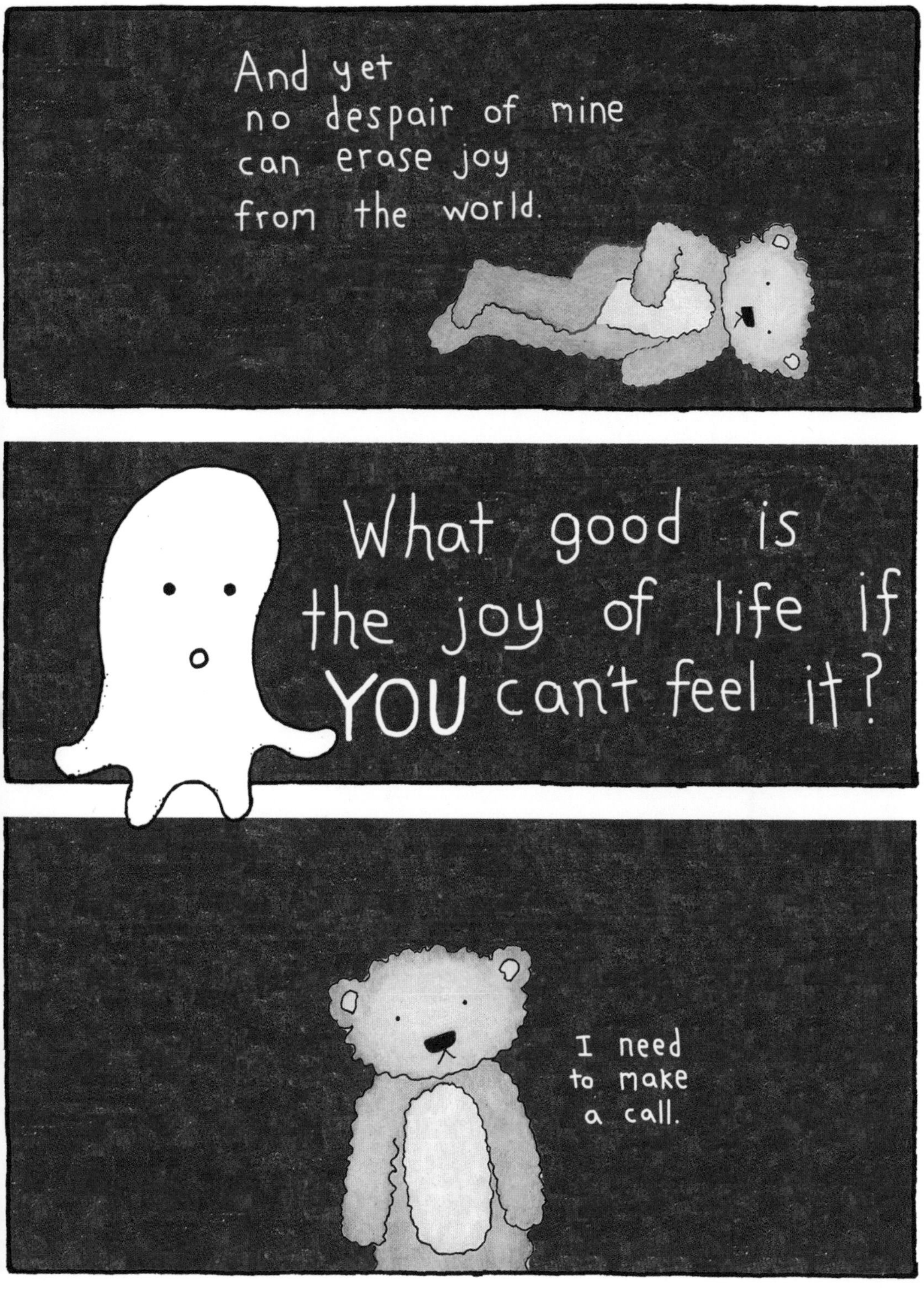

And yet
no despair of mine
can erase joy
from the world.

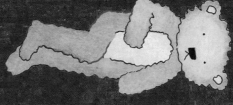

What good is
the joy of life if
YOU can't feel it?

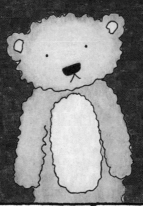

I need
to make
a call.

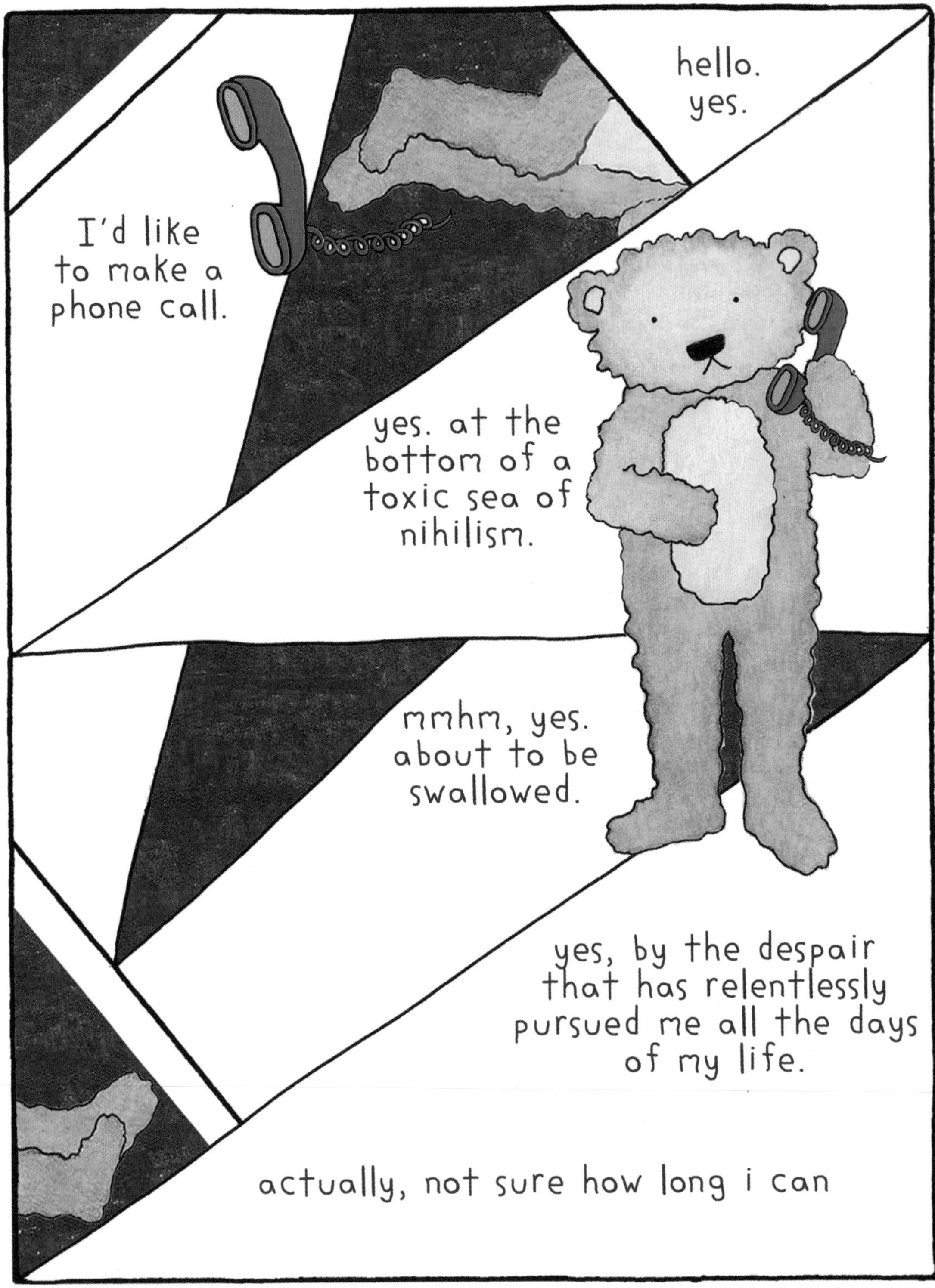
hello.
yes.
I'd like to make a phone call.
yes. at the bottom of a toxic sea of nihilism.
mmhm, yes. about to be swallowed.
yes, by the despair that has relentlessly pursued me all the days of my life.
actually, not sure how long i can

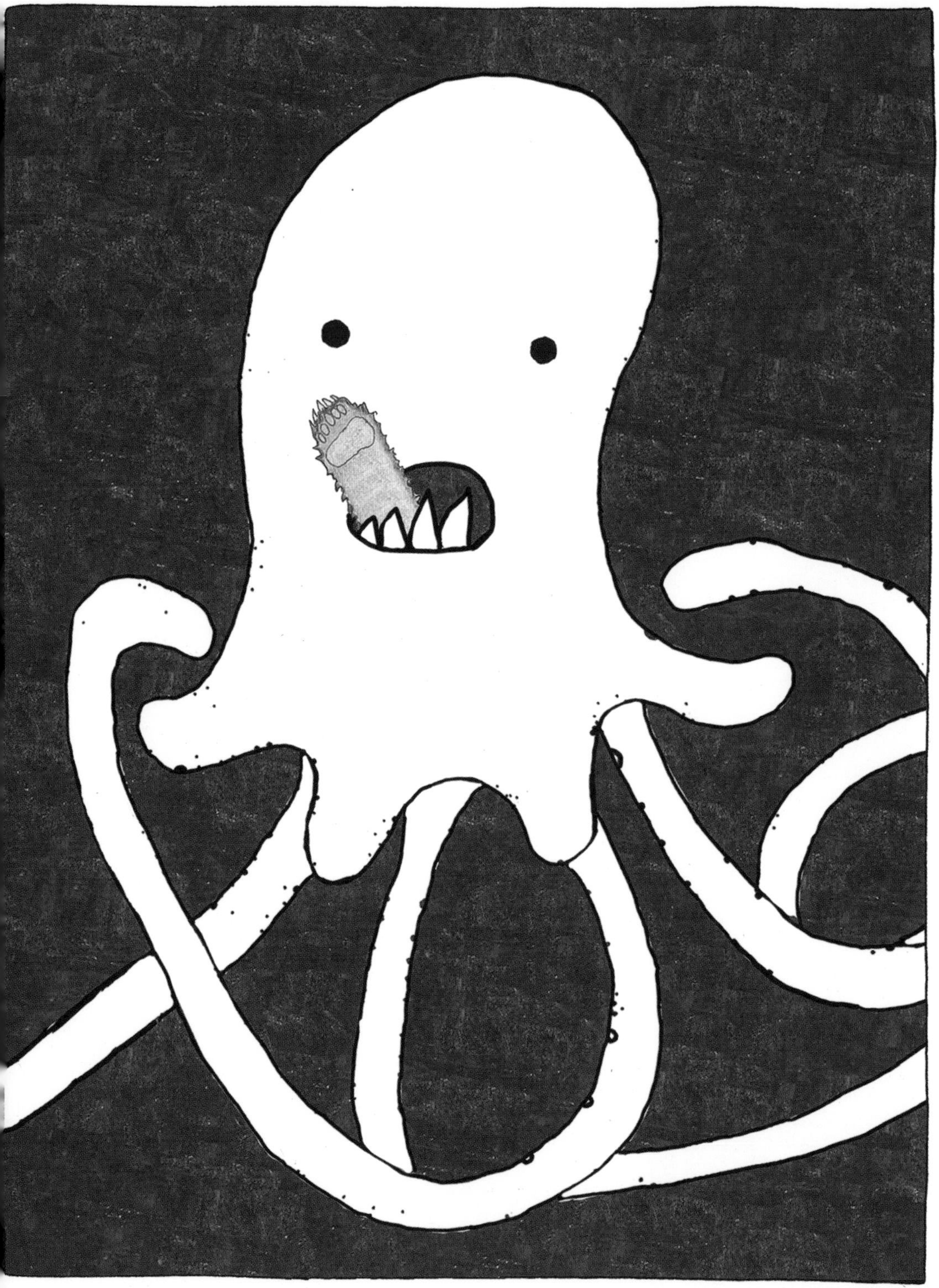

wait

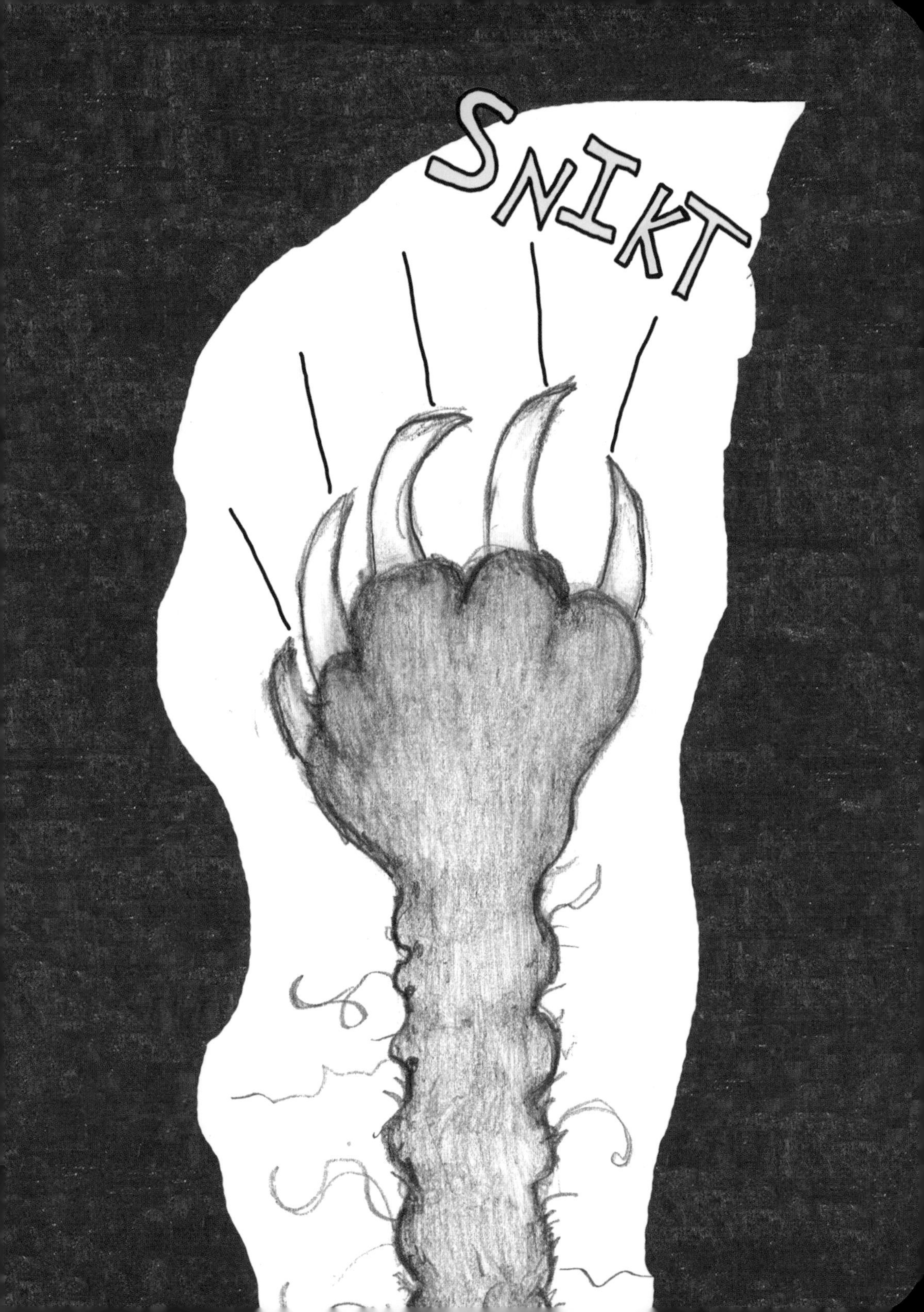
SNIKT

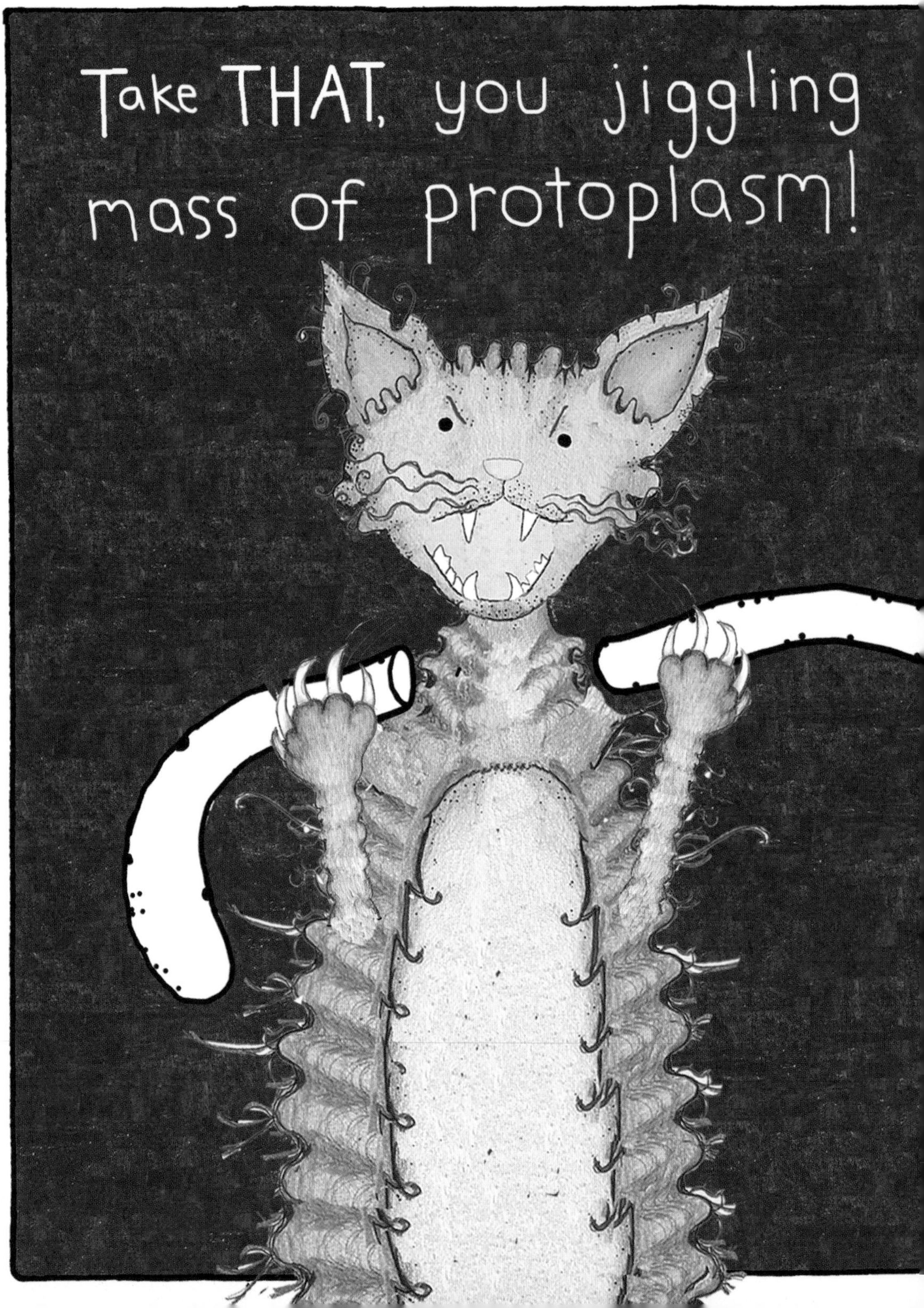
Take THAT, you jiggling mass of protoplasm!

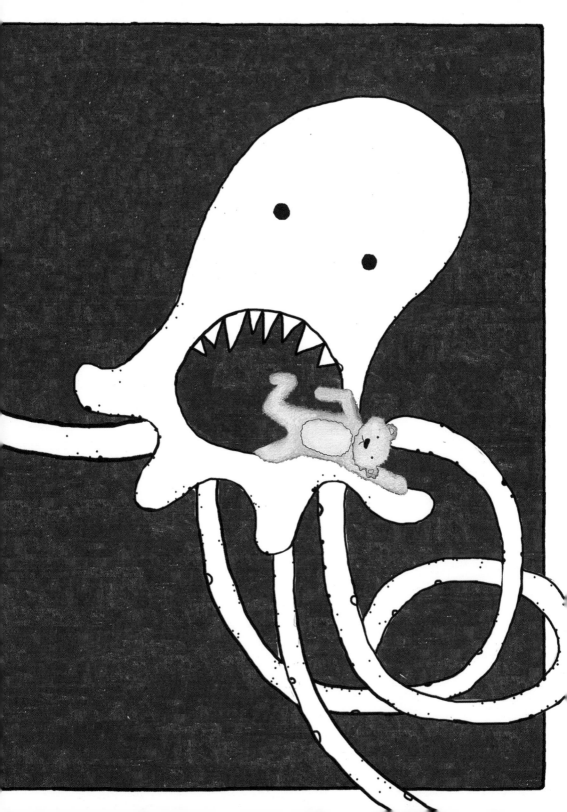

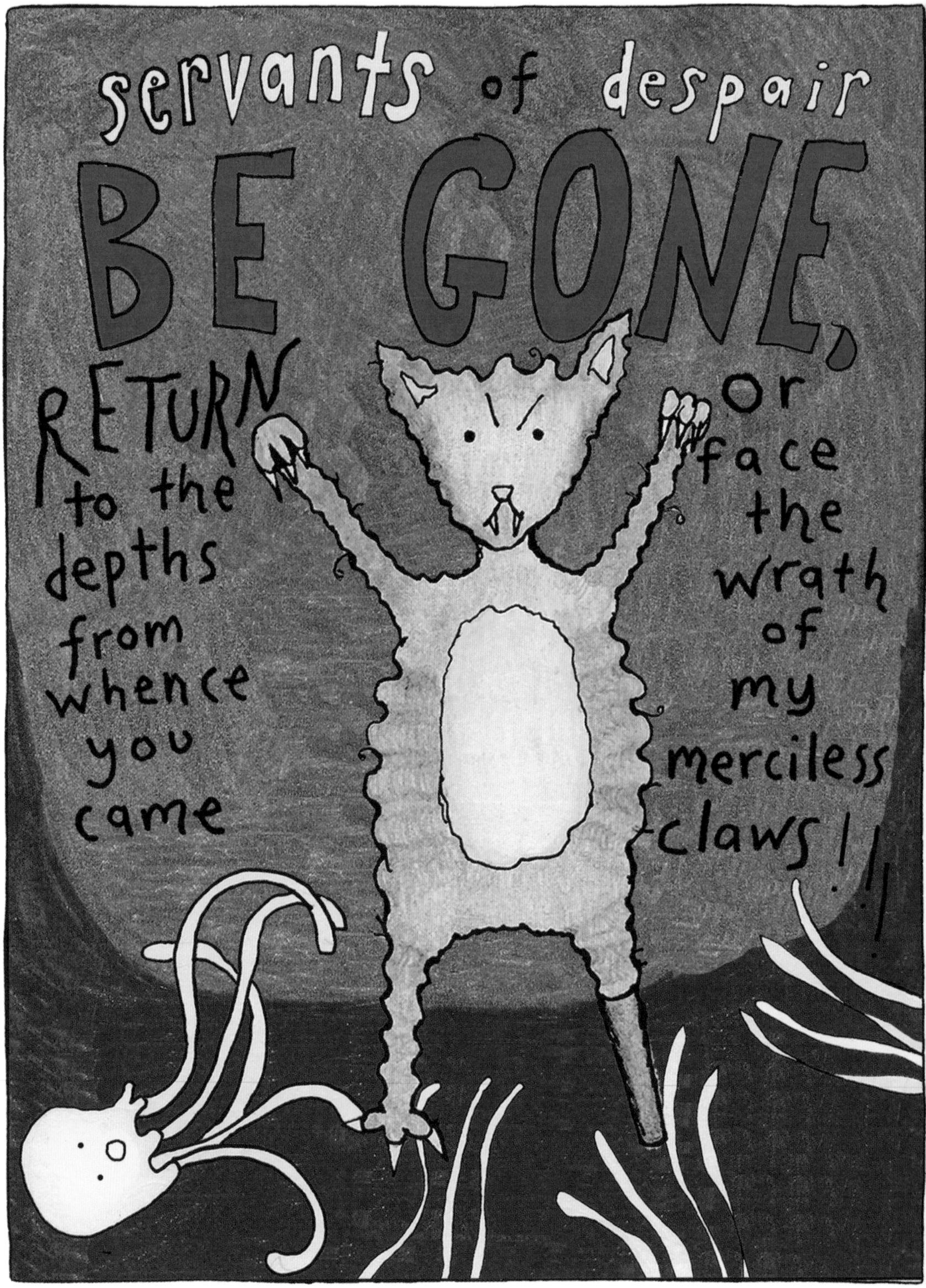
servants of despair
BE GONE,
RETURN to the depths from whence you came
or face the wrath of my merciless claws!!!

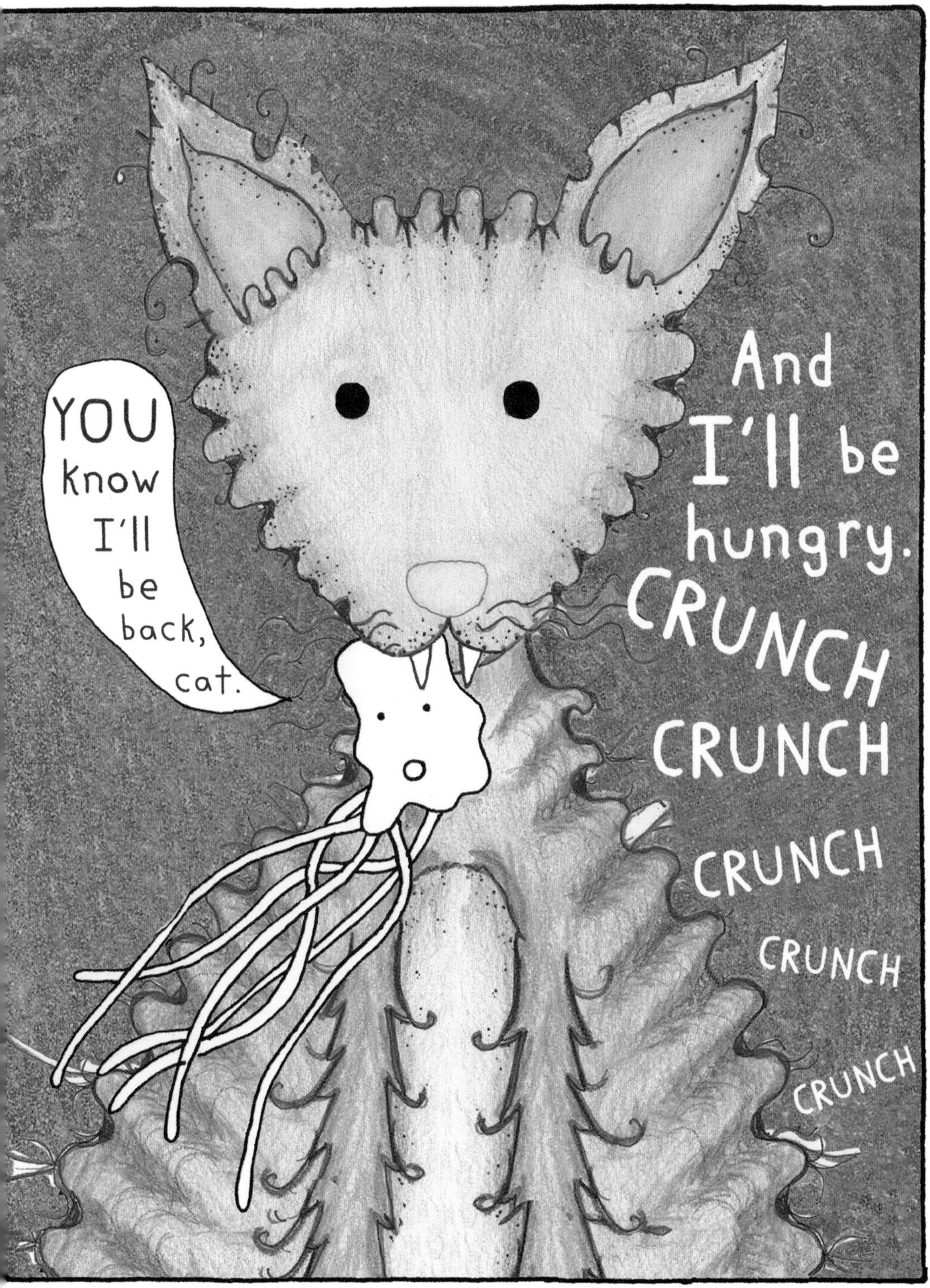
YOU know I'll be back, cat.
And I'll be hungry.
CRUNCH
CRUNCH
CRUNCH
CRUNCH
CRUNCH

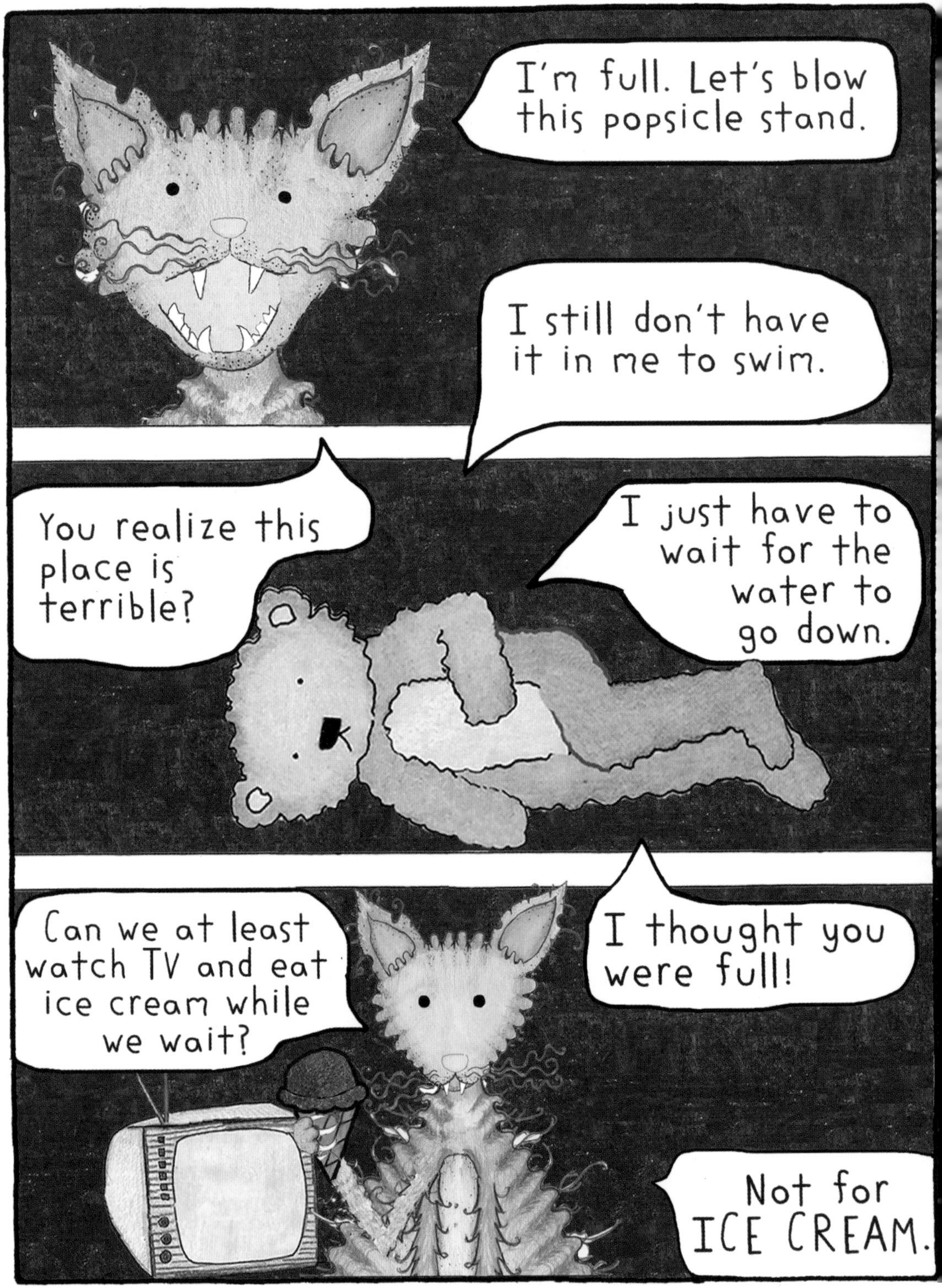
I'm full. Let's blow this popsicle stand.
I still don't have it in me to swim.
You realize this place is terrible?
I just have to wait for the water to go down.
Can we at least watch TV and eat ice cream while we wait?
I thought you were full!
Not for ICE CREAM.

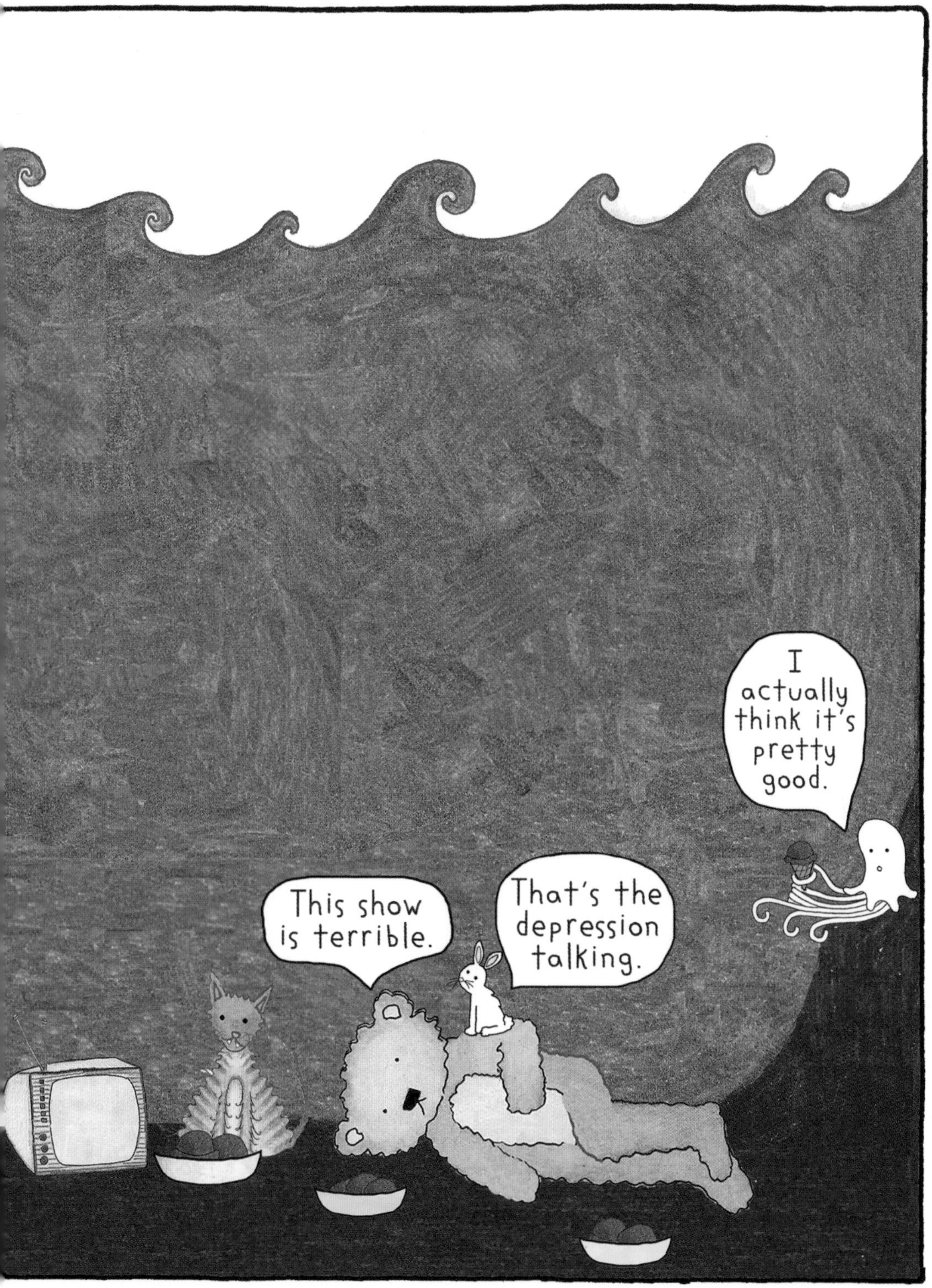
This show is terrible.
That's the depression talking.
I actually think it's pretty good.

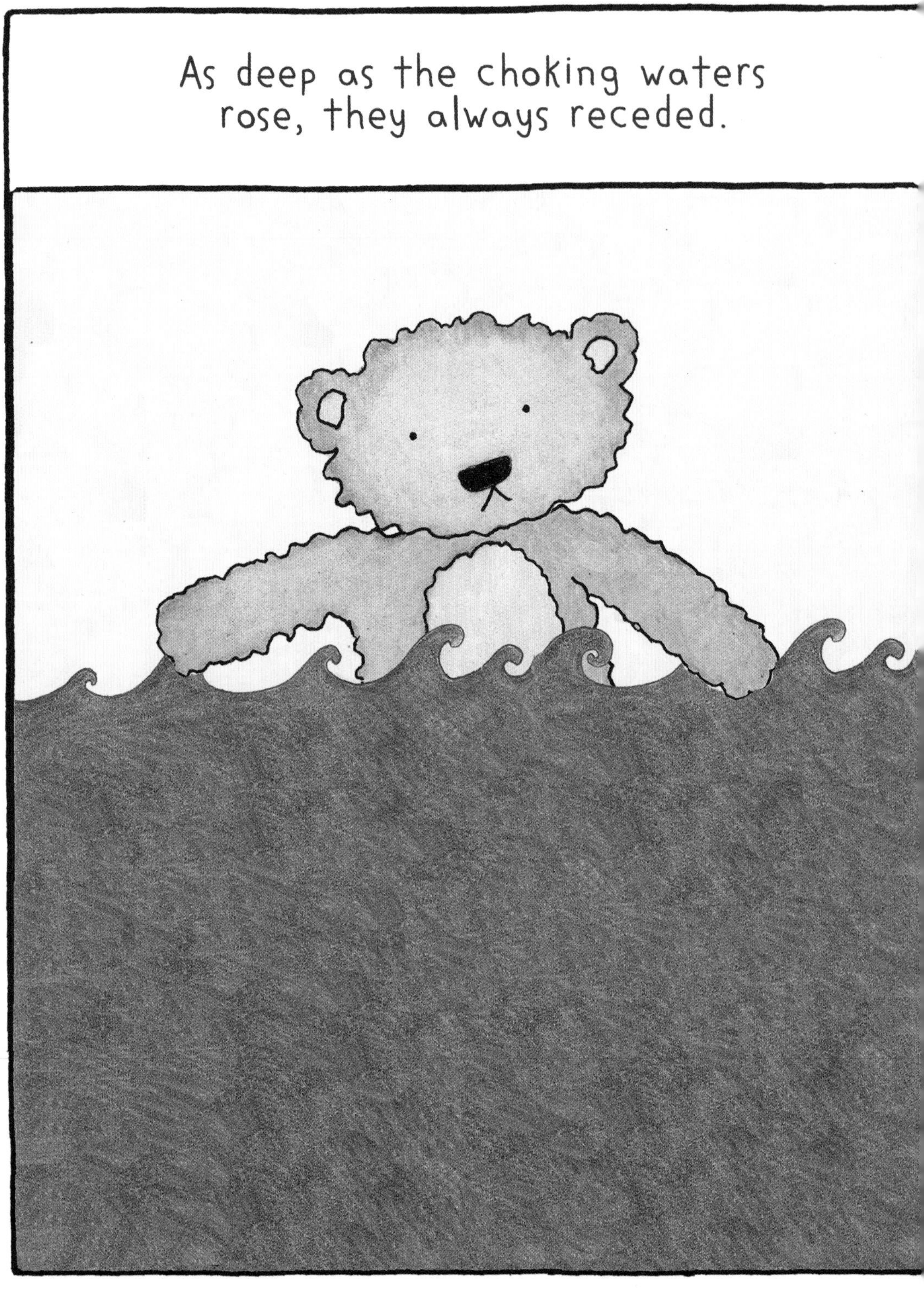
As deep as the choking waters rose, they always receded.

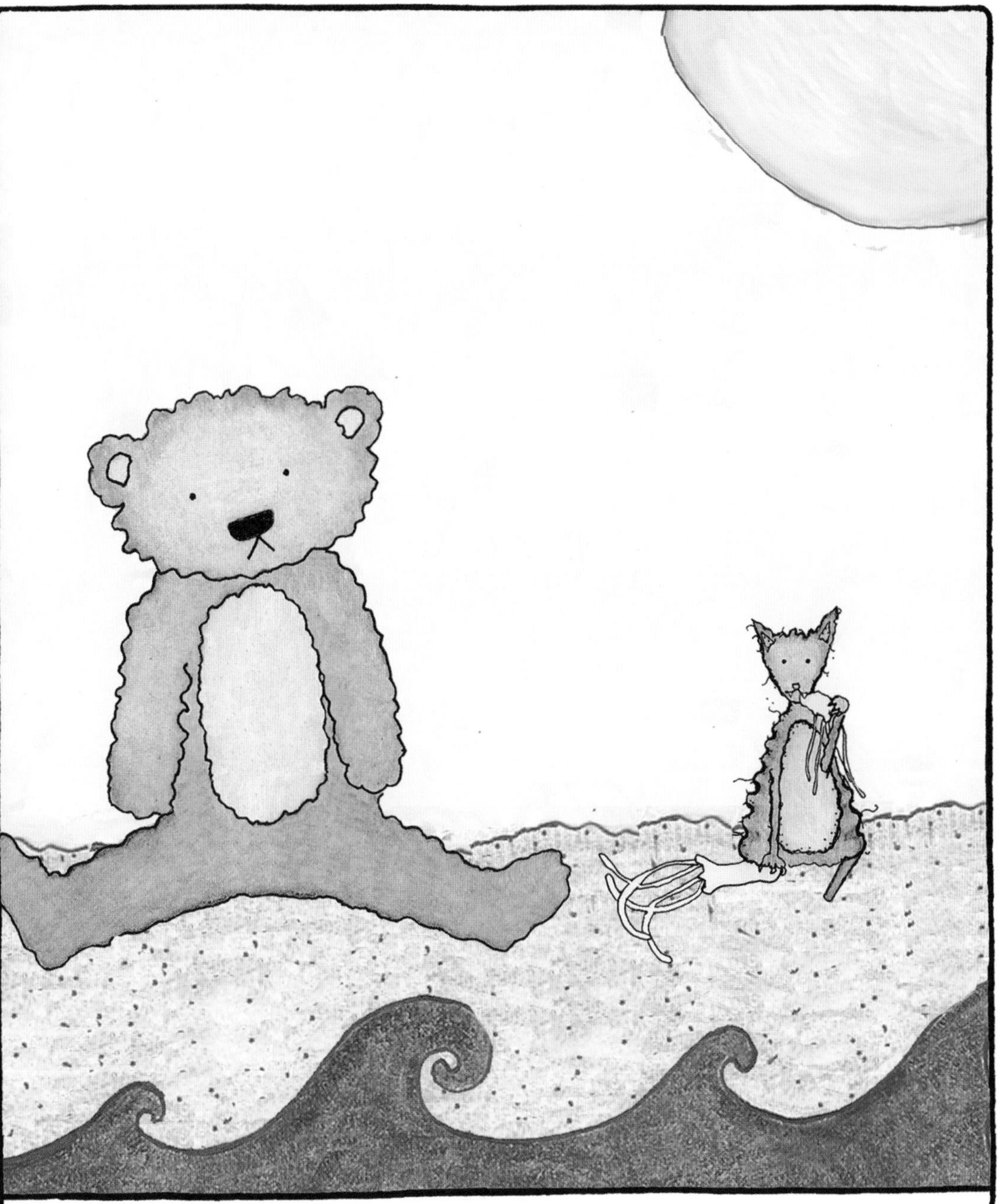

And Theodore felt the sun on his fur.

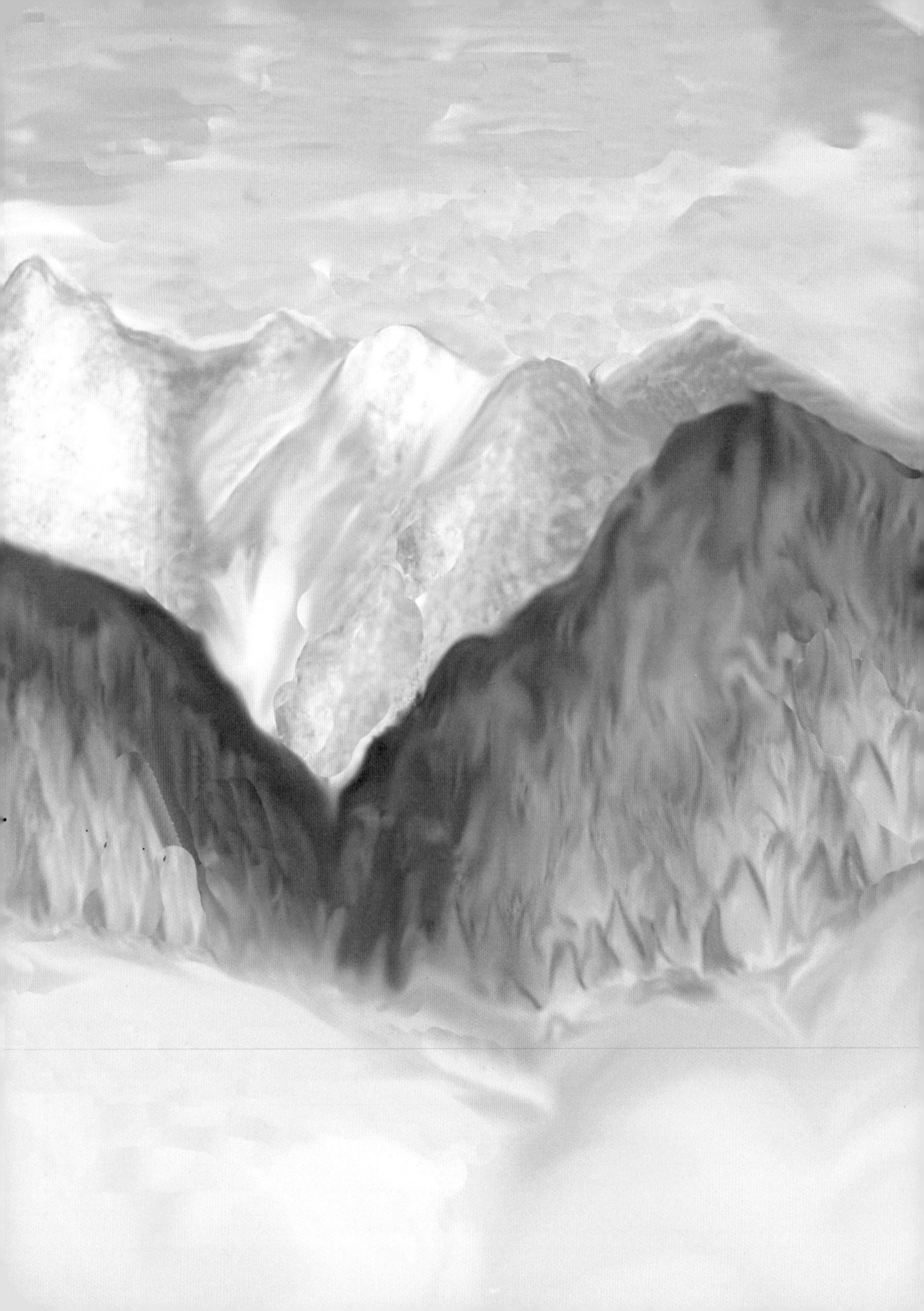

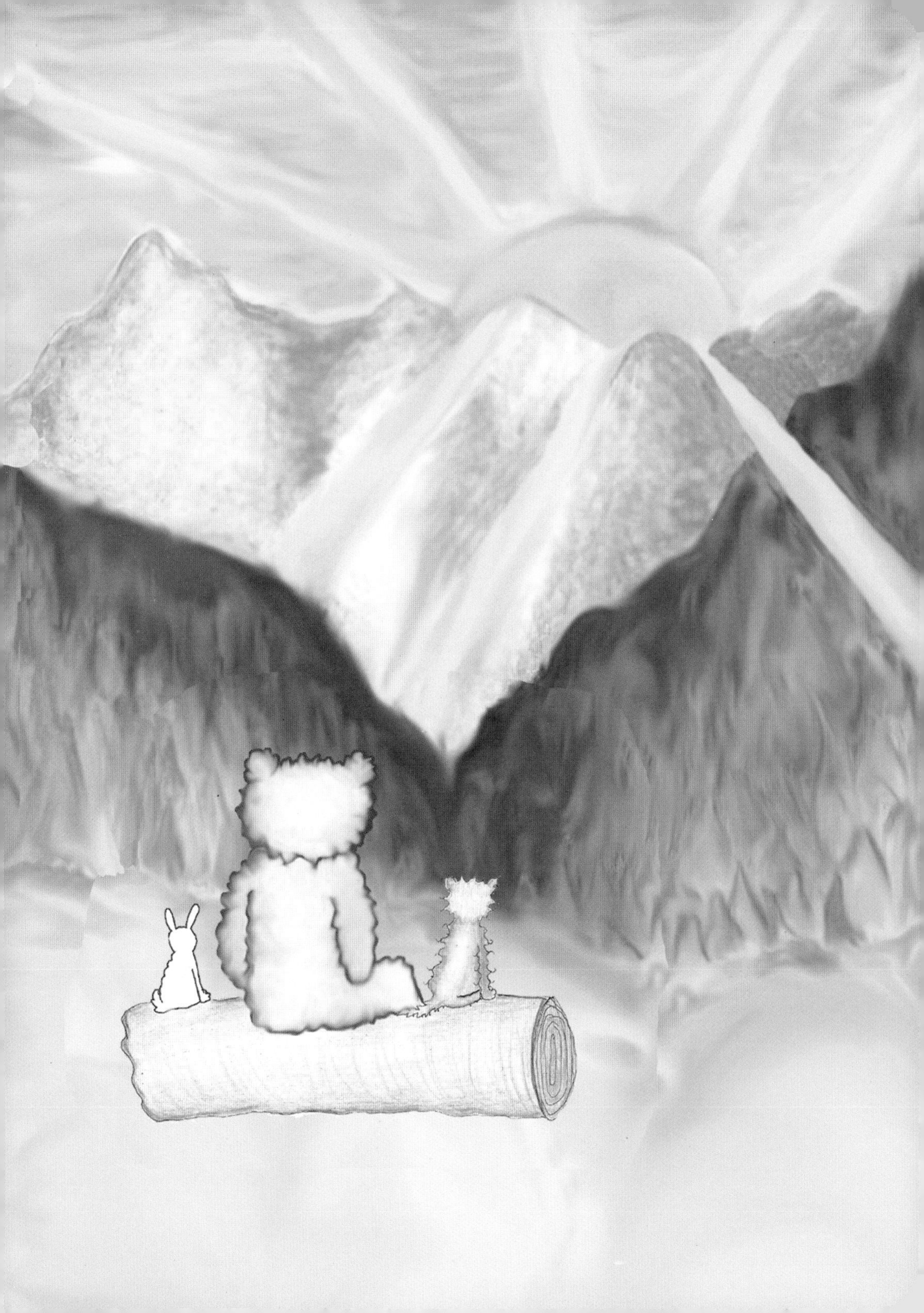

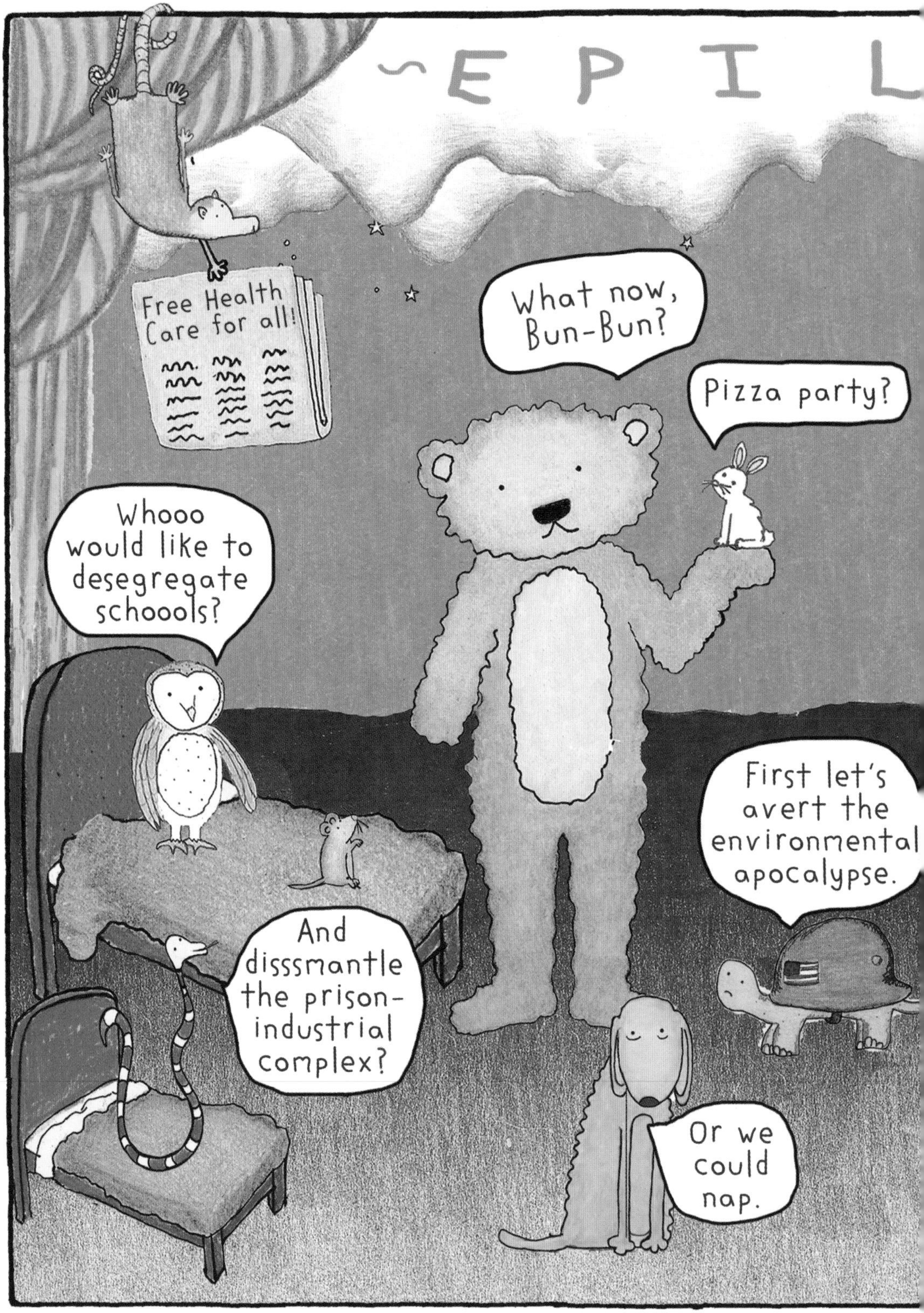
~E P I L
Free Health Care for all!
What now, Bun-Bun?
Pizza party?
Whooo would like to desegregate schoools?
First let's avert the environmental apocalypse.
And disssmantle the prison-industrial complex?
Or we could nap.

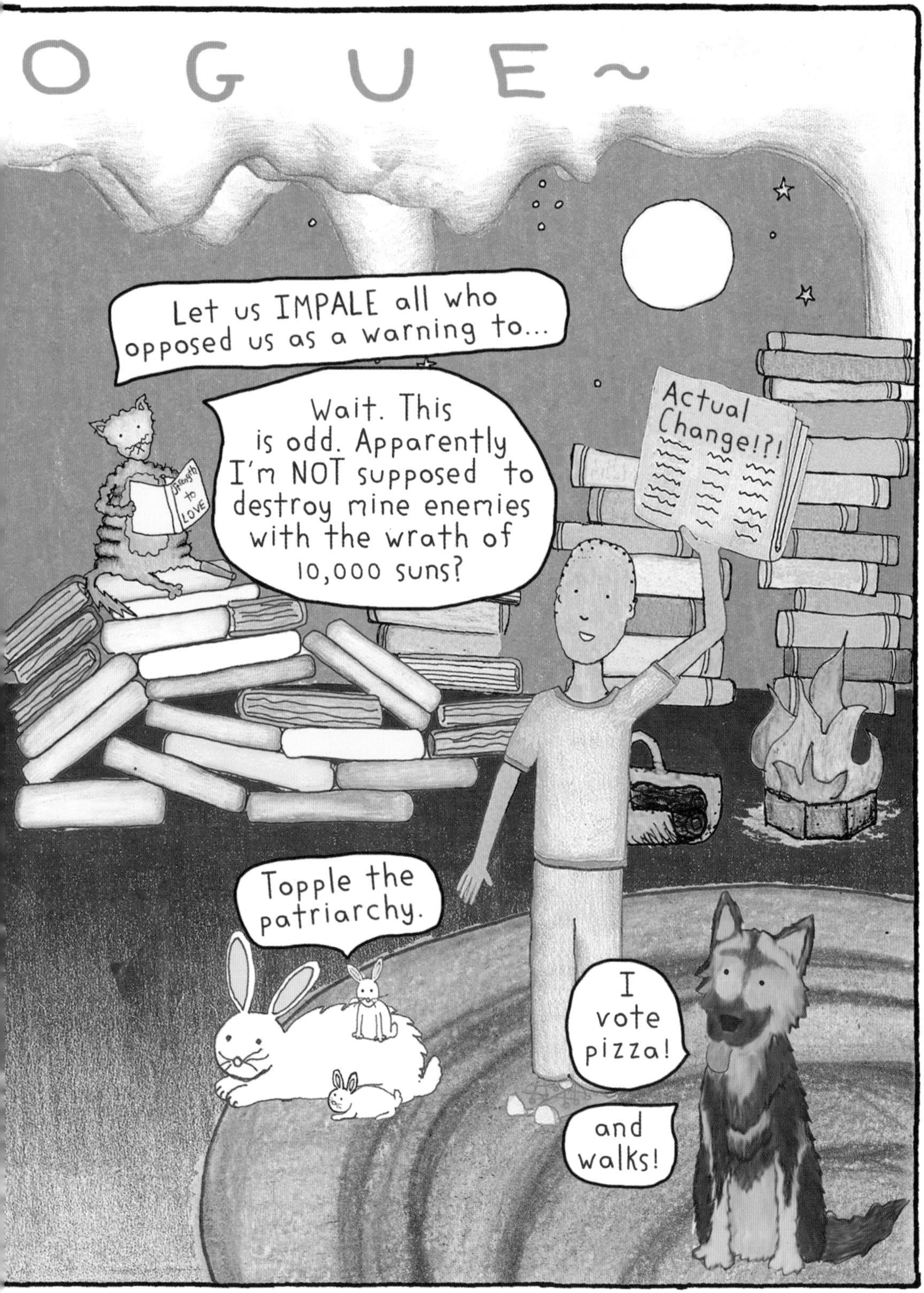
O G U E ~
Let us IMPALE all who opposed us as a warning to...
Wait. This is odd. Apparently I'm NOT supposed to destroy mine enemies with the wrath of 10,000 suns?
Strength to LOVE
Actual Change!?!
Topple the patriarchy.
I vote pizza!
and walks!

Afterword

This book began as a scribble on a scrap of binder paper—a tiny cartoon I drew for the amusement of a friend in a grad school fiction-writing class. (At the age of 26, I was probably too old to be passing notes. In my defense, the classes were three hours long, and doodling helped me sit still.) The little cartoon was titled "Bipolar Bear." It had two panels. In one, a manic bear declares, with expansive hand gestures, "I'm the king of the forest!" In the other panel, the bear sits in a dark cave, thinking: *berries make me sad.*

The cartoon was based on personal experience. Except in my case, it was not berries that filled me with melancholy. It was the carrots in my crisper. In the midst of a depressive episode, I had trudged out of my dimly lit room, seeking solace in a snack. There wasn't much in the fridge. I contemplated a lonely bunch of carrots. They were dry and slightly shriveled. I considered the fact that they had once been young, robust carrots—full of potential and hope. Now they would endure the fate of all living things: wilting, decomposition, death.

Carrots make me sad, I thought.

Then I laughed at myself. Then I returned to my room for a good bout of crying. Then I slept for ten hours. Then I called my mom.

She suggested that it might be time to see someone about my mood.

The psychiatrist at the campus counseling center listened to my elaborate metaphors for my state of being: I felt the weight of an iron wall crushing my chest. I felt like a scarecrow stuffed with garbage. I felt like I was walking through pea-soup fog. When I mentioned that I had a family history of bipolar disorder, the psychiatrist asked me if I had ever experienced a time when I had an extraordinary amount of energy, little need for sleep, or an ecstatic mood. I told him about the month in college when I slept three hours a night and had a series of euphoric realizations about the nature of the universe. After a slew of follow-up questions, the psychiatrist delivered a diagnosis: *bipolar disorder, major depressive episode.*

He prescribed medication. Though I was trudging through each day like a zombie slug and barely able to string a sentence together, I was reluctant to take the pills. I was afraid that they would rob me of my sparkling personality.

Instead, the meds restored me to functioning. I poured my newfound energy into short stories and a fledgling novel. When I had writer's block, I drew children's books for my little brother (seventeen years my junior). The books starred angst-ridden animals: a lonely giant squid, a socially anxious possum, a snail with low self-esteem, and a burro who wants to be a unicorn. All of the books have the same plot: the animal protagonist experiences angst, then reads philosophy or consults a wise creature, then experiences an epiphany.

I decided to expand my bipolar bear cartoon into an angst-ridden-animal book and worked on the project whenever I was too depressed to write fiction. (The meds only made the depression go away for a while. It always came back. This is the unfortunate reality of chronic disease.) My life unfolded: I graduated from the MFA program, got married, became a college English instructor, and moved back to my homeland of California. My husband and I decided to start trying for a baby. In anticipation of a pregnancy, I cut down on my meds. The depression returned with a vengeance.

So I worked on *Bipolar Bear*.

I was excited at the prospect of becoming a mother, but I had a secret fear that pregnancy would cause hormonal changes that would lead to postpartum psychosis. Stanford Hospital had a special clinic that focused on prenatal and postpartum psychiatric health. I called the clinic to confirm that they accepted my insurance and made an appointment. The Stanford psychiatrists were helpful. They assured me that my medication wasn't super risky to take during pregnancy, and with the lowered dose, chances of birth defects were slim. I returned home and resumed drawing bears.

Then a letter from my insurance company came in the mail. The letter informed me that my $650 Stanford appointment had not been covered. My husband and I were barely scraping by, and the $650 bill was nearly a month's rent—a major financial blow.

I called the number on my insurance card. I enunciated my identification information to a computerized voice. I waited on hold, listening to tinny music. I paced. The tinny hold music went on and on. When I finally connected with a person, I learned that I had pressed the wrong extension. I needed to start over. My sojourn through the phone labyrinth went on for a good part of the afternoon. Eventually, I spoke with a representative and learned that the Stanford clinic was an out-of-network provider. As I had not yet reached my deductible, I was on the hook for the bill.

I may have done some crying.

When I returned to drawing bears, it occurred to me that an inextricable part of any mental illness is dealing with health insurance bureaucracy. I decided that my bipolar bear should have to face the Labyrinth of Health Insurance Claims. This made the children's book a good deal longer. It also made it something other than a children's book. As the book grew in length and scope, I contemplated the faceless insurance bureaucracy. Who benefited from the system? The customer service agents I spoke to on the phone weren't getting rich. From chatting with my psychiatrist, I knew that providers loathe the labyrinth. Was it really only a handful of top executives who profited from the misery of millions? I lacked an outlet for my anger, so I made my bipolar bear confront a lair of fat-cat health insurance CEOs and devour them all. My husband and I had just adopted a hideous kitten with bat-like ears and a rat-like tail. Friends regularly asked us if our cat might actually be a possum. Our homely kitten became the inspiration for Theodore's fat-cat CEO nemesis, Baroness Von Stinkleshanks.

My life continued to unfurl. I had a beautiful baby. My first book, a novel-in-stories titled *When Mystical Creatures Attack!*, got published. (The book is about an idealistic English teacher who struggles with bipolar disorder. Write what you know.) I had another beautiful baby. I taught. I wrote short stories and essays and began another novel. Whenever I was down, I returned to *Bipolar Bear*. Ten years after I'd begun the project, I finally finished the book. I eagerly sent it off to my agent.

She said there was no way she could sell it. It was way too weird.

I was, of course, devastated. I surrendered to despair for a week. Then I amicably split up with my agent. I began sending out queries, certain I could find an agent who shared my conviction that there was a rich, untapped market for graphic novels about health insurance bureaucracy and existential despair told via children's book–style drawings of forest creatures.

While I waited for the expressions of interest to come rolling in, a depressive episode inspired me to scrap the book's happy ending. I decided to give Theodore a brutal relapse and to make him ponder my own gnawing question: What is the point of my healing journey if the sickness always, always, comes back?

When I came out of the depression, I decided I owed it to the reader to hazard an answer. I created a philosophical debate between Theodore and his depression (as embodied by an enormous ghostfish). The ghostfish tells Theodore that his life has no meaning. Theodore gives a rousing speech declaring himself to be an existentialist who, despite the absurdity of life, makes his own meaning in the face of despair.

Then it occurred to me that when I am severely depressed, I am not capable of making my own meaning. I am not even capable of getting off of the linoleum. When depression is very, very bad, I cannot believe in any good thing inside myself. My crumb of hope is the knowledge that even if despair overwhelms me entirely, my despair cannot erase joy from the world. When I can't register kindness, kindness still exists. The truth is true whether or not I believe in it. So I had Theodore grandly proclaim: "It is true that I can no longer taste food or hear music or remember kindness or know love. But my despair does not erase them from the world. Even when I cannot feel the sun, it still remains."

Isn't that poetic?

Problem is, poetic speeches don't make depression go away. Getting wound up in an argument with your own depressed thoughts just traps you in your head. I realized the ending of my book should reflect the fact that a person in a deep depression should not waste time arguing with a nihilistic ghostfish. A person in a deep depression should call a friend.

There is a very old book called *Pilgrim's Progress*. It was written in 1678. It was a big hit during its time. The book is an allegory of the soul, in which a man named Christian (they weren't very subtle back then) goes on an arduous journey that represents human life on earth. Sins and virtues are represented as characters—Christian encounters personages named Sloth, Hopeful, Presumption, and so on. At one point in the story, Christian gets stuck in The Slough of Despond. It is not the avatar of faith or reason or even love or hope that gets him out of the slough.

It's Help.

I am a bit of a hypocrite for having Theodore respond to his own despair by calling for help. I hate asking for help. I struggled with mental illness for ten years before I got up the courage to see a therapist. I still try to white-knuckle my way through the bad times in order to stave off the humiliation of asking for help.

In *A Man Without a Country*, Kurt Vonnegut asks his son for the meaning of life. His son says: "We're here to get each other through this thing, whatever it is."

The awful truth is that no one gets through life without help. We are all flawed and broken. I wish the truth were more dignified, but the human condition appears to involve depending on other humans. The good news is that sometimes you get a turn to be the helper. Everyone, at some point, has the chance to throw a rope to a struggling friend. Maybe you'll even have the chance to be a really big helper. Perhaps you will help dismantle the Labyrinth of Insurance Claims, or abolish Debtor's Prison, or restore voting rights. It would be wonderful if somebody averted the environmental apocalypse. The clock is ticking on that one.

Theodore has come to the end of his journey, but we are still here.

Let's help each other through this thing, whatever it is.

—**Kathleen Founds**

How to Get Help

National Alliance on Mental Illness HelpLine: 800-950-6264
The HelpLine can give you referrals for treatment, info about mental health conditions, and techniques for dealing with symptoms.

National Suicide Prevention Lifeline: 988 (previously 800-273-8255)
The person on the other end of the line knows how to help out when things are very, very bad. You can also text TALK to 741741, the Crisis Text Line, to text with a trained crisis counselor.

My degree is in fiction writing. I am qualified to write depressing short stories, not to dole out advice about depression. But, in case it is helpful, I put some mood disorder–related resources on my website: www.kathleenfounds.com.

How to Help Out

Here are some organizations fighting the good fight.

Restoring Voting Rights
Organization: When We All Vote

Abolishing Debtor's Prison
Organization: Fines and Fees Justice Center

Dismantling the Labyrinth of Health Insurance Claims
Organization: Healthcare-NOW

All of the above organizations are wonderful, but what I most recommend is getting involved at the local level. Research the issue you care about, and find a local group that works on it. Go to a meeting. There, you will have a chance to meet a bunch of weirdos who care about the same stuff you do. This will make you feel less lonely. Also, there might be snacks.

Acknowledgments

It took a lot of encouragement to keep going on this strange and unwieldy project. I couldn't have done it without the support and encouragement of: Yuri Anderson, Wendy Root Askew, Victoria Banales, Michele Bigley, Jeffrey Billet, Tomiko Breland, Michael Burkhard, Nikia Chaney, Serena Coleman, Vanessa Diffenbaugh, Karen Joy Fowler, Hannah Von Benedikt-Fowler, Emily Nisco-Frank, Abigail Morton-Garland, John Garland, Mary Gaitskill, Lorie Gearhart, Carolyn Gonzalez, Ruth Gutierrez, Gideon Lewis-Kraus, Maribel McClain, Elizabeth McKenzie, Annarose McQuaid, Sara Michas-Martin, Liza Monroy, Adrianne Myers, Adela Najarro, Micah Perks, Gail Root, Enid Ryce, Melissa Sanders-Self, Deb Sandweiss, George Saunders, Paula Saunders, Susan Sherman, Anna Sochynsky, Karen Spicher, Dr. Susan Squier, Lizz Stearns, Sheryl Stewart, Daniel Torday, Peggy Townsend, Daniel Blue Tyx, Laura Nikstad Tyx, Jenn Updyke, Vauhini Vara, Kate Warehouse, Naomi Waters, Tobias Wolff, Jill Wolfson, and Jan Wright. Thanks to Chuck and Carol for their unflagging support. Thanks to Faye and Donna for enthusiasm and babysitting. Thanks to Summer Star, for believing in the bear and contributing clever details. Thanks to Mom and Dad, for instilling the confidence that kept me going. Thanks to David, Laura, Jenny, Ness, Michael, and Matthew, for the Foundsian exuberance. Thanks to Violet and Lila, for coloring companionship. Thanks to Dave, for being a super-dad while I spent five hours a day drawing bears.